READER'S DIGEST
1,001
HOME
REMEDIES

Published by The Reader's Digest Association, Inc.
London • New York • Sydney • Montreal

READER'S DIGEST
1,001 HOME REMEDIES

Trustworthy treatments for everyday health problems

Project Staff

Consultants
Pamela Mason BSc MSc Ph.D MRPharmS
Sheena Meredith MB BS

Project editor
Rachel Warren Chadd

Designers
Austin Taylor
Jane McKenna

Proofreader
Ron Pankhurst

Indexer
Hilary Bird

For Vivat Direct

Editorial director
Julian Browne

Art director
Anne-Marie Bulat

Managing editor
Nina Hathway

Picture resource manager
Sarah Stewart-Richardson

Pre-press technical manager
Dean Russell

Book production manager
Claudette Bramble

Senior production controller
Katherine Tibbals

Origination
FMG

Printing and binding
Arvato Iberia, Europe

For Reader's Digest USA

Editor in chief and publishing director
Neil Wertheimer

Editor
Marianne Wait

Designer
Rich Kershner

1,001 HOME REMEDIES Published in the United Kingdom by Vivat Direct Limited (t/a Reader's Digest), 157 Edgware Road, London W2 2HR

1,001 HOME REMEDIES is owned and under licence from The Reader's Digest Association, Inc. All rights reserved.

Reprinted in 2010

Adapted from **1801 Home Remedies** published by The Reader's Digest Association, Inc., USA.

We are committed both to the quality of our products and the service we provide to our customers. We value your comments, so please do contact us on **08705 113366** or via our website at **www.readersdigest.co.uk**
If you have any comments or suggestions about the content of our books, email us at gbeditorial@readersdigest.co.uk

Any references in this book to any products or services do not constitute or imply an endorsement or recommendation.

MEDICAL ADVISORS

Carolyn Dean, M.D., N.D. Consultant, Integrative Medicine, City Island, New York

Mitchell A. Fleisher, M.D. Clinical Instructor, University of Virginia Health Sciences Center and the Medical College of Virginia; Family Physician, Private Practice, Nellysford, Virginia

Larrian Gillespie, M.D. Retired Assistant Clinical Professor of Urology and Urogynecology, Beverly Hills, California

Chris Kammer, D.D.S. Center for Cosmetic Dentistry, Madison, Wisconsin

Chris Meletis, N.D. Chief Medical Officer and Director of Education Affairs, Pearl Clinic Professor of Natural Pharmacology, National College of Naturopathic Medicine, Portland, Oregon

Lylas G. Mogk, M.D. Henry Ford Visual Rehabilitation & Research Center, Grosse Pointe and Livonia, Michigan

Zorba Paster, M.D. Professor of Family Medicine, Dean Medical Center, University of Wisconsin-Madison

Ricki Pollycove, M.D., M.H.S. Clinical Faculty, University of California School of Medicine; Private Practice of Gynecology, San Francisco, California

David B. Posner, M.D. Chief of Gastroenterology, Mercy Medical Center, Baltimore, Maryland; Assistant Professor of Medicine, University of Maryland School of Medicine

Adrienne Rencic, M.D., Ph.D. Attending Dermatologist, Mercy Medical Center, Baltimore, Maryland; Clinical Instructor, University of Maryland Medical System

Kevin R. Stone, M.D. Orthopedic Surgeon and Founder and Chairman of The Stone Foundation for Sports Medicine and Arthritis Research and the Stone Clinic, San Francisco, California

Cathryn Tobin, M.D. Pediatrician, Private Practice, Markham, Ontario

Contributors

Bookside Press Editors
Edward B. Claflin
E. A. Tremblay

Writers
Matthew Hoffman
Eric Metcalf

Researchers
Janel Bogert
Elizabeth Shimer

Illustrators
Harry Bates
Inkgraved Illustration:
Cindy Jeftovic

Contents

PART ONE   28
EVERYDAY AILMENTS

Here are effective treatments for more than a hundred common health complaints – simple remedies, mostly based on ingredients that are readily available or already to hand in your home.

SPECIAL FEATURES

Do-it-yourself healing in these colourful pages includes remedies, recipes and effective, simple exercises for relieving common aches and pains.

PART TWO
20 TOP HOUSEHOLD HEALERS 384

A selection of the most effective remedies to stock at home and details of their myriad uses – to short-circuit a migraine, soothe sunburn, ease arthritis pain and much more …

About this book

Y ou're about to discover more than 1,000 home remedies you can use whenever you need to treat an everyday health problem – acne or nausea, insomnia or wrinkles – and just about everything in between.

But before you do, turn to *Using Home Remedies*, where you'll find advice on using self-treatments safely and effectively. See page 19 for instructions about growing five useful medicinal plants. And for cautions regarding specific herbs and supplements, turn to our four-page guide starting on page 434.

Part One, *Everyday ailments*, offers home remedies for more than 100 common conditions listed in alphabetical order. A home remedy is basically anything you can use at home that doesn't require a prescription. You probably have many of the ingredients in your cupboards already: bicarbonate of soda, for example (use it in place of talcum powder to neutralize body odour), mustard (add it to a warm footbath to ease a headache) or tea bags (hold a wet one against a mouth ulcer to relieve the sting). Some, such as arnica ointment, are sold in health-food shops; others, like camomile tea, are sold in supermarkets.

A few of the remedies, such as fish oil supplements for angina, should be used under your doctor's supervision because they could interact with other medications you may be taking. We highlight such instances.

Part Two describes *20 Top Household Healers* – herbs, foods and other staples worth keeping on hand for potential use in many of the remedies in this book. Find out what vinegar, yoghurt, Epsom salts and ginger are good for, and discover omega-3 fatty acids, the 'good' fats found in fish (and supplements) that not only protect your heart, but also help to treat arthritis, menstrual cramps and even depression.

This book was a hugely enjoyable project for those who worked on it – not only in terms of discovering new remedies, but also trying them out. We hope you enjoy the book too, and find many of its suggestions helpful now and in the future.

The Editors

Using home remedies

People have always turned to what they could find round about them to cure their ills – whether healing muds and salts, plants or common foodstuffs. Some plants were thought to have magic powers, often based on the shape of their roots or leaves. But simple scientific observation eventually led to the identification of what actually worked. This was vital – some substances that are perfectly safe when used externally can be fatal if eaten. This is true today. Don't forget that home remedies and herbs, like pharmaceutical drugs, can contain powerful compounds – and just because something is 'natural' does not necessarily make it 'safe'.

Nearly every family has some home 'cures' that have been passed down from generation to generation, their origins lost in the mists of time. Who was the first grandmother to serve peppermint tea to a sick grandchild? Why did that herdsman decide to pick dock leaves and rub them onto nettle stings? Who was the first cook to discover that chicken soup could help you to recover from the common cold?

Considering how often favourite home remedies have been used to cure everyday ailments and relieve pain, it's a pity we can't thank the people who discovered them. But we can benefit from the tips that they passed on.

More than a thousand remedies

Home remedies begin at home – and that's often where the secrets stay. But when you open this book you are effectively accessing thousands of households and discovering myriad remedies that have been handed on over generations.

Some of these remedies – including a sore throat cure, a hiccup stopper, a soother for aching muscles and a way to relieve insect stings – arrived in the post. These home cures have all been included in the relevant chapters.

That was just the beginning. We also unearthed acupressure treatments of Chinese doctors, the healing methods of tribal shamans, centuries-old European folk cures and those used by American pioneers. We were given the top home remedies endorsed by herbalists, homeopaths, naturopathic doctors and masseurs, specialists in cardiovascular medicine and favourite GPs. Our search took us through history, from the age of Hippocrates to the battlefields of the First World War – and the gardens and allotments of 21st century herbal practitioners.

Choosing the best

Though the net was cast wide, the final choice of the best home remedies was a carefully selective process. Lots of traditional home remedies didn't make it into the book because they were just too weird or revolting. The asafoetida bag, once a valued cure for colds, smells so disgusting that those who once used it remember it with horror. Other old remedies are so odd, superstitious or complex that they are only worth mentioning for curiosity's sake. An Appalachian cure for warts, for example, was to rub a potato onto the wart, put the potato in a sack and leave the sack at a fork in the road.

Every remedy in this book was carefully reviewed by our board of advisors to ensure that they are safe for you to use as recommended.

Of course, any remedy that does no harm might also do some good, especially when administered by someone who has a gentle, healing touch and cares for the patient. But once we had discarded the strangest, least credible, most complicated or potentially risky, we were left with the terrific remedies that you'll find in this book – more than a thousand of them – that have helped to heal millions of people. Each remedy was then reviewed by our board of advisors – including doctors, qualified specialists and naturopathic healers – to ensure that they are safe for you to use as recommended.

All within reach

As you read about the home remedies in this book – and start to use them yourself – you'll probably begin to remember tried-and-trusted healing methods from your own family's past. But we've become so used to blood tests, X-rays, potent prescription drugs and all the other trappings of modern medicine that we tend to forget, or neglect, our amazing legacy of home cures. Time tested remedies are just as useful today as they ever were. The tricks you learnt from your parents and grandparents, like dabbing bicarb on a bee sting, putting a soothing cool wet tea bag on tired eyes, or applying a warm cooked cabbage leaf to draw out a boil, aren't replacements for high-tech treatments, of course. But you can count on them to make you feel better fast – and, in many cases, to prevent small problems from turning into bigger ones.

There's something very satisfying about watching a burn heal almost like magic when you apply a dab of aloe vera gel. Or when you inhale the scent of lavender and feel anxiety melt away. But sweet nostalgia isn't the reason doctors continue to advocate home treatments. They recommend them because they work.

There's something almost magical about watching a burn heal when you follow your grandmother's advice and apply a little aloe vera gel.

Did you know that at least 25 per cent of the drugs in your medicine cabinet contain active ingredients that are similar or identical to those found in plants? The active substance in aspirin – one of the world's most widely used medications – was first derived from white willow bark. The decongestant ephedrine is based on chemicals in the ephedra plant. The heart drug digitalis is derived from the foxglove. The cancer drug paclitaxel comes from the Pacific yew tree. In fact, big drug companies often send teams of scientists to remote locations to hunt for medicinally promising chemicals.

Finding out what works

In current medical practice, traditional healing techniques are sometimes neglected but, by and large, they have not been forgotten. Physiotherapists use the same hot and cold treatments that were popular among Native American tribes – treatments that often work better than drugs but with none of the side effects. A cut from a kitchen knife may heal faster when you apply antiseptic ointment. But coating it with honey does just the same thing and may work even more quickly. (As with any cut, be sure to wash it thoroughly in plenty of running water before applying anything to it.)

Molly Hopkins, a 60-year-old landscape designer, discovered first-hand that alternative treatments can work better than conventional medicine. 'I used to get sinus infections every time I caught a cold and then I had to take antibiotics,' she says. A friend, who's a family doctor, told her to start taking echinacea at the first sign of sniffles. 'I haven't had a serious cold since – and no sinus infections at all,' she says.

Most of us use traditional cures for minor aches and pains, but doctors at top research institutions are beginning to realize that they can also help with serious health problems. Take diabetes, for example. Hundreds of thousands of Britons need to have daily injections or oral drugs to keep their blood sugar levels stable. But people who eat a clove of garlic every day may be able to lower their blood sugar naturally, and with it their doses of medicine. Depression is another condition that often requires medication, but studies show that the herb St John's wort may be as effective as drugs for mild to moderate cases.

Many of the most popular home remedies, such as yoghurt for fungal infections or camomile tea for insomnia, have been used for generations. Others – what you might call 'future traditions' that will hopefully be passed on to our children and grandchildren – are being developed all the time.

• Creams containing the herb arnica help bruises to heal faster and with less pain because they contain natural painkilling and anti-inflammatory compounds.

• A blend of honey and yoghurt creates a natural bleach that can help to lighten the brown liver spots that commonly appear on the backs of our hands as we age.

• Researchers at one US children's hospital recently found that duct tape, that do-it-all household standby, can make warts disappear in just a few days.

The commonsense approach

While this book contains a wealth of comforts and cures, there's nothing like good judgment when it comes to using any home remedy. Sometimes you need to be on the lookout for signs of more serious problems. Clara Boxer made the sort of mistake doctors worry about. She is a fifty-something accountant and had been suffering from occasional light-headedness, usually in the morning when she got out of bed. She read on the internet that ginger is a good remedy for feeling dizzy. So she stocked up on ginger supplements at her local health-food shop and took them for a few weeks. Then one morning she stood up in the bath, passed out and fell and broke her wrist.

Fortunately, the accident and emergency doctor who treated her managed to establish why the accident had happened in the first place. Ginger is in fact a traditional remedy for vertigo, a type of dizziness often associated with inner-ear disturbances. But Clara didn't have vertigo. What she had was orthostatic hypotension, a sudden drop in blood pressure sometimes caused by high doses of blood pressure medication. Her GP reduced her prescribed dose and the dizziness went away.

Even though most home remedies are safe, people sometimes take them for the wrong reasons.

Even though most home remedies are safe, people sometimes take them for the wrong reasons. Or they diagnose themselves when they really need a doctor. Some conditions are easy to recognize and treat at home. You don't need a battery of tests if your gums bleed for a couple of days or you get the occasional tummy upset. But it isn't always easy to tell what is minor and what isn't.

That is why it can be important to check with your doctor before taking herbs or other supplements, or to tell your doctor what you're already taking before he or she prescribes any other medicine. Supplements can alter the effects of both over-the-counter (OTC) and prescription drugs. For example, people who take vitamin E along with blood-thinning drugs may have an increased risk of internal bleeding.

Even if a herbal tea or capsule seems completely innocuous – stinging nettle for arthritis, for example, or dandelion to lower blood pressure – if you're taking it regularly to treat a health problem, it's a good idea to let your doctor know. Some herbs aren't as effective as people claim and you don't want to make the mistake of undertreating a potentially serious problem. Even if a supplement is safe and does just what the manufacturer says it does, it won't do you any good if you take it for a condition you don't actually have.

Proceeding with some cautions

Traditional cures have been used every day for thousands of years, so they probably work or people wouldn't use them. But there are always risks of side effects, interactions with drugs or simply using the wrong remedy. The home remedies in this book are supported by anecdotal evidence of their efficacy – and in many cases by scientific studies – and they have been carefully screened for safety by our medical advisors. Be sure to observe the '*Alert*' notices that appear after certain remedies, and be aware that there are certain times when you must be especially careful, such as when:

• **You are pregnant** Do not take any herbs, supplements or over-the-counter medications without first talking to your midwife or doctor. Many of these can affect the health of your baby, particularly if taken in large doses.

• **You are taking prescription medicine** Talk to your doctor about possible interactions between your prescribed medi-cation and any herbs, supplements or over-the-counter drugs recommended in this book. The cautions on pages 434–437 give some guidelines about drug, herb and supplement inter-actions and some additional warnings. But you should also tell your doctor about any other supplements or medications that you take at the same time – particularly if you have a chronic condition such as diabetes or heart disease.

• **You know you are allergic to a food or medication** People with allergies should be extra cautious: make absolutely sure that the substance to which you're allergic is not one of the ingredients in whatever it is you're proposing to take or use on your skin. For example arachis oil, found in some laxatives and skin moisturizers, is a purified peanut oil and potentially dangerous for anyone with a peanut allergy. Watch out for 'cross-reactivity' between foods, plants and herbs as well. In other words, if you're allergic to shrimp, chances are you'll react to crab and lobster, too. And people who are sensitive to ragweed often react to eating melon, while those with birch pollen allergy may react to apple peel.

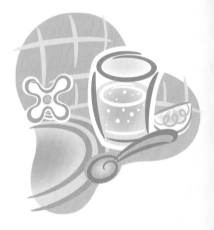

• **You have a serious health condition** Pay special attention to the 'Should I call the doctor?' panel found in each chapter. The purpose of home remedies is to help you to deal with everyday ailments and improve your overall health – not to mask serious conditions that require medical treatment.

• **You are treating a child or infant** Some herbs, supplements and home remedies are not appropriate for children or babies. Unless a remedy is specifically recommended for children, ask your GP or health visitor for advice before treating your children. And buy over-the-counter products designed for children rather than for adults (children's paracetamol syrup, for instance, instead of standard paracetamol).

Growing medicinal plants

Several of the plants recommended in this book are both pretty and easy to grow. Some have the advantage of being delicious in cooking or in salads. Best of all, if you've grown them yourself, you can guarantee their freshness and purity.

Many herbs and medicinal plants can be grown from seed. Some are started indoors in trays and transplanted after the last frosts. Others don't like to be moved and are sown where you want them to grow. Woody herbs, such as lavender and rosemary, are best propagated from cuttings. Dip healthy shoots from the current year's growth in rooting hormone and stick them in a pot of compost.

You don't need lots of space for herbs: many will grow happily in hanging baskets, window boxes and all sorts of pots. If you have a garden, herbs and bulbs can be popped in between flowers and shrubs in a border. But keep them away from busy roads, or you'll be getting an unhealthy dose of exhaust residues along with those beneficial ingredients. Avoid pesticides for the same reason.

Whether planted in a border or a pot, most herbs need good drainage – though peppermint doesn't mind damp soils. Herbs tend to prefer poor soils to rich ones. Think wild thyme on a Mediterranean hillside and you'll get the picture.

Aloe vera

Buy a couple of small plants from a garden centre and keep them indoors on a sunny windowsill. A kitchen or a heated conservatory are fine – but don't let the plants dry out or get cold. They will die if the temperature falls below 5°C (40°F).

How to use *Cut one of the fleshy leaves and squeeze the gel onto minor cuts or burns. The gel dries and forms an invisible bandage keeping bacteria out and moisture in.*

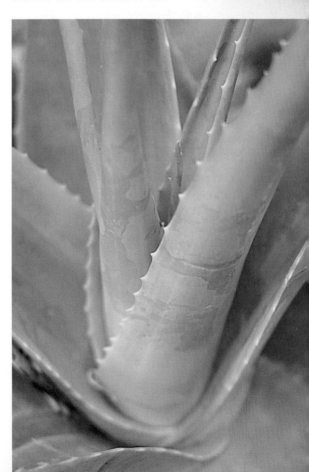

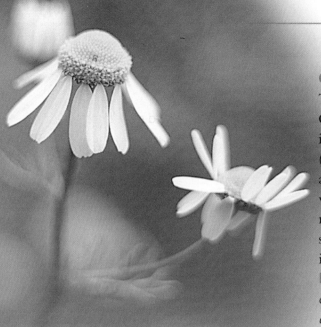

German camomile, the most popular form, is an annual. Sow the seeds where they are to flower when all danger of frost has passed. Scatter the seeds, tamp down and keep damp. Camomile likes a well drained, partially shaded spot.

How to use *Pick the flowers in full bloom and spread them on a muslin cloth on a rack in a warm dry place, or hang them upside down over a paper bag to catch the falling petals. Camomile tea calms stomach upsets and eases anxiety.*

Cumin and caraway

Cumin and caraway produce masses of seeds with a distinctive aniseed flavour. They taste terrific in spicy or fragrant dishes, and do wonders for the digestion. Both can be sown outdoors in a sunny position once danger of frost has passed.

How to use *Harvest the seeds at the end of summer. They can be ground in a pestle and mortar or used whole. Put a teaspoon of either type, or mix the two, in a cup of boiling water, steep for 10 minutes, strain and drink before meals.*

Garlic

This is most satisfying to grow. Before Christmas, break up a plump, healthy bulb into individual cloves and plant them 5cm (2in) deep in rows about 15–20cm (6-8in) apart and forget about them. Each clove will grow into a bulb and they will be ready to dig up in July or August. Keep the stems on (so you can plait them) and hang in a warm airy place to dry.

How to use *Peel the cloves and add to recipes or eat them whole. Eating a clove or two a day during the colds and flu season will help to boost immunity.*

Peppermint

This aromatic plant loves rich moist soil in sun or light shade. It grows easily from seed or runners and spreads fast. To keep it under control, grow it in a bottomless pot sunk into the soil. Or grow it in a container, but be sure to keep the soil well watered.

How to use *Use the leaves fresh or dried in digestive infusions and mouthwashes. Add the leaves to a steam inhalation for treating colds or flu.*

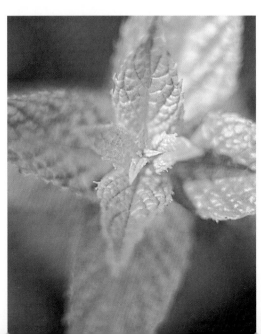

Herbal healing

When James Duke slipped a disc in his upper back in the early 1990s he tried all the things his doctor recommended: rest, ultrasound and hefty doses of anti-inflammatory drugs. But he didn't stop there. He took liquorice to settle his stomach, milk thistle to protect his liver from the aspirin, and echinacea before surgery to protect against infection.

James Duke is a botanist expert on medicinal herbs, and author of *The Green Pharmacy*. He is one of millions of people who appreciate the healing powers of plants. According to the World Health Organization, about 80 per cent of the world's population relies on herbs as their main medicinal source. Herbs are cheaper than drugs, and in many cases they're just as effective and often safer.

About 80 per cent of the world's population depends on herbs as their primary source of medical care.

When you're used to clicking open a child-proof cap and taking a convenient capsule, the idea of dealing with dried leaves can be a bit daunting. But it shouldn't be. Nearly all herbs are available in capsule or liquid forms, with dosage instructions printed on the label. You can also buy loose herbs – leaves, seeds, stems or whatever part of the plant contains the active ingredients – at many health-food shops and brew them into aromatic, appetizing, healing teas.

You can easily grow your own herbs in the garden or in pots on a windowsill. The usual harvesting method is to snip the stems, rinse the herbs with water and then hang them upside down to dry. When the leaves feel brittle but aren't so dry that they crumble, pick them and store them in a dark container. Packing jars to the lid keeps out oxygen and helps to maintain freshness. If you're growing herbs for their medicinal flowers, harvest the flowers just after the plant blooms.

Most herbal teas involve adding 1 rounded teaspoon of dried herb (or a tablespoon of fresh) to a cup of boiling water. Infuse for about 10 minutes, let cool, then strain and drink. Teas made from bark, seeds or roots need to steep longer. Start with small amounts of a therapeutic herbal tea – say, one to three cups a day. Only use larger amounts under the supervision of a qualified herbalist or a herb-friendly doctor.

Other supplements

'Supplements' used to mean standard vitamins and minerals that people took to give their diets a boost. Today, pharmacy shelves sag under the weight of amino acids, natural hormones and antioxidants, to name just a few.

For a long time, doctors dismissed the claims (sometimes extravagant) of supplement makers. There are, undeniably, some dubious products on sale that make outrageous promises, ranging from instant weight loss to an overnight boost in virility. On the other hand, even the most old-fashioned doctors have realized that some supplements have earned their place alongside conventional drugs.

Glucosamine is a good example. It was initially dismissed by the medical profession but studies over the last 15 years have shown that it does in fact help the body to repair damaged cartilage. Rheumatologists and orthopaedic specialists now often recommend it to people who need relief from arthritic joints.

Lycopene is another supplement singled out for scientific attention. An antioxidant found in tomatoes and sold in supplement form, it may help to lower a man's risk of prostate cancer. Coenzyme Q_{10}, a chemical naturally produced by the body, improves the heart's pumping ability in people with congestive heart failure. Fish oil capsules may lower levels of both cholesterol and also inflammatory chemicals that increase the risk of heart attack. The list goes on.

Even the most old-fashioned doctors have realized that some supplements have earned their place alongside conventional drugs.

Buying supplements

You don't have to spend long online to realize that many of the claims about supplements are exaggerated, to say the least. There is much confusion about the law as regards supplements – even some manufacturers and nutritional therapists are baffled by it. Part of the problem is that supplements are covered by either food or medicine legislation, neither of which is necessarily appropriate. Most supplements are classed as foods, so they don't have to undergo the rigorous testing and scrutiny that drugs receive, and manufacturers aren't allowed to promise specific health benefits on the labels. They are allowed to describe potential benefits, though – such as 'promotes healthy cholesterol' or 'aids digestion'. Medicinal

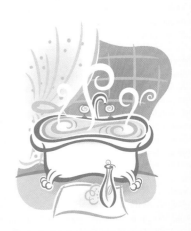

benefits can only be claimed on products that have a special licence from the Medicines and Healthcare products Regulatory Agency (MHRA). Licensed vitamin supplements have a PL (Product Licence) number on the packaging.

Even if a herb or supplement has been proven to be safe and effective, there's no guarantee that the particular product you're buying contains the active ingredients in the right amounts. Here's some advice to help you choose and use good products.

Buy reputable brands When independent laboratories analyse supplements, they sometimes find nothing very useful at all. Supplements may contain little or even none of the listed active ingredients. And the amounts of those ingredients can vary unpredictably from pill to pill. Established manufacturers have their reputations to protect so will try to ensure that their products contain what is stated on the labels.

Buy standardized herbal extracts Whenever possible, buy herbal supplements with the word 'standardized' on the label. This indicates that each pill or capsule contains a specified amount of the active ingredient.

Take the correct dose Be sure to read labels and package inserts carefully and never exceed the recommended doses on herbal remedies or supplements. The same applies, of course, to over-the-counter medications.

Understanding BP This stands for British Pharmacopeia, a commission appointed by the government that works closely with the Medicines and Healthcare products Regulatory Agency (MHRA). 'BP' on a label means the product contains the right amount of the right active ingredient of the right quality. It applies to all products intended for medicinal use. Products like vitamins that are not sold for medicinal purposes do not have to comply with the British Pharmacopeia but can carry the letters BP if they are of the required quality.

Aromatherapy: healing scents

As you stroll through a herb garden, it's hard to resist the temptation to pick a few leaves, crush them between your fingers and enjoy the fragrance. We now know those scents are not only pleasant but often therapeutic. Captured in essential oils, the fragrances pass directly to nerve centres in the brain, where they produce a wide range of responses. Essential oils can help to relieve anxiety and depression, tame our reactions to stress and enhance energy. Research shows that the scents of certain herbs – such as lavender, bergamot, marjoram and sandalwood – actually alter brain waves, inducing relaxation and sleep.

Today we can get these benefits from commercially prepared, highly concentrated essential oils. A plant may contain as little as 1 per cent fragrant oil, but when that oil is extracted and distilled, the scent is intense.

You can enjoy the healing benefits of essential oils in several ways – inhaling the scent, soaking in water that contains an oil or massaging it onto your skin. To inhale the fragrance, just put a drop or two of essential oil on a handkerchief, or a few drops on a lightbulb ring, or use a vapourizer or diffuser.

An oil used for bathing or massage should be diluted in a 'carrier' oil. To make a massage oil, add 8 to 12 drops of essential oil to 8 teaspoons of a cold-pressed plant oil such as almond, grapeseed or sunflower oil. For bathing, the usual mix is 10 to 30 drops of essential oil in 20 teaspoons of a carrier.

Essential oils can help to relieve anxiety and depression, tame our reactions to stress and enhance energy.

Essential oils are highly concentrated and must not be taken internally. Some people have an allergic reaction to oils, so take care when trying out a new oil. Also, because essential oils can pass through the skin into the bloodstream, they should not be used by pregnant women. Talk to a qualified practitioner before applying essential oil if you have sensitive skin, epilepsy, high blood pressure or if you've recently had an operation.

To make sure you buy high-quality essential oils and store them properly, you may want to get some advice from an aromatherapist. Many oils can be stored for years without losing their fragrance, though some citrus oils – like orange and lemon – need to be kept in the fridge. Store oils in sealed dark bottles away from sunlight, and preferably in a cool place.

What is homeopathy?

If you haven't come across homeopathy before, you might be wary of the strange little bottles marked with 'c's and 'x's on the shelves of health-food shops. But there's no need to fear these remedies. The homeopathic mixtures recommended in this book are extremely safe, and many are widely respected as healing agents – even if it's impossible to explain why they work. Imagine taking a single drop of any drug – say, a liquid decongestant. Dilute that drop with 10 drops of water. Shake the mixture well, take out a single drop, and dilute it with another 10 drops of water. Repeat the process a few times, and what's left? According to the laws of science, not much. But according to homeopathy, the highly diluted mixture is among the most powerful drugs you can take.

You can see why homeopathy, a branch of medicine that was developed by a German physician more than 200 years ago, hasn't won unanimous support from mainstream medics. Nevertheless many homeopaths are also conventional doctors, and the experience of millions of patients – and several scientific studies – suggest there's something to it.

Here are the basics. Working from a list of more than 2,000 substances, homeopaths give sick patients a substance that in large doses would mimic the symptoms of their disease but, in very tiny amounts, theoretically relieves their symptoms. Most of the remedies used in homeopathy come from herbs or minerals, such as St John's wort for depression, comfrey for wounds or bruises and eyebright for tired sore eyes. But many are diluted with so much water that they contain little or even none of the active ingredient.

An analysis of 107 scientific studies of homeopathic medicines found that 77 per cent of them showed positive effects.

Most experts say that homeopathy violates a basic principle of pharmaceutical science: the smaller the dose, the *smaller* the effects. Yet researchers who study homeopathy have come up with some intriguing results. A study of 478 flu patients, for example, found that 17 per cent of those treated with homeopathy improved, compared to just 10 per cent of those taking placebos. In 1991, the prestigious *British Medical Journal*, in an analysis of 107 scientific studies of homeopathic medicines, found that 77 per cent of them showed positive effects.

It has been suggested that the process of diluting and shaking the solutions somehow 'potentizes' the remaining water and changes its chemical properties. But no one really knows how – or whether – homeopathy actually works. As the doses of active ingredients are so small, however, there's no harm in trying it. You can buy homeopathic remedies in health-food shops, but you should consult an experienced homeopath. Different remedies are used for each symptom you are experiencing, and the remedies as well as the doses may change depending on your mental and emotional state at the time.

The doses used in homeopathy are confusing at first. You'll usually see them listed as x or c on the label. A 1x remedy has been diluted once, using 1 part of the active ingredient in 10 parts water. A 2x solution contains 1 part of the active ingredient in 100 parts water, and a 3x solution contains 1 part of the active ingredient in 1,000 parts water. The c solutions are even more dilute; they may not contain even a single molecule of the original active ingredient.

Homeopathy isn't a substitute for a doctor's care. Most homeopaths spend at least an hour with new patients. They take a complete health history, review symptoms and decide whether or not homeopathy is appropriate for the patient – and whether he or she needs to see a conventional doctor.

Mind-body medicine

Many of the health conditions in this book suggest remedies that involve meditation, progressive relaxation, yoga or tai chi. Whatever form they take, relaxation and meditation techniques have proved their power. One of the most well-studied practices is transcendental meditation, or TM. In exploring the benefits of TM, Harvard researcher Dr Herbert Benson measured the physical responses of students who sat quietly with their eyes closed and repeated a word or phrase (called a mantra) over and over again. The 20-minute 'exercises' were done once or twice a day. Dr Benson discovered that the profound calm induced by TM could reduce blood pressure as well as slow down heart rate and breathing. Many of the stress-relief benefits of meditation also help to increase immunity and combat problems such as anxiety and depression.

All kinds of meditation and relaxation techniques can be done at home at any time and with minimal preparation, so they are suitable for many health conditions, from anxiety and high blood pressure to psoriasis and menstrual problems.

If you have never tried meditation, start with a simple 20-minute exercise. Just sit in a comfortable, upright position with your back straight, your head upright and your body relaxed. With your eyes closed, concentrate completely on your breathing. Take deep steady breaths feeling the rise and fall of your abdomen, not your chest. Focus on a word or sound, such as 'peace' or 'om', and repeat it over and over again. Whenever your attention wanders, bring it back to your word or sound and your breathing again. After about 20 minutes stop, open your eyes and stretch. Take it slowly when you first stand up and begin to move around again.

If you have difficulty meditating, you might want to have classes from an instructor who practises TM, yoga or tai chi. Classes are often advertised at health clubs, community centres or adult education centres.

Teaming up with professionals

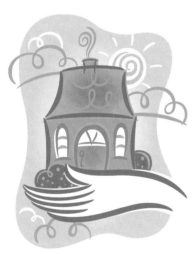

We may spend millions of pounds a year on herbs and supplements but we haven't given up on conventional medicine. What most of us want is the best of both worlds – cutting-edge techniques of modern medicine *and* the natural home treatments that earlier generations depended on.

This approach, known as complementary medicine, makes sense. If you have heart disease or diabetes, for example, you want the most advanced care you can get. But there's a lot you can do yourself at the same time – not only to relieve symptoms and feel better, but also to give nature a hand and help your body to reverse the condition or recover more quickly.

Don't hesitate to talk to your doctor about the remedies you use at home. You may even discover that your GP has his or her own favourites, such as massaging away a headache or soothing a rash with an oatmeal bath. After all, conventional medicine and home remedies aren't the adversaries they're sometimes made out to be. Each has strengths and weaknesses – and both work best when used together.

If you like the idea of 'natural' healing methods which involve non-suppression of symptoms and non-interference with the body's natural defence systems, consider seeing a naturopathic doctor. The letters ND after a name mean that a naturopath has acquired a national diploma after a four-year degree course. Naturopaths have similarly rigorous training in diagnostic skills as conventional doctors.

The remedies: a final word

This book contains a huge number of remedies from a wide variety of sources, including traditional folk remedies. Many of the traditional 'recipes' we found for teas, elixirs and tonics called for specific measurements. One grandmother may have specified, for instance, 2 teaspoons of honey, 24 cloves of garlic or 3 handfuls of fresh parsley. But in many cases the exact amounts aren't critical to the success of the remedy. So the quantities that you find in this book may differ somewhat from those in home remedies that you may have gleaned from your own family.

What most of us want is the best of both worlds – cutting-edge techniques of modern medicine *and* the natural home treatments that earlier generations depended on.

For each 'recipe', however, we've included the ingredients that are most likely to provide some direct health benefits and left out those that are ineffective or that could cause problems.

Whenever possible, we recommend ingredients available from local sources such as supermarkets, pharmacies, health-food shops or medical supply stores. Many products are now available online.

Of course, many of the remedies in this book don't require any special ingredients at all – just the right food, exercise or hands-on healing. Temporary relief, or even a cure, may be as near as your kitchen cupboard or medicine cabinet.

If one remedy doesn't work for you, try another. If it does work, make sure you pass it on to a loved one or friend so that they might one day benefit from it too.

NHS direct offers advice and information online – **www.nhsdirect.nhs.uk** – and by telephone, 24 hours a day. You can call the helpline – **0845 46 47** – at local call rates for advice from a nurse about what to do when you are ill, and both services can give information about specific health conditions and support organizations, as well as your local NHS services including doctors, dentists, opticians and pharmacies.

PART ONE

EVERYDAY AILMENTS

When you itch, ache, or sting, when you're coughing, sneezing or otherwise suffering, it's **deeply comforting** to know that there are thousands of **effective remedies** that can help. And you don't need a doctor's prescription for any of them. Just stock your cabinets with a few **healing essentials** (see The Top 20 Household Healers, page 384), then raid your **refrigerator**, plunder your **larder**, harvest your **garden** and rob your **garage** to find what else you need. Some of the remedies, like simple acupressure techniques, are literally **at your fingertips**. Something ailing you? Find out how to **soothe** it with oatmeal, **pamper** it with peppermint, **banish** it with bicarbonate of soda or **tame** it with tea bags. From bad breath to bug bites, head lice to heartburn, shingles to splinters, here are treatments for more than a **hundred health complaints**.

Acne

If scientists can decipher the human genome why, you might ask, can't they find a way to eradicate acne? With no sign of a cure on the horizon, it's up to you to deal with the outbreaks of spots that can damage your looks and your self-esteem long past adolescence. When a pimple rears its ugly head, there are several over-the-counter products that can help. But then, so too can simple natural remedies.

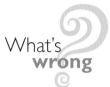

What's wrong

Your skin is producing too much sebum – a natural oily lubricant – and the excess is blocking your pores. There are two kinds of acne. The most common form, acne vulgaris, occurs on your face, chest, shoulders or back as blackheads, whiteheads or red spots. Cystic acne occurs as painful cysts or firm, painless lumps. Hormone fluctuations caused by puberty, taking contraceptive pills, periods, pregnancy or the onset of the menopause often increase sebum production, which can trigger an outbreak of acne. Other culprits include certain types of make-up, sunbathing and stress. Acne is usually hereditary.

Eradicate spots now

• The first avenue of assault is an over-the-counter cream, lotion, liquid or gel formulated with **benzoyl peroxide** – the Oxy range or PanOxyl, for example. These work by mildly irritating the skin, which encourages dying skin cells to flake off. This in turn helps to reopen blocked pores. Benzoyl peroxide also kills the bacteria that infect blocked pores.

• **Alpha-hydroxy acids** (AHAs), such as glycolic acid, slough off the outermost layer of dead skin cells, which helps to keep pores clear and unblocked. Look for any skin cream, lotion or gel that contains glycolic acid.

• At the first hint of a pimple, get out an **ice cube, wrap it** in a piece of cling film and hold it to the area affected at least twice a day – every hour if you can, but for no longer than five minutes each time. The cold will reduce the redness and ease the inflammation.

• Take **aspirin** or **ibuprofen**. These painkillers are anti-inflammatory and can help to calm an acne outbreak. Take the recommended adult dose up to four times a day. (Do not take aspirin regularly for more than a few days without checking with your doctor, and never give aspirin to a child under 16.)

Alternative acne treatments

• Apply a drop of **tea-tree oil** to blemishes three times a day to discourage infection and speed up healing. Research has found that 5 per cent tea-tree oil is as effective against acne as a 5 per cent benzoyl peroxide solution.

• For acne that flares up before a menstrual period, drink 1 to 2 cups of **chasteberry tea** a day. Some studies show that this herb helps to regulate female hormones, but give it two or three months to work. And don't drink lots more of the tea to improve the results – it may make your skin worse.

● Apply **vinegar** or **lemon juice** to pimples using a cotton wool pad. The acids present in lemon juice and all vinegars can help to flush out pores. **Toothpaste** smeared on an outbreak is also reputed to work well – try applying it before you go to bed.

● A folk remedy for healing pimples is to use a mixture of **spice and honey** on them. Mix 1 teaspoon of powdered nutmeg with 1 teaspoon of honey and apply it to the pimple. Leave it on for 20 minutes, then rinse off. There's no scientific proof that this helps, but honey does have antiseptic properties.

● Apply **aloe vera.** One study found that 90 per cent of skin sores were completely healed with aloe vera within five days. Buy a product containing aloe vera, or squeeze the gel from the middle of a freshly cut leaf and apply it to the skin.

Keep your skin clean – but not too clean

● You may think that keeping your skin clean will prevent blocked pores. But overcleansing can cause acne by stimulating the sebaceous glands to produce more oil. **Avoid granulated cleansers.** And **don't use a flannel,** which is **abrasive** and may also harbour bacteria. Instead, use disposable cleansing pads.

● Make a skin cleanser by adding 1 teaspoon of **Epsom salts** and 3 drops of **iodine** to 125ml water. Bring to the boil, let cool and apply on a clean cotton wool ball.

● Men: **clean your razor** with surgical spirit after use to stop any bacteria being harboured.

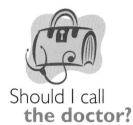

Should I call the doctor?

Getting a pimple now and then is not a major problem. But if your blemishes don't respond to over-the-counter treatments within three months or your skin becomes severely inflamed with painful, fluid-filled lumps and a reddish or purplish cast, then see your doctor. You should also seek medical advice if your skin is always red and flushed, even if acne isn't present; you may have the beginnings of rosacea (see page 328), a skin condition characterized by persistent redness, pimples and enlarged blood vessels.

To squeeze or not to squeeze

If you have to attack your spots, follow this dermatologist-approved method, suitable for whiteheads. Clean the area and sterilize the tip of a needle by holding it in a naked flame for 3 seconds or wiping it with surgical spirit. Then gently nick the surface of the pimple. Drain it with cotton wool and clean it with 20 vol hydrogen peroxide solution. Don't squeeze or pick the spot – you'll make it worse. To deal with blackheads, buy a blackhead extractor, available online and from some chemists. Soften the blemish with a hot-water compress for 10 minutes before you use the device.

Age spots

Age spots, or liver spots, are flat areas of brown pigment that often occur on the backs of the hands. The best way to prevent them – and to protect yourself from skin cancer, too – is by using plenty of sunscreen. If it's too late and you already have age spots, look for an over-the-counter fading cream or apply a simple, natural bleaching agent. Bear in mind that it can take several months to see an improvement. And from now on, make sure you never leave the house without proper sun protection.

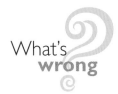

What's wrong

Despite their name, these flat or rounded brown spots that can appear on the face or backs of the hands aren't caused by age. They are simply areas of excess pigment, which result from years of exposure to sunlight. Because it takes decades to see the sun damage, many people don't notice the marks until later in life, but people who have had significant sun exposure can develop them in their twenties and thirties. Some drugs can make you more vulnerable to sun damage and related age spots. These include diuretics, tetracycline and drugs for diabetes and high blood pressure.

Lighten up

- A stain lightening cream called **Fade Out** contains a 2 per cent solution of the bleaching agent hydroquinone. (Darker spots may need a stronger solution, but for that you will need a prescription from a dermatologist.) Before you use Fade Out, carefully read the manufacturer's directions.
- Apply the juice of a **lemon** to the spots at least twice a day. Lemon juice is mildly acidic and may be strong enough to take off the skin's outer layer and remove or lighten age spots.
- Blend **honey and yoghurt** to create a natural bleach that can lighten age spots. Mix 1 teaspoon of plain yoghurt and 1 teaspoon of honey. Apply, allow to dry for 30 minutes, then rinse. Do this once a day.
- Coat your spots with **aloe vera gel**, taken straight from the leaves of a living plant, if possible. Cut the leaf and squeeze it to extract the gel. The plant contains chemicals that slough away dead cells and encourage the growth of new, healthy ones. Apply the gel once or twice a day.
- A folk remedy for removing age spots is to wipe them with buttermilk. This contains lactic acid, which gently exfoliates sun-damaged skin and pigmented areas.

Go undercover

- Camouflage age spots with a **cosmetic concealer** – sold in department stores and pharmacies. Some are enriched with oils to moisturize your skin as well. Ask a sales assistant to help you find the right shade for your skin – usually slightly lighter than your own skin tone – and show you how to apply it.

The power of prevention

● **Avoid the sun** as much as possible during peak hours – from 10am to 4pm in summer or in hot climates, and from 10am to 2pm for the rest of the year.

● Every day, 30 minutes before you go outside, apply **sunscreen** to your face and the backs of your hands. Make sure it has a sun protection factor (SPF) of at least 15. The most effective sunscreens for guarding against age spots contain zinc oxide or titanium dioxide. If you are going to be outdoors for any length of time, reapply every two hours.

● **Wear a sunhat** with a wide brim of at least 10cm (4in). This will keep the sun off your face and neck and help to stop age spots from developing in those areas. Choose a hat with a cotton lining – woven straw hats don't give much protection.

● After you've been out in the sun, apply some **vitamin E** oil. Vitamin E is an antioxidant and may help to prevent age spots by neutralizing skin-damaging free radical molecules. But smooth it on only *after* sun exposure as vitamin E itself produces free radicals when it's exposed to sunlight.

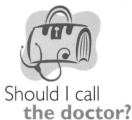

Should I call the doctor?

Age spots, which usually look like dark, smooth freckles, are generally harmless. However, if a spot starts to tingle, itch, change size or colour or bleed, you should see your doctor. Some skin cancers, like melanoma, can look like age spots. If home remedies don't work on your age spots, your GP may recommend a dermatologist who may get rid of them using laser treatment or by applying liquid nitrogen. This treatment is unlikely to be available on the NHS.

Allergies

Itching, sneezing, sore or irritated eyes and a runny nose – these are all common symptoms of hay fever and other allergies. Take anti-allergy medication if you wish – but take it *before* an allergy attack for the best results – or try one of the natural antihistamines suggested below. You'll also want to tackle pollen, house dust mites, pet dander and other microscopic menaces that send your immune system into overdrive.

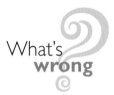

What's wrong

Allergic symptoms are signs that the immune system is overreacting to normally harmless substances such as pollen (which causes hay fever), dust, pet dander (tiny flakes of dried saliva, skin and hair) or mould. Usually, the immune system ignores these 'triggers' and focuses on protecting you from real threats, such as viruses or bacteria. But when someone has an allergy, the immune system cannot distinguish certain harmless substances from dangerous ones. Triggers can be ingested (such as wheat and peanuts), absorbed through the skin (such as plants or base metals), inhaled (such as mould or pollen) or received by injection (such as a penicillin jab). Sensitivity to allergens tends to be inherited.

Nature's antihistamines

• **Nettle** contains a substance that works as a natural antihistamine. Capsules of the freeze-dried leaf are sold in health-food shops. Take 500mg three times a day.

• **Ginkgo biloba** has become renowned for its memory-boosting properties, but it can also be an effective allergy fighter. Ginkgo contains substances called ginkgolides, which can halt the activity of certain allergy-triggering chemicals (platelet activating factor, or PAF). Take up to 240mg a day.

• **Quercetin**, the pigment that gives grapes their purple hue and puts the green in green tea, inhibits the release of histamine. Take one 500mg capsule twice a day. (*Alert* Do not take this if already taking nettle, as nettle contains quercetin.)

Try something fishy

• **Omega-3 fatty acids** help to counter inflammatory responses in the body, such as those triggered by allergies. Salmon, sardines, fresh tuna and mackerel are good sources of these fats. If you prefer the idea of fish oil capsules, take a supplement that provides 1000mg combined EPA/DHA (eicosapentaenoic and docosahexanoic acids) a day.

• **Flax seed oil** (or linseed oil) is another excellent source of omega-3 fatty acids. Take 1 tablespoon of flax seed oil a day. You can add it to salad dressing or a glass of juice or blend it into a smoothie, but avoid heating it.

Try these simple soothers

• To soothe red, itchy, swollen eyes, dampen a flannel with **cool water** and place it over your eyes as often as you wish.

• **Saline nasal sprays** have long been used to clear nasal mucus and can also help keep your nasal passages moisturized. But a recent study has shown that some nasal sprays contain a preservative that can actually damage the cells of your sinuses, so it may be safer to make your own. Dissolve half a teaspoon of salt in 250ml of warm water. Fill a bulb syringe, lean over the sink and gently squirt the saline into your nose.

Protect yourself from hay fever symptoms

• **Shelter** indoors before a **thunderstorm** – and for up to three hours afterwards. Storms are preceded by high humidity, which makes pollen grains swell, burst and release their irritating starch, triggering a hay fever attack.

• When you have to go out, wear **wraparound sunglasses** to keep the pollen away from your eyes.

• If you don't mind how you look, **wear a face mask** when you know you might be exposed to pollen. DIY stores sell effective and inexpensive small air filter masks designed for people working in dusty environments.

• You can also protect yourself outdoors with a 'pollen trap.' Dab a little **Vaseline (petroleum jelly)** just inside your nostrils – the theory is that the sticky layer will trap spores that are wafting around before you inhale them.

• **Keep the windows closed** when travelling by car and if the car is fitted with an air conditioner, choose the 'recirculate' setting so as not to draw pollinated air into the car. Some cars can be fitted with pollen filters – ask for details at your local garage or dealer.

• **Wash your hair** before going to bed so you don't transfer a headful of dust and pollen to your pillow.

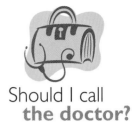

Should I call the doctor?

If a person's tongue, face, hands or neck swell rapidly, he or she has difficulty in breathing – with or without wheezing – and rapidly develops urticaria or hives (raised red or white weals), then dial 999. These are signs of anaphylactic shock, a potentially fatal allergic reaction – for example, to a bee sting, peanuts or shellfish. Generally, allergy symptoms tend to be merely miserable and uncomfortable. However, if over-the-counter remedies don't do the trick or no longer work for you, or if you can't work out what it is that you're allergic to, then it is advisable to go and see your doctor.

Don't give up gardening

If you enjoy gardening, you might consider creating a hay-fever-friendly environment for yourself. Grow insect-pollinated plants such as geraniums, iris and clematis. Consider replacing the lawn with attractive paving – as mowing the grass creates clouds of pollen and spores. Don't grow any new hedges and don't cut existing ones yourself. Do away with compost heaps, which produce mould spores. Ask Asthma UK (www.asthma.org.uk) for a free copy of their Low-Allergen Garden pamphlet. This is full of practical advice about creating the type of garden that won't exacerbate your hay fever.

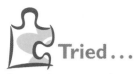

Deal with dust mites

- **Dust mites,** nasty little flesh-eating monsters too small to be seen by the naked eye, inhabit your carpets, curtains and bedding. Their faeces can be a significant cause of allergies. To starve mites of the dust they eat – which is mostly made of shed skin cells – **cover your mattress, divan base and pillows** with covers made specifically to repel allergens. These covers are sold in pharmacies and department stores.
- **Vacuum your carpets** regularly. If you can afford one, buy a vacuum cleaner that uses a double bag and a HEPA (high-efficiency particulate air) filter. These machines can filter out even microscopic allergens. If you have an attractive wood or tile floor underneath your carpets, think about getting rid of the carpets altogether.
- **Change your sheets** once a week and wash them in very hot water – at least 60°C – to kill the mites.
- **Clear away clutter,** which can gather dust and harbour dust mites.
- If you don't have **a dehumidifier,** it's a good idea to get one. Keeping the air in your home dry will significantly reduce the population of dust mites, which die when humidity levels fall below 45 per cent.

Reduce reactions to animal allergens

- **Keep your pet out of the bedroom.** Allergic reactions can be triggered by animal fur, dead skin, dried saliva and dander – particles of scurf from the coats of animals. All of these allergens linger even when the animal leaves the room.
- Some dogs are perfectly happy in a traditional **outdoor**

When a kiss is <u>not</u> just a kiss ...

Avoiding known food or drug allergens may sound easy, but sometimes you can be exposed in less-than-obvious ways. Take the case of a young woman who had a life-threatening allergic reaction to shellfish simply when she kissed her boyfriend. He had eaten prawns an hour before he kissed her good night. Almost immediately, her lips swelled up, her throat began to close, she started wheezing, hives appeared, her stomach cramped and her blood pressure plummeted. She survived, but the lesson is clear: if your partner is severely allergic to a particular food, you must give it up as well. No one knows whether simply brushing your teeth or rinsing your mouth out would do any good, so it is better not to take the chance at all.

A military manoeuvre against allergies

This remedy was found effective in tests carried out by the US army. Eat honey made in your immediate neighbourhood and, if you can get hold of it, chew the honeycomb it comes in, too. The theory is that by eating honey produced by local bees, you can desensitize your immune system to local pollens. Starting two months before the hay fever season, eat 2 tablespoons of the honey a day, and chew the beeswax for 5 to 10 minutes. Continue until the hay fever season is over.

kennel. If you are allergic to your dogs, that might be the kindest solution for both of you.

- **Give your pet a bath once a week.** Bathing can remove up to 85 per cent of pet dander. You can use plain water or a proprietary pet shampoo.

Clear the air

- **Modern air filters** can capture air-borne allergens and may bring some relief from allergies to mould, pollen and pet dander though one study showed that they only significantly reduced cat allergens in uncarpeted homes. HEPA filters tend to work best. If you use an HEPA filter in your bedroom, keep the door closed so that it can effectively filter just the air in that room.

- Studies show that vigorous household cleaning significantly reduces dust, mould, dander and other common allergens. So give your home **a thorough clean** twice a year – once in spring and again in autumn. Wash every scrubbable surface with diluted bleach, from the insides of cupboards to the kickboards at the bottoms of kitchen base units. Clean furniture with a damp cloth. If your allergies are severe, you may want to pay someone to do the cleaning.

- Basements and cellars are havens for moulds, mildew and dust mites, especially if they become wet in rainy weather. **Run a dehumidifier** all the time in a damp basement – and empty its reservoir regularly.

- A tumble dryer can throw out masses of fine particles of lint and dust. **Make sure the tumble dryer's hose is properly sealed** and ideally vents outdoors, so that it doesn't send allergy-triggers floating through the house.

Angina

Anyone consulting a doctor with angina symptoms is likely to be given a prescription for nitroglycerine (also known as glyceryl trinitrate). But rather than causing an explosion, nitroglycerine tablets can help patients to deal with the onset of attacks, easing the chest pain and tightness by increasing the supply of blood and oxygen to the heart. As the slogan for travellers' cheques goes – don't leave home without them. But in addition to medication, there are plenty of ways to cope with angina attacks, reduce their frequency or even prevent them from happening at all.

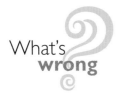

What's wrong

That crushing, squeezing chest pain is telling you – loudly – that your heart isn't getting enough oxygen-rich blood. The most likely cause is the build-up of a fatty substance called plaque that is blocking the arteries that serve the heart. Angina pain often begins below the breastbone and radiates to the shoulder, arm or jaw. It may be accompanied by shortness of breath, temporary nausea, lightheadedness, irregular heartbeat and anxiety.

Immediate measures

● If you're standing, walking around or exercising when an attack occurs, **sit down and rest** for a few minutes.

● If you're lying down or resting when the telltale pressure presents itself, **change your body position** by sitting or standing up. That takes pressure off the nerve in your heart that is signalling pain. Angina that occurs when you are resting is a sign that you may be at much higher risk of a heart attack, so contact your doctor as soon as possible.

● If the attack comes on when you're emotionally excited or anxious, try to **calm yourself**. Like physical stress, mental stress can increase your heart's demand for oxygen. Do your heart a favour by learning yoga, tai chi, meditation or some other stress-relieving technique that you can practise regularly.

Help your heart with foods and supplements

● Several studies have shown that **a clove of garlic a day** can lower high cholesterol and there is evidence that garlic also reduces the tendency of blood to clot – another heart benefit. Eat it raw for maximum effect. If you can't stand the smell, take garlic capsules instead. Choose capsules that supply 4000mcg of allicin and take 400mg to 600mg a day.

● **Folic acid and vitamin B_{12}** are vitamins that lower raised levels of homocysteine, a substance in the blood that can increase your risk of heart disease. The best source of these vitamins may be dietary – some studies have questioned the benefits of supplements. Eat plenty of meat, fish or eggs for B_{12}

and leafy vegetables and citrus fruits for folic acid. Other research suggests that you can cut your risk of heart disease by taking 400mcg of folic acid and 0.5mg of vitamin B_{12} a day. (*Alert* If you have coronary heart disease, check with your doctor before taking folic acid and Vitamin B_{12} supplements.)

- Omega-3 fatty acids protect the heart and blood vessels and may help protect against angina. They are found in **fish oil capsules**, though if you eat oily fish – such as mackerel or sardines – twice a week, you need not take capsules. Check with your doctor before taking the supplements to be sure they won't interact with medications you are taking. Look for a supplement that provides 1000mg combined EPA/DHA (eicosapentaenoic and docosahexanoic acids) a day. This may mean taking a capsule labelled as 3000mg fish oil or more.

The power of prevention

- Work out an **exercise programme**, with your doctor's guidance; regular exercise can help to ward off angina pain.
- **If you smoke, quit.** The nicotine in cigarettes constricts the arteries, triggering angina or making it worse. And stay away from smoky environments, too.
- **Give up coffee**. Coffee has been linked to raised homocysteine levels, which increase the risk of angina attacks.
- After eating a large meal, rest or **engage in a quiet activity.** When you consume a heavy meal, the body diverts extra bloodflow to the digestive tract to aid digestion; so the heart receives less oxygen and is more vulnerable to an attack.
- **Don't stay outdoors in cold weather.** Cold air stimulates muscular reflexes that can cause angina.
- **Avoid sudden physical exertion,** such as running to catch a bus or lifting a heavy object.
- Try to **maintain a healthy body weight**. Eat five portions of fruit and vegetables a day and plenty of wholegrain cereals and starchy foods such as potatoes, pasta and rice. Cut down on fatty foods, particularly fried foods, biscuits and chocolate; and choose skimmed or semi-skimmed milk. Eat lean meat in preference to fatty cuts and fish at least twice a week. Keep spreads and oils to a minimum and vary them – olive oil for salad dressings and a polyunsaturated fat spread, for example. A moderate intake of red wine may also be helpful.

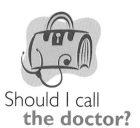

Should I call the doctor?

Many people who experience angina for the first time think that they're having a heart attack. While angina does not completely block the flow of blood to the heart, as a heart attack does, it's a warning that should not be ignored. If you think you might have angina, see your doctor as soon as possible. If you have chest pain that lasts for 15 minutes or is accompanied by shortness of breath and nausea, dial 999 straight away. While waiting for the ambulance to arrive, take 300mg soluble aspirin immediately (usually one tablet, but check the packet).

Anxiety

If it feels as if the causes of your anxiety are all around you, take heart: so are the cures. There are herbs and oils to add to a soothing warm bath, worry-calming teas and even some classic comfort foods. For those times when you feel anxious, here are some ways to be kind to yourself and lessen the worries.

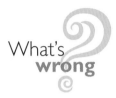

What's wrong

Anxiety is a reaction to a threat or danger that is vague or even unknown. You feel worried, but you are not quite sure why. It can manifest itself via any number of symptoms. including sweating, tummy churning, rapid heart beat, shivering, irritability, poor concentration, shallow breathing and unwanted thoughts or behaviour.

Soak away your cares

● A **warm bath** is one of the most pleasant and reliable ways to soothe your senses. To enhance its effects, add some **lavender oil** (or dried flowers if you have them) to the tub and soak to your heart's content. Although no one knows what gives this wonderfully scented herb its ability to calm, lavender has been used for around 2,000 years to relax and soothe the nerves. If you have no time for a bath, try dabbing a little lavender oil on your temples and forehead and sitting quietly for a few minutes.

Breathe slowly and deeply

● **Regulating your breath** can help to bring your anxiety swiftly under control. To slow and deepen your breathing, sit down, put one hand over your abdomen, and slowly inhale so that your belly expands under your hand but your shoulders do not rise. Hold your breath for four or five seconds, then very slowly exhale. Repeat until you feel calmer.

Sip something soporific

● An old-fashioned remedy for insomnia, drinking a glass of **warm milk** really works – and at any time of day. Milk contains tryptophan, an amino acid used in the production of the brain chemical serotonin, which enhances feelings of well-being. Bananas and turkey are also rich in tryptophan.

● **Hops**, which give beer its distinctive flavour, have a long history as a sedative. In fact, workers who harvested hops used to suffer from sleepiness known as hop-pickers' fatigue. Place 2 teaspoons of the dried herb in a cup of very hot water, and drink up to three cups a day of this 'anti-anxiety tea'.

- **Three flowers** used to make relaxing teas are Seville (bitter) orange blossom, lavender and lime tree. Any of these sweetly scented teas taken at bedtime will help to encourage a good night's sleep.

Don't make the symptoms worse

- Limit yourself to a single cup of **coffee, tea or cola drink** per day. Studies suggest that people with anxiety symptoms may be especially sensitive to caffeine.
- **Watch your intake** of wine, beer and other alcoholic drinks. While they seem to subdue anxiety at first, when the alcohol wears off, anxiety can actually increase.

Speed up and slow down

- **Aerobic exercise** is a great anxiety reliever. Taking a brisk 30 minute walk spurs the release of endorphins, chemicals that block pain and improve your mood.
- Whether it's meditating, praying, pruning the roses or watching your goldfish, do some sort of **meditative activity** for 15 minutes several times a day.

Try a natural anxiety soother

- A pleasant smell *isn't* something you can expect from the herb **valerian**, but if you are looking for relief from anxiety, you might forgive the stench. Research suggests that the active ingredients in valerian attach to the same receptors in the brain that are affected by the anti–anxiety drug diazepam, better known as Valium. Take 250mg twice a day and up to 500mg before bedtime.

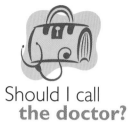

Should I call the doctor?

Prolonged, severe anxiety can take a serious toll on your physical health. Seek help if you're anxious for most of the time, can't sleep or concentrate, turn to alcohol, drugs or food to quell your anxiety, or feel as if you might harm yourself or others. It is worth noting that anxiety symptoms can mimic those of serious conditions, such as hyperthyroidism, hypoglycaemia (low blood sugar) and heart attack, or occur as a side-effect of some medications. So it is advisable to discuss your symptoms with a doctor.

Anxiety or panic attacks

Unlike general worry, anxiety attacks come on suddenly and with overwhelming force. The heart begins to race, the blood pressure rises, it becomes a struggle to breathe and the victim may feel dizzy or faint. The symptoms can even be confused with those of a heart attack. Anxiety attacks are most likely to occur after a period of unusual stress, such as a death or divorce. The best way to handle them is to see them for what they are: harmless, if frightening, emotional states. Remind yourself that you're not in any danger; it is only a panic attack, and it will soon end. Stay as calm as you can, try to regulate your breath, as described above, and let the attack run its course.

Beat anxiety with positive thinking

If you repeat a statement to yourself often enough, you start to believe it. This is a useful tool for dealing with challenging situations. Try these – or make up some of your own.

Meeting strangers: *'This is a valuable opportunity to get to know someone I've never met before.'*

Beginning a new job: *'I am capable of doing this job, and I can master the skills that will allow me to succeed.'*

When challenged: *'It doesn't matter whether others think I am right or wrong as long as I make the best judgment I can and express my views honestly.'*

Dealing with setbacks and insecurity: *'I have overcome hurdles like this in the past, and I know I can do it again.'*

Making a public speech or presentation: *'I have something important to say that everyone in this room wants to hear.'*

When faced with rejection: *'I have been given the chance to try new alternatives and take a different path, and I am prepared for new challenges.'*

● Take a **B-complex multivitamin** each day. Studies show that B vitamins are natural stress-reducers – the body requires vitamin B_6 to make serotonin, for example – and not getting enough of the vitamins can contribute to anxiety.

● **5-hydroxytryptophan (5-HTP)** can replenish your supply of serotonin, an anxiety-calming brain chemical. The 5-HTP in your body comes from the amino acid tryptophan, but small quantities are also found in the seeds of an African plant, *Griffonia simplicifolia*. Supplements of 5-HTP are made from extract of the plant or produced synthetically. You can buy them in health-food shops or online. Take 50mg three times daily with meals. But consult your doctor if you're also taking any prescription antidepressant, such as Prozac, Lustral or Seroxat as these drugs also affect serotonin receptors, and the combined effect could be dangerous. Do not drive or do hazardous work until you determine how 5-HTP affects you. It can cause drowsiness in some people.

Arthritis

If you suffer from joint pain, join the club. So many people have osteoarthritis, you'll soon be offered advice not only by your doctor, family and friends but also by the plumber and your next-door neighbour. Anti-inflammatory drugs – prescription and over-the-counter – can ease the pain, and most people will want to take them. But relief from arthritis doesn't end there. There are plenty of other measures that sufferers can take to achieve their goal of easy-moving, pain-free days.

Pain removers

- Take **glucosamine and chondroitin sulphate** supplements to reduce pain and slow down cartilage loss. Evidence suggests that this combination can be effective for people with mild to moderate arthritis. Follow the dosage directions on the label, and persevere: it may take a month or more before you begin to feel the benefits.
- Take a ½ teaspoon of **powdered ginger** or up to 35g (about 6 teaspoons) of fresh ginger once a day. Research shows that ginger root helps to relieve arthritis pain, probably because of its ability to increase blood circulation, and thus ferry inflammatory chemicals away from painful joints.
- Take two 400mg doses of **SAM-e** (S-adenosylmethionine) a day. Supplementing with SAM-e, a chemical found naturally in all cells of the body, has been shown to help relieve arthritis pain by increasing blood levels of proteoglycans – molecules that seem to play a key role in preserving cartilage by helping to keep it 'plumped up' and well oxygenated. SAM-e also appears to reduce inflammation. Research has found the supplement as effective as anti-inflammatory drugs such as ibuprofen in fighting arthritis pain.

If you get good results with 800mg a day, reduce the dose to 400mg a day after two weeks. SAM-e has few side-effects, although it can cause dyspepsia and nausea. It seems to be safe to take with most prescription and OTC drugs, but if you are taking drugs prescribed for bipolar disorder (manic depression) or Parkinson's disease, you should consult your doctor *before* taking SAM-e supplements.

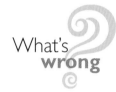

What's **wrong**

There are more than 100 types of arthritis, but the most common type is osteoarthritis. Symptoms include painfully stiff, swollen joints in any part of the body. The pain is the result of wear and tear on cartilage, the gel-like shock-absorbing material between joints. When cartilage wears away, bone grinds against bone. Although you can develop osteoarthritis at any age, it usually occurs in people over 45, and is more common among women. Other forms of the disease are rheumatoid arthritis and psoriatic arthritis.

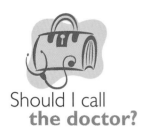

Should I call the doctor?

Since you can't be sure what kind of arthritis you have, or whether your symptoms suggest another condition entirely, it's best to discuss any joint stiffness, swelling, redness or pain with your doctor. If you've already been diagnosed with arthritis, see your doctor if you notice a new or different type of swelling in your joints.

Seek heat relief and cold comfort

- **Applying heat** to a painful joint can provide significant relief. For heat sources, you can use electric blankets and hand warmers, heating pads or hot packs. Warm the achy joint for 20 minutes. Simply taking a hot bath can also be soothing.
- **Cold treatments** can work well when joints are inflamed. Wrap ice cubes in a towel or flannel and hold against the sore joint. Alternatively, you can use a bag of frozen peas.

Wear gloves to bed?

- If you frequently have stiff, swollen hands in the morning, try **wearing a snug-fitting pair of gloves** to bed. They may help to keep the swelling in check. But stop if you find that wearing gloves to bed only makes morning stiffness worse.

Oil your aching joints

- Eat more **oily fish.** Many people who supplement their diets with omega-3 fatty acids – found in oily fish such as mackerel, pilchards, salmon and sardines – discover that pain and stiffness are lessened. These substances seem to discourage inflammation in the body.
- You can also take the oils alone or in capsule form. Research at Cardiff University has shown that the omega-3 fatty acids in **cod liver oil** can slow and may even reverse the destruction of cartilage that leads to osteoarthritis. The recommended dose is 2000mg of an omega-3 supplement three times a day, with meals. But check with your doctor first before taking **fish oil supplements** if you are taking blood-thinning drugs, have high cholesterol or are diabetic.
- As an alternative to fish oil capsules, take 1 tablespoon of **flax seed (linseed) oil** a day. It's loaded with the same type of omega-3s. Take the oil straight from a spoon, mix it with orange juice or add it to your salad dressing.
- If you like **nuts**, indulge. They also contain beneficial oils.

Rub on relief

- **Eucalyptus oil** can be effective. Put a few drops on the skin and rub it in, but don't use the oil under a heating pad or hot compress, as the additional heat can cause it to burn or irritate the skin.

Rheumatoid arthritis

A more serious form of arthritis, rheumatoid arthritis, occurs when the immune system attacks rather than defends the body. Along with joint pain and swelling, rheumatoid arthritis can cause fatigue, poor circulation, anaemia and eye problems. Here are some coping strategies.

• Start a food diary to identify what you were eating when your symptoms flared up. You may find that your body's inflammatory response goes into overdrive when you eat certain foods, such as wheat, dairy produce, citrus fruit, eggs or tomatoes.

• Try becoming vegetarian – under your doctor's supervision. In a one-year study, people with rheumatoid arthritis who followed a vegetarian diet that was also free of eggs, gluten (a protein in wheat), caffeine, alcohol, salt, refined sugar and milk products had less pain and swelling in their joints after just one month. And they were able to start eating dairy products again after the first three months with no adverse effects.

• Research has found that gamma-linolenic acid (GLA) supplements can help to lessen the pain and inflammation of rheumatoid arthritis. The best sources are borage seed oil, blackcurrant oil and evening primrose oil. Recent studies suggest that the greatest relief is gained by taking at least 1.4g GLA per day. But you should consult a medical herbalist before taking this level of GLA; for over-the-counter GLA supplements, the usual recommended dose is much lower at 0.24g.

• Some doctors believe a brief (one or two days) fast can ease rheumatoid arthritis pain. The theory is that fasting gives the overworked immune system a much-needed rest. Check with your doctor first, especially if you take prescription medications.

• **Capsaicin** is a substance that gives chilli peppers their 'heat'. It is also the active ingredient in some products designed for ongoing joint pain. Capsaicin is a counter-irritant: it irritates nerve endings, diverting the brain's attention from arthritis pain. You will need to see your doctor for chilli creams such as Axsain and Zacin, as they are available only on prescription. Other counter-irritants can be bought over the counter: try Algipan rub, Ralgex cream or the delightfully-named Fiery Jack cream or ointment.

Keep those joints moving

• Whether it's walking, swimming, cycling or yoga, begin a **gentle exercise regime**. The better your physical condition, the less pain and stiffness you'll have. If you have arthritis in your ankle, knee or hip, you might need to walk with a stick – at least to begin with – to help stabilize the joints. If your joints are swollen and inflamed, don't work through the pain. Instead, take a day off.

DO-IT-YOURSELF HEALING
ARTHRITIS

Exercise is probably the most important thing you can do to keep joints from becoming overly stiff. Each of these gentle exercises can be repeated at least 3 to 5 times but be sure to stop if you feel intense or sudden pain.

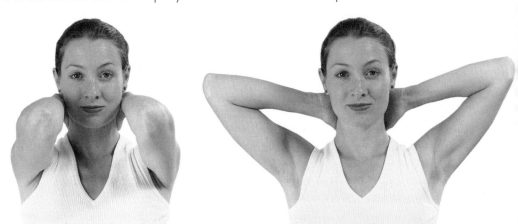

SHOULDER STRETCH The following stretches will help to increase shoulder mobility while relaxing the neck and shoulder muscles.

1 *Stand upright with your fingers interlocked behind your neck and your elbows pointing straight ahead.*

2 *Slowly bring your elbows back, breathing in deeply as you do so. Hold for about 5 seconds, then breathe out and bring the elbows forward again until they touch.*

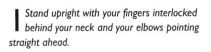

KNEE EXERCISE
Strengthening the quadriceps muscles at the front of your leg will give your knees the support they need.

Sit in a hard-backed chair with a rolled-up towel under your knees.

1 *Straighten one leg, without locking the knee, and hold for 3 to 5 seconds.*

2 *Lower the leg back down and repeat with the other leg.*

FINGER EXERCISES

If you have arthritis in your hands, the following exercises will help to improve finger flexibility so that you can grip and hold objects more easily.

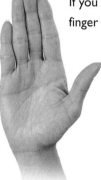

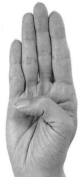

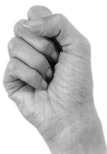

1 *Hold one hand upright with the palm open and fingers relaxed, as if you were stopping traffic.*

2 *Bring your thumb across the palm as far as you can, reaching for the base of your little finger. Hold for 3 seconds, then bring the thumb back to normal position and spread your fingers as much as possible.*

1 *Make a loose fist, with your thumb outside the curl of your fingers.*

2 *Hold for 3 seconds, then open the fist. Straighten and spread your fingers.*

ANKLE EXERCISE

To maintain flexibility in swollen ankles, do the following exercises when you're sitting comfortably in a straight-backed chair with your feet flat on the floor.

1 *With heels resting on the floor, lift the balls of your feet.*

2 *Pivot your toes back and forth slowly, using your heels as fulcrums.*

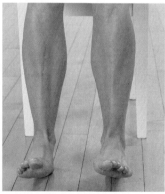

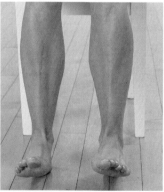

3 *Now put the balls of your feet on the floor and lift the heels.*

4 *Gently pivot your heels left and right.*

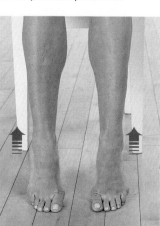

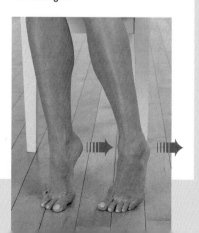

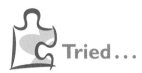

Tried...

People with arthritis have long worn copper bracelets to 'draw out the pain'.

**...&
true**

Researchers in Australia have found that people who wear copper bracelets and also take aspirin experience less pain than people who treat their pain with aspirin alone.

• Talk to your doctor or physiotherapist about how to start a **weight training** programme. Strong muscles will help to support your joints and absorb shock.

Try to measure up

• If you have hip or knee arthritis, ask your doctor to **measure the length of your legs.** One in five people with arthritis in these joints has one leg that is slightly longer than the other. Your doctor may be able to refer you to a podiatrist to have corrective shoes made for you.

Listen to the weather forecast

• Many people with arthritis find that their pain is triggered by **changes in the weather.** If you are one of them, it's not just your imagination: a sudden increase in humidity and rapid drop in air pressure affect bloodflow to arthritic joints. When storms are forecast, try turning on a dehumidifier to dry the air.

The power of prevention

• **Maintain a healthy weight** to help to prevent osteoarthritis of the knees. No matter what your current weight, losing just 5 kilos (10lb) and keeping it off for 10 years will halve the risk of arthritis affecting your knees.

• If walking is part of your exercise programme, make sure you **don't cover the same ground every day.** Varying the kind of terrain you walk on will prevent you from repeatedly stressing the same joints in the same way.

• Invest in good **walking shoes.** The softer heels will lessen the impact of walking on your foot, ankle, leg and hip joints. Flat, supportive shoes are generally considered best for knees.

• Recent clinical studies have shown that **vitamin C** and other antioxidants can help to reduce the risk of osteoarthritis and its progression. Antioxidants prevent bone breakdown by destroying free radicals – harmful oxygen molecules that cause tissue damage. Take 500mg of vitamin C every day.

• Take **zinc** supplements. One long-term study of nearly 30,000 women found that those who took zinc supplements reduced their risk of rheumatoid arthritis. Taking too much zinc may cause other health risks, however, so limit your intake to one 15mg dose a day and take it with food.

Asthma

For severe asthma attacks – the kind of tightness, wheezing and shortness of breath that can be really frightening – most people do as their doctor recommends. Often, that means quick action with a prescribed inhaler. If this is what you do, and it works, don't give it up. If you use a preventer inhaler, you should continue to use it as prescribed, as this will cut down your risk of attack. There is no cure for asthma, but there are lots of ways to reduce or even eliminate the symptoms. Certain simple lifestyle changes can help most asthma sufferers to breathe more easily.

Ease breathing during an attack

• When an asthma attack occurs, try to **stay calm.** Panic can make your symptoms worse. This visualization trick may help. Close your eyes. As you inhale, see your lungs expand and fill with white light and feel your breathing become easier. Repeat this exercise twice more, then open your eyes.

• In an emergency, drink a strong cup of **coffee**, two 330ml cans of cola or a Red Bull or Lipovitan (both of which are high in caffeine). Caffeine is chemically related to theophylline, a medication for asthma. It helps to open the airways.

Combat constriction with supplements

• Practitioners of traditional Chinese medicine have been using the herb **ginkgo** to treat asthma for centuries. One recent study suggests that this herb interferes with a protein in the blood that contributes to airway spasms. If you want to try it, buy supplements labelled ginkgo biloba extract, or GBE, and take up to 250mg a day.

• **Magnesium** may make you feel better. Much research suggests that magnesium relaxes the airways. The recommended dose is 300mg a day for men and 270mg for women.

Counter inflammation

• **Omega-3 fatty acids**, found in oily fish such as tuna, salmon and mackerel, work much like a class of asthma drugs called leukotriene inhibitors. These drugs stop the actions of body

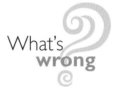

What's wrong

An asthma attack can occur when an irritant – usually a common substance like smoke, cold or dry air, pollen, mould or dust mites – meets a pair of sensitive lungs. Hormonal fluctuations, stress and anger can also trigger an attack. Sometimes there's no apparent cause. Your difficulty in breathing occurs because the bronchioles (air passages in the lungs) go into spasms. This can cause coughing and tightness in the chest. The spasms trigger the release of histamine and other chemicals that cause inflammation and the production of airway-clogging mucus.

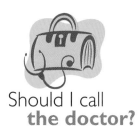

Should I call the doctor?

If you experience asthma symptoms for the first time, you must consult a doctor. Get someone to take you to the nearest A&E department if you can't speak without gasping for breath, develop a bluish cast to your face or lips, find it extremely difficult to breathe or become confused or exhausted. If you are already being treated for asthma, you probably already have medication that you can take at the onset of an episode. Even so, see your doctor if you notice that you need to use your medication more often, or if your symptoms worsen even after you take it.

compounds that cause inflammation in the airways. Take six 1000mg fish oil capsules a day in divided doses. Talk to your doctor first if you are taking anticoagulant drugs.

● **Evening primrose oil** is rich in an essential fatty acid called gamma-linolenic acid (GLA), which is converted by the body into anti-inflammatory substances. Take 1000mg three times a day. Take with meals to enhance absorption.

● **Bioflavonoids**, compounds that give fruits and vegetables their bright colours, have powerful anti-inflammatory and anti-allergenic properties. **Quercetin**, one of the best-known bioflavonoids, inhibits the release of histamine. Take 500mg of quercetin three times a day, 20 minutes before meals.

● **Turmeric**, the yellow cooking spice used to flavour Indian curry dishes, is a powerful anti-inflammatory. The compounds it contains inhibit the release of COX-2 prostaglandins, hormone-like substances involved in inflammation. Mix 1 teaspoon of turmeric powder – found on the spice rack in supermarkets – in a cup of warm milk and drink this up to three times a day. Turmeric capsules and tinctures are also available in health-food stores.

Keep a record

● In a diary, **make a note of everything you eat** for a month. Also record your asthma symptoms. Although food allergies are rarely associated with asthma, occasionally there is a connection. Check your diary against your symptoms to see if anything you're eating increases the frequency or severity of your attacks.

● If you take asthma medication, **get a peak-flow meter**, available from pharmacists or on prescription from your doctor. This device measures the speed at which air leaves your lungs – an indication of how well you're breathing. By reading your 'peak flow' at certain times, you can tell how well a medication or remedy is working. You can also use it during an asthma attack to determine its severity and decide whether you need medical attention.

The power of prevention

● **Don't smoke**, and stay away from people who do. Tobacco smoke irritates the airways.

Practise abdominal breathing

This simple deep-breathing trick can help reduce the severity and frequency of your asthma attacks. When an attack starts, you naturally become more anxious as it gets harder to breathe. This produces a 'clenching' response that can further restrict your airways. But if you've practised this breathing technique ahead of time, you can use it to help yourself breathe more freely.
• Lie on your back on a carpet or mat and place a book on your stomach.

• Inhale gently and deeply, but not by expanding your chest. Instead, expand your abdomen. Keep an eye on the book. If it rises, you're breathing in the right way.
• Just when you think you've reached full capacity, take in a little more air. See if you can raise the book a little higher.
• Exhale gradually, slowly counting to five. The more you exhale, the more relaxed you'll feel.
• Repeat at least five times.

• Don't huddle around a **fireplace** or wood-burning stove.

• In cold weather, **wrap a scarf** around your nose and mouth to help warm up chilly air before you inhale it.

• **Be alert** for unusual asthma triggers, such as **highly-scented foods** or the **strongly perfumed sample strips** bound into magazines, and do what you can to avoid them. It's also a good idea to open the window when cooking with strong smelling foods such as garlic or onions.

• **Try eating smaller, more frequent meals**, and don't eat before you go to bed. The upward migration of stomach acids that cause heartburn can also trigger asthma attacks.

• About 5 per cent of people with asthma are allergic to nonsteroidal anti-inflammatory drugs (NSAIDs) such as aspirin and ibuprofen. For these people, taking the drugs can trigger an attack. If you are one of them, use an **aspirin-free pain reliever** like paracetamol instead.

• Consider the **Buteyko method**, a complementary therapy for controlling the symptoms of asthma and other breathing related disorders. It is based on the belief that breathing related disorders result from chronic over-breathing (hyperventilation). It involves very specific breathing exercises as well as dietary and lifestyle changes. (See **www.buteyko.com** for more information.)

Athlete's foot

This irritating fungal infection is not confined to athletes. It can be picked up by anyone walking barefoot on damp floors in changing rooms, bathrooms or at the swimming pool. Once it takes hold, you have to be tough with it. The more you treat your feet and dry your toes, the better. Use these remedies to soothe the itching and fight the fungus that causes it. And follow our prevention tips so it doesn't strike again.

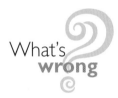

What's **wrong**

Athlete's foot is caused by a fungus called *tinea pedis*. This stealthy intruder, which targets the nails, skin and hair, causes skin to redden, crack, burn, scale and itch. When the fungus invades the area between the toes, the classic symptom is itchy, flaking skin. Sometimes tinea stays between the toes. But it may also appear on the soles and sides of the feet and even spread to the toenails. Severe cases of athlete's foot can be accompanied by oozing blisters. Warm damp floors are a common breeding ground for tinea, but it loves any warm, moist places. So the feet, often confined in sweaty shoes and socks, make an ideal breeding ground.

Treat the infection fast and intensively

- When you visit the pharmacy for an over-the-counter remedy, look out for creams and ointments that contain **miconazole** or **clotrimazole**, such as Canesten AF or Daktarin. Massage a small amount into the affected area two or three times a day. And don't make the mistake of stopping the cream when your symptoms subside. Use it for at least two weeks after the problem appears to have cleared up in order to eradicate the fungus permanently.

- Some cures are found in the kitchen cupboards. Simple **bicarbonate of soda** can relieve the itching and burning between your toes or on your feet. Add enough water to 1 tablespoon of bicarb to make a paste. Rub in the paste, then rinse and thoroughly dry your feet. Finish off with a dusting of **cornflour**.

- For a soothing foot soak, add 2 teaspoons of **salt** per 500ml of warm water. Soak your feet for 5 to 10 minutes. Repeat this soak at frequent intervals until your feet have completely healed.

- **Tea** contains tannic acid, a natural astringent that works wonderfully to dry out sweaty feet. Steep five tea bags in a litre of boiling water for 5 minutes. Leave to cool to lukewarm, then soak your feet in this tea bath for 30 minutes.

- Here are some other suggestions for topical applications – some a little strange but others less so. They all come from athlete's foot sufferers who have tried their cures and swear by them: **surgical spirit**, apple cider **vinegar**, **garlic powder**, **hair spray** and raw **honey**. Apply any one of these three or four times a day.

Don't allow the fungus to spread

The tinea fungus that causes athlete's foot can also cause uncomfortable itching in the groin. So, when you have athlete's foot, be careful not to infect your groin area. Be sure to wash your hands thoroughly after touching your feet. And don't pull your underwear on over your bare feet. Put on your socks first. If you wear tights, put on a pair of socks, don your knickers, take the socks off and then put on your tights.

- A further tip to speed up healing is **go barefoot** whenever possible (but not on wet floors or you risk passing on the infection).
- Wash your socks or tights in **very hot water,** or microwave washed socks, to kill the fungus and prevent any recurrence.

Fight fungus with food

- Plain **yoghurt** containing live acidophilus bacteria is an instant remedy for athlete's foot. These friendly microorganisms keep the fungus in check. Simply dab the yoghurt on the infected areas, let dry and rinse off. (But don't use flavoured yoghurts!)
- Add a few drops of **mustard** oil or a sprinkling of mustard powder to a footbath. Mustard will help to kill the fungus. Soak your feet in the bath for up to half an hour.

Seek herbal relief

- The oil of the Australian tea tree is a potent antiseptic. It alters the environment of the skin, making it harder for tinea to do its nasty work. For a soothing, healing treatment, mix **tea tree oil** with the same amount of **olive oil** and rub the combination into the affected area twice a day. The olive oil helps to tenderize skin toughened by athlete's foot so the tea tree oil is better absorbed.
- Alternatively, mix **tea tree oil** with **aloe gel**, another skin softener. Mix three parts tea tree oil to one part aloe gel and rub this ointment into the infected area twice a day. Give this treatment six to eight weeks to work.
- The heavenly scented herb **lavender** also has antifungal properties. Make a massage oil by adding three drops of lavender oil to one teaspoon of a suitable carrier oil (any vegetable oil will do). Rub into the infected skin every day.

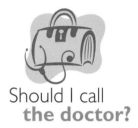

Should I call the doctor?

Give home treatments at least three weeks to work. If your symptoms are severe, however, see your doctor or a chiropodist. Left untreated, a fungal infection can cause the skin to crack, which allows infection-causing bacteria to gain entry. You should also see your doctor as soon as possible if you see signs of a more serious infection such as skin that is angry red and tender to the touch or oozing. Other warning signals are swelling of the foot or leg accompanied by a fever, or red streaks radiating from the infected area.

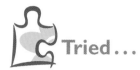

Tried...

Some people claim that they've used their own saliva to cure athlete's foot.

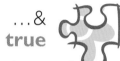

**...&
true**

Studies in animals suggest that saliva does appear to have antibacterial and antifungal powers. For example, when the salivary glands of rats are removed, their wounds heal more slowly, and a dog's saliva kills bacteria that can cause infections in newborn puppies. Human saliva contains substances called histatins, shown to have antifungal activity.

• **Calendula** has been valued for centuries as a topical treatment for wounds and skin conditions. This herbal healer is said to have both antifungal and anti-inflammatory powers. Rub calendula ointment, available in pharmacies and health-food stores, on the affected areas, especially between your toes.

The power of prevention

• After a bath or shower, **dry your feet thoroughly**. You could also try using a hair dryer on a low setting particularly between your toes.

• Wear clean **cotton socks**. Natural fibres absorb moisture best. If your feet sweat a lot, then change your socks two or three times during the day to keep your feet sweat-free. And, as mentioned earlier, be sure to wash them in **very hot water** to kill any tinea fungus spores. The 60° setting on the washing machine will do the trick.

• Wear shoes made of canvas or leather, which **allow your feet to breathe**. Avoid rubber and plastic, which hold moisture in and can cause feet to sweat.

• Don't wear the same shoes two days in a row. It takes at least a day for shoes to dry out. If your feet sweat heavily, **change your shoes** twice a day.

• Dust the insides of your shoes with **antifungal powder** or spray. To kill fungus spores, spray some **disinfectant** on a cloth and wipe out the insides of your shoes after you take them off.

• **Wear flip-flops** in places where other people go barefoot, such as gyms, health clubs, changing rooms and around swimming pools.

• If your toenails are thick, yellow, crumbly and brittle, you probably have a fungal nail infection, which can lead to athlete's foot. **Get rid of the toenail fungus** – with either an over-the-counter antifungal medication or a visit to your GP or chiropodist – and you'll reduce your chances of getting athlete's foot.

Back pain

'Ow, my back hurts!' How many of us wish we never had to utter those words again? Take it easy for a couple of days while taking some ibuprofen or (prescribed) naproxen sodium to ease swelling and relieve the pain. Also try the fast-acting solutions below – especially ice and heat – for immediate relief. Then, as soon as possible, slowly get moving again. When your back is feeling moderately better, do the stretching and strengthening exercises starting on page 58 – every day without fail – and in four to six weeks your back should be back in action.

Ice first, heat later

• As a pain reliever, **ice** works really well. It temporarily blocks pain signals and helps to reduce swelling. Several times a day, place an ice pack wrapped in a towel on the painful area for up to 20 minutes. Alternatively, you can use a bag of **frozen peas**. During the first few days of home treatment, apply the ice pack as often as necessary. Later, you may still want to use ice after exercise or any physical activity.

• After about 48 hours, switch to **moist heat** to stimulate blood flow and reduce painful spasms. Dip a towel in very warm water, wring it out, then flatten and fold it. Lie on your stomach with pillows under your hips and ankles. Place the towel across the painful area, cover the towel with cling film, then put a heating pad – set on medium – on top of the film. Leave it on for up to 20 minutes. You can repeat this three or four times a day for several days.

Rub in some relief

• Ask a partner or close friend to **massage** the aching area. If you want to use a cream or ointment sold as a 'back rub', then do so, but with care – these topical creams tend to cause skin irritation after a few applications. For a simple back-massage aid, stuff several tennis balls into a long sock, tie the end of the sock, and ask your partner to roll it up and down your back.

• Rub on an old-fashioned liniment. Choose a cream containing methyl, diethylamine or glycol salicylate. All are similar and have pain relieving properties. Examples include

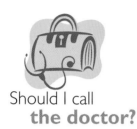

Should I call the doctor?

Before you try any home remedies or exercises, see a doctor to find out whether you have a common type of lower back pain or a medical problem that requires specialist treatment. A good physiotherapist or chiropractor can help to stop the back spasm by applying traction and gentle manipulation. Also see the doctor if pain comes on suddenly, radiates down your leg to your knee or foot or if it's accompanied by fever, stomach cramps, chest pain or laboured breathing. Doctors often view back pain as a wake-up call, and may recommend an exercise programme to stabilize and strengthen the spine and help prevent future problems.

Algesal cream, Radian B Muscle Lotion and Heat Spray, Deep Heat Maximum Strength Cream and Ralgex Heat Spray and Stick. The creams, known as counter-irritants, stimulate nerve endings in the skin, distracting you from deeper pain. When you use them, you're also giving yourself a massage – and the hands-on pressure combined with the surface action provides a double benefit. (*Alert* Do not use a liniment if you are also using heating pads or hot compresses on the area.)

● Your doctor may be prepared to prescribe a cream that contains **capsaicin** – the heat-producing substance in hot chilli peppers. Applied to your skin, capsaicin depletes nerve endings of a neurochemical called substance P. Researchers have found that substance P is essential for transmitting pain sensations to the brain, so when there's less substance P in circulation, the pain is reduced. You may have to use the cream for several weeks to feel the full effect. Stop using it if you begin to feel any skin irritation. (*Note* The creams – under the brand names Axsain and Zacin – are available on prescription only.)

Try these herbal soothers

● Take up to 500mg of **bromelain** three times a day on an empty stomach. Derived from pineapples, this enzyme promotes circulation, reduces swelling and helps your body to reabsorb the byproducts of inflammation. To achieve a strong therapeutic effect, look for a strength of at least 2000 MCU (milk-clotting units) per gram. (*Alert* Because bromelain is a blood thinner, it should be avoided by anyone taking anti-coagulant drugs.)

● Try taking one 250mg capsule of **valerian** four times a day. Some scientists claim that this herb's active ingredient interacts with receptors in the brain to cause a sedating effect. Although sedatives are not generally recommended, valerian is much milder than any pharmaceutical product. (Valerian can also be made into a tea, but the smell is so strong – reminiscent of overused gym socks – that capsules are vastly preferable.)

Perfect your posture

● Look for the **posture that puts the least stress** on your back. Stand up straight with your weight evenly balanced on both feet. Tilt your pelvis forwards, then back, exaggerating the

Fast relief from the doctor

Doctors used to prescribe muscle relaxants for quick relief, but these drugs are rarely prescribed anymore. They tend to make people tired and contribute to poor muscle tone and coordination, which is just the opposite of what you really need for back-pain relief. These days, if you visit your doctor or hospital to be treated for intense pain, you are more likely to be given a short course of powerful painkillers or anti-inflammatory drugs, to stop muscle spasm and relieve the pain.

movement. Then settle into the position that feels most comfortable. Now 'work your way up' your back, focusing on one area at a time. First concentrate on the area near your waist, then your chest area and finally your neck and shoulders. Try to feel which position is most comfortable and least stressful. This is the position to maintain when you're standing, walking and beginning or ending any exercise.

- **When you're sleeping,** lie on your back or your side (*unless* you have sciatica). If you're more comfortable on your back, place a pillow under your knees as well as under your head to relieve pressure on your lower back. If you prefer to sleep on your side, place a pillow between your legs. If you have sciatica, the recommended position is on your stomach.
- If you like to sit up in bed to read or watch television, buy a **large foam wedge** that supports your upper body in a comfortable position. For added comfort – and to keep your neck in the proper position – use a foam or inflatable neck support when you are sitting up.
- When you are sitting on a chair at the office or at home, keep your feet flat on the floor, with your hips slightly higher than your knees. Use a **lumbar support** behind your lower back. The lumbar roll is a chair's-width foam cylinder about 12cm (5in) in diameter. You can improvise with a rolled-up towel, but the foam version is lighter, easier to position and usually has straps that attach it to the back of the chair.
- Try and stay out of the car, but if you must drive, place a **foam wedge** behind your lower back.
- If you're accustomed to walking around with **a wallet** in your hip pocket, **take it out** whenever you're sitting. Even though it feels like a small lump, it's big enough to tilt your backside, throwing your spine ever so slightly out of alignment.

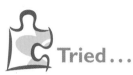

Tried...

In days gone by, a mustard poultice was a favourite remedy for sore backs and aching joints.

...& true

Like capsaicin and other counter-irritants, mustard delivers a warm, tingling sensation that can distract you from deeper pain. To make a poultice, mix one part powdered mustard with two parts flour, adding water until you have a paste. Spread it on an old teatowel, then fold the cloth over and apply it like a compress to your skin; the mustard paste will seep through. Mustard can burn if left on for too long, so remove it if you feel skin discomfort. Don't use a mustard poultice more than three times a day. (**Alert** Protect the skin with petroleum jelly when using a mustard poultice.)

DO-IT-YOURSELF HEALING
BACK PAIN

The following exercises from Dr Kevin Stone, an orthopaedic surgeon based in San Francisco, California, have been designed to improve flexibility and strengthen the muscles that play a role in supporting your spine – in your abdomen, along your back and around your trunk.

1 *Lie with your hands palm down on the mat, directly under your shoulders, in a push-up position, with your lower body completely relaxed.*

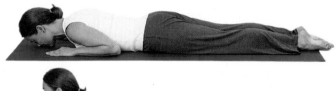

2 *Keeping your hips in place and legs relaxed, slowly raise your upper body until you can feel the stretch in your back. Return to starting position. Repeat 10 times.*

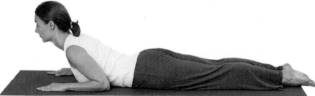

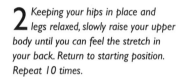

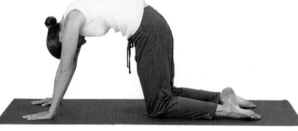

1 *Kneel on all fours with your knees hip-width apart.*

2 *Keeping your stomach muscles tensed, arch your back, stretching as a cat does. Hold for 5 seconds, then release. Repeat.*

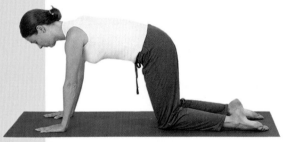

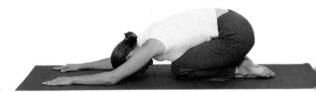

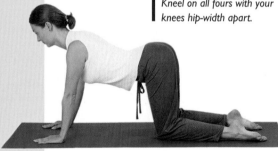

3 *Now hollow your spine slightly, hold for 5 seconds, then release. Repeat.*

4 *Finally, sit back on your heels and reach your arms in front of you for a nice stretch.*

Lie on your back with your knees bent. Slowly pull your right knee towards your chest until you can feel a stretch in your lower back. Count to five, then slowly lower the leg. Switch legs. Repeat 10 times, alternating right and left.

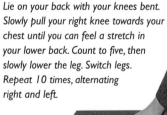

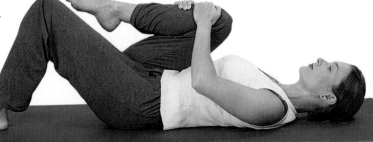

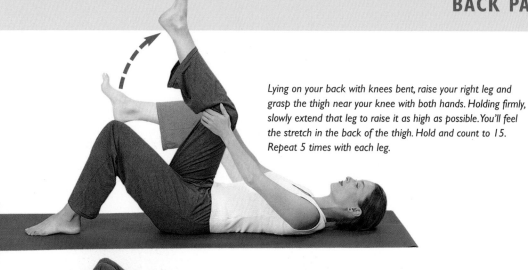

Lying on your back with knees bent, raise your right leg and grasp the thigh near your knee with both hands. Holding firmly, slowly extend that leg to raise it as high as possible. You'll feel the stretch in the back of the thigh. Hold and count to 15. Repeat 5 times with each leg.

1 Lie on your back with your knees bent and your arms out to the sides.

2 Keeping your knees bent, slowly drop them to the right, using your right hand to gently pull the top knee towards the mat. Hold and count to five. You'll feel the stretch in your back and hips. Return your knees to the starting position, then repeat on the other side. Alternating, repeat 10 times.

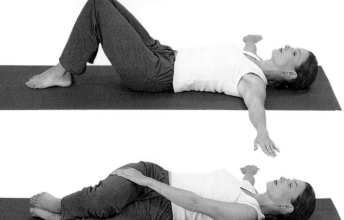

1 Lie on your stomach with a rolled-up towel under your forehead. Without moving the rest of your body, contract the muscles in your buttocks as if you were pressing your pelvis down into the mat. Slowly count to five, then relax. Repeat 10 times.

2 Keeping your hips pressed into the mat, raise your right arm and, at the same time, your left leg. Keep your balance by tensing your stomach muscles. Lower the arm and leg to the mat, then lift the left arm and the right leg. Alternating lifts, repeat 20 times.

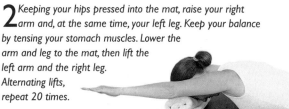

NOTE: Do these exercises on an exercise mat. Alternatively, you can use a well-padded carpet or rug. Try to perform the recommended number of repetitions but be sure to stop if you feel unusual discomfort or sharp pain.

Sciatica: when back pain affects your legs

The roots of the sciatic nerve lie near the base of your spine. They pass through a tunnel in your pelvis called the sciatic notch, then come together like separate lanes merging into motorways – the two large sciatic nerves that lead all the way down your legs. When the sciatic roots are pinched – by pressure from a herniated disc, for instance – sensations of pain, tingling or numbness may extend all the way from your buttocks to your legs, feet and toes.

About half the people who have sciatica achieve good results from most of the treatments recommended for lower back pain. If you have sciatica and don't get relief with these treatments, however, you should keep your doctor informed. And contact your doctor straight away if your foot is dragging or if you stumble when you walk or if you start to have trouble controlling your bladder or bowels. You may need urgent treatment in hospital and possibly surgery.

● When you're standing at the sink doing dishes, or waiting in a bus queue, **raise one foot higher than the other**. In the kitchen, keep a low sturdy box or a couple of old books by the sink, and put up a foot while you're standing there. Waiting in a queue, use a step or curb. (Think of the traditional brass rail in a public house, which serves the same purpose.) Periodically change position by putting up the opposite foot. This shifting of weight gives alternating back muscles a chance to relax.

Rise and shine

● Each morning **before you get out of bed**, lie on your back and slowly stretch your arms overhead. Gently pull your knees to your chest, one at a time. To get up, roll to the edge of your bed, turn on your side, put your knees over the edge, and use one arm to push yourself up as you let your feet swing to the floor. Once you're on your feet, put your hands on your buttocks and lean back very slowly to stretch out your spine.

Bad breath

Suppose you conduct a 'breath test' as you make your way to an important meeting, and you fail. Don't worry – the following quick fixes can help to minimize your horrible halitosis. If your gums, tongue and teeth are harbouring odour-causing bacteria, you'll want to adopt some rigorous daily hygiene habits to inhibit them. That's when special rinses, attention to toothpaste and regular brushing and flossing can begin making bad breath good.

Take emergency measures

● A dry mouth is a haven for the bacteria that cause bad breath. So find a tap and swish the **water** around in your mouth. Water will temporarily dislodge bacteria and make your breath a bit more acceptable.

● At the end of your business lunch or romantic dinner, munch the sprig of **parsley** that's left on your plate. Parsley is rich in chlorophyll, a well known breath deodorizer with germ-fighting properties.

● If you can get hold of an **orange**, peel and eat it. The citric acid it contains will stimulate your salivary glands and encourage the flow of breath-freshening saliva.

● If there are no oranges in sight, **eat whatever is available**, except known breath-pollutants such as garlic, onions or a stinky cheese. Eating encourages the flow of saliva, which helps to remove the unpleasant, odour-causing material on the surface of your tongue.

● Vigorously **scrape your tongue** over your teeth. Your tongue can become coated with bacteria that ferment proteins, producing gases that smell bad. Scraping your tongue can dislodge these bacteria so you can rinse them away.

● If you have a metal or plastic spoon to hand, you can use it as an effective **tongue scraper**. To scrape safely, place the spoon on the back of your tongue and drag it forwards. Repeat four or five times. Scrape the sides of the tongue as well, with the same back-to-front motion. But don't push the spoon too far back in your mouth as you may activate your gag reflex and cause yourself to vomit.

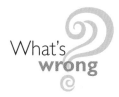

What's **wrong**

People back away from you whenever you talk to them. Or someone has told you frankly that you have bad breath. The most obvious and immediate cause is eating a dish laced with peperoni, onions, garlic or blue cheese. But there are plenty of other possible causes. Perhaps you're a smoker; or could it be that you don't brush your teeth or floss often enough? Gum disease is another common cause of bad breath. If you have an abscessed tooth or a sinus infection, your unpleasant breath is almost certainly a side-effect. Other suspects include certain prescription drugs, a chronically dry mouth or too many cups of coffee.

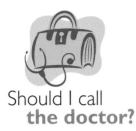

Should I call **the doctor?**

While all of us have bad breath from time to time, good oral hygiene should keep it to a minimum. But bad breath that lingers for more than 24 hours can also be a sign of gum disease, intestinal problems or a more serious condition. If you brush and floss diligently, but can't banish bad breath on your own, see your doctor or dentist. You should also see a doctor if your breath smells sweet or fruity, as this could be a sign of diabetes.

Raid the spice rack

• **Cloves** are rich in eugenol, a potent antibacterial. Simply pop one into your mouth and dent it with your teeth. The pungent aromatic oil may burn slightly, so keep the spicy clove moving. Continue to bite until the essence permeates your mouth, then spit it out. Don't use clove oil or powdered cloves; they are too strong and can cause burns.

• Chew on **fennel**, **dill**, **cardamom** or **anise seeds**. Anise, which tastes like liquorice, can kill the bacteria that grow on the tongue. The others will help to mask the odour of halitosis.

• Suck on a stick of **cinnamon**. Like cloves, cinnamon is effective as a mouth antiseptic.

Choose your fresheners

• Most popular branded products advertised as breath-fresheners are rarely, if ever, effective in the long term. But it appears that a **chlorine dioxide** rinse, such as Eliminator Mouthwash (available online), can combat the sulphur compounds responsible for bad breath.

• Use a toothpaste that contains **tea tree oil**, a natural disinfectant. If you can't find it in the pharmacy, look for it in health-food shops (Holland & Barrett have their own brand).

The power of prevention

• Use an **oral irrigator** (such as Powerfloss), which is a hand-held gadget that rapidly pulses a small jet of water into your mouth, to flush out the bad bacteria. It can go deeper than a brush or floss can reach.

• Carry a **toothbrush** with you and brush after every meal. Brushing thwarts the development of plaque, the soft sticky film that coats the teeth and gums. It is not necessarily good advice

How to sniff out bad breath

Just how bad is your breath? To find out, perform a 'sniff test' on dental floss after you have pulled it gently between your teeth – but make sure you choose only an unwaxed and unflavoured variety. Another alternative is rubbing a flannel across the tongue and smelling it. If you are worried about your breath, talk to your dentist or hygienist. They will also be able to advise you on mouth hygiene and will check to see whether gum disease or poor mouth hygiene are likely causes.

to brush *immediately* after a meal: if you have consumed anything potentially erosive, like cola or citrus fruit, this can cause added damage to dental enamel. In this instance, brushing an hour after a meal is better.

- Keep **chewing gum** in your pocket or bag. Chewing a stick of gum, especially after meals, will stimulate saliva flow and clear away food debris.

- To keep your toothbrush free of bacteria, store it, head down, in a lidded plastic tumbler of **hydrogen peroxide**. Rinse the brush well before you use it.

- If you wear **dentures**, it's possible that they are absorbing the bad odours in your mouth. Always soak them overnight in an **antiseptic solution**, unless your dentist has advised you otherwise.

- **Don't skip meals.** When you don't eat for a long period of time, your mouth can get very dry. It becomes a perfect breeding ground for bacteria.

- Some things can sour your breath even when there are no bad bacteria. These include cigarettes, alcohol, onions, garlic and especially strong cheeses such as Camembert, Roquefort and other blue cheeses. In situations where sweet breath is a must, use the commonsense approach – **just say no**.

- Ask your doctor if a **medication** could be fouling the air you expel. Any drug that dries out your mouth, thereby depriving it of saliva, is suspect. These include over-the-counter antihistamines, decongestants, diet pills and also prescription medications for depression, rheumatoid arthritis and high blood pressure.

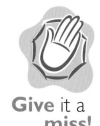

Give it a miss!

It's a common misconception that minty mouthwashes or breath mints will make your breath fresh. However, most mouthwashes contain alcohol, which dries up saliva. When you use them, you actually make your breath worse afterwards. And mint sweets are just a cover-up; they actually feed the odour-producing bacteria with more sugar.

VERSATILE GARGLES

Gargling isn't only useful for freshening bad breath – though a quick swish round with clove tea (quickly made with 1 or 2 teaspoons of bruised cloves steeped in a cup of boiling water) does that quite well. Depending on what you gargle with, gargling is also a wonderfully simple and remarkably effective way to kill germs, soothe a scratchy throat – even stop heartburn.

Like most home healing techniques, gargling has a long tradition. Those who practise the ancient Indian healing system known as Ayurveda believe that a mouth rinse of vegetable oil improves sleep and boosts brainpower, whitens the teeth and rejuvenates the gums. Closer to home, mainstream doctors now believe that germ-killing gargles and mouthwashes may help to prevent cardiovascular disease. It appears that the germs that cause bad gums (gingivitis) can enter the bloodstream and trigger clots that cause heart attacks and strokes.

Gargles help to clear away mucus and cellular debris that irritate the mouth and throat. And the ingredient or ingredients that you add to the water act on inflamed tissues, helping to soothe areas irritated by dry or polluted air – or by an afternoon of cheering at the local football pitch.

Making gargles need not be time-consuming or complicated. All you really need is hot water and a few ingredients that you may already have to hand.

Soothe a sore throat

For a sore throat, it's hard to beat a gargle of **lemon juice in water**. The astringent juice helps to shrink swollen throat tissue and creates a hostile, acidic environment for viruses and bacteria. Just mix a teaspoon of lemon juice into a cup of hot water. Of course, there's also simple **salt water**. Use ¼ teaspoon of salt in a cup of hot water and add 1 tablespoon of 20 vols hydrogen peroxide to kill germs.

There are plenty of other sore throat gargles. Try this effective old-style remedy: pour ½ cup of hot water over a teaspoon of powdered **ginger**; add the juice of half a **lemon** and a teaspoon of **honey**. Ginger has anti-inflammatory properties, while honey coats the throat and is also mildly antibacterial. Honey is also used in this hedgerow gargle: put 10g dried **blackberry leaves** into 100ml (3½ fl oz) water. Bring rapidly to the boil and allow to infuse for 15 minutes. Strain, sweeten with honey and use as a mouthwash or gargle twice a day. Blackberry leaves, loaded with tannins, are both antiseptic and antifungal.

Gargling with the herbal germ-killer **goldenseal** (1½ teaspoons of goldenseal tincture in 250ml (9fl oz) water) kills viruses and bacteria as it soothes inflamed throat tissue. Another remedy is **wheatgrass juice**. The best method is to buy wheatgrass and juice your own (available online from www.wheatgrass-uk.com).

A gargle and rinse with this chlorophyll-rich liquid may ease throat pain. Held in the mouth for 5 minutes or so, wheatgrass juice is said to help revitalize weak gums and stop toothache.

Head off heartburn

For occasional heartburn, try a **saltwater gargle** (¼ teaspoon of salt in a cup of warm water). The briny solution helps to rinse away and neutralize acids in the throat, relieving the burning sensation and promoting fast healing of irritated mucous membranes. If you have chronic heartburn, see a doctor. You may have a stomach ulcer or a hiatus hernia. Chronic acid reflux, in which gastric juices seep upwards, can damage the oesophagus.

Disinfect to destroy

Even the healthiest mouth is home to millions of bacteria, which produce waste products that give rise to unpleasant odours and spur the growth of dental plaque – the sticky coating that rots teeth and irritates gums. If brushing and flossing don't seem to be keeping oral bacteria in check, ask your dentist about gargling each day with a 50/50 solution of **water and 20 vols hydrogen peroxide**. For even greater germ-killing punch, try chlorhexidine mouthwash. Hydrogen peroxide and chlorhexidine are sold over the counter in pharmacies.

Clobber the cold virus

Next time you feel a sniffle, try gargling with a dash of **Tabasco sauce in water**. Hot sauce fans swear it's the fastest way to open blocked airways. If you can't take the heat, try **echinacea**, the herbal virus-killer. Add 2 teaspoons tincture of echinacea to a cup of water and gargle three times a day. This will ease throat pain and give your immune system the boost it needs to fight the infection.

Lay into laryngitis

There's no substitute for giving your voice a rest and boosting your intake of fluids. But you may be able to speed up the healing process by gargling with **myrrh** (a teaspoon of tincture in a cup of water). Highly astringent, myrrh is superb at combating inflammation. It is antiseptic, too. Gargle six times a day – a bit of an effort, maybe, but well worth it.

Gargling basics

- Mix a fresh gargle for every use. It is better to waste a bit pouring it away than to leave it in your glass, where it might become contaminated with bacteria.
- Use the hottest water you can comfortably tolerate. Cold gargles are ineffective.
- Don't swallow the gargle. Spit it out.

Bedwetting

Children don't wet the bed on purpose – and that's important to remember, especially on those mornings when you're faced with sopping sheets, again. One thing is certain: the problem can't be 'solved' through punishment. It does help to keep a sense of humour about the situation, which will undoubtedly pass. And try these techniques in the meantime.

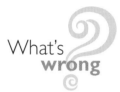

What's wrong

Nothing, usually. When you're bringing up a child, bedwetting comes with the territory. In fact, in Britain, at least 15 per cent of children over the age of five don't heed nature's call during the night. The most likely reason is that your child is not waking up when his or her bladder is full – and this is only a problem because the child is producing a lot of urine in the night or has a bladder that's somewhat low on capacity.

Keep those 'wee hours' drier

● Restrict your child's fluid intake for an hour before bedtime. In particular, cut out cola drinks or hot chocolate that may contain **caffeine**, which irritates the bladder.

● If your child usually drinks a mug of **milk** at bedtime, try to stop the practice for a week or two and see if it helps. A few children are allergic to the proteins in milk, primarily casein and whey, and the allergy can cause bedwetting.

● Make sure your child **goes to the toilet** before he or she goes to bed. It won't stop the bedwetting, but there will be less stored urine, which means less urine to wet the bed.

● Make the pre-bedtime routine **calm and quiet.** Rough, active play or even an exciting television programme increases the risk of bedwetting. Read a story or leave the child to read alone in bed.

● If the child is seven or older, consider buying a **bedwetting alarm.** This is a battery operated sensor that emits a buzzing or ringing sound when it detects moisture. It conditions children to recognize the need to urinate and wake up before they have to go. Don't give up if the alarm hasn't solved the problem after a week or two; most children respond within two months.

Limit the damage

● Put a **waterproof mattress protector** on your child's bed (supermarkets sell packets of padded disposable ones). Not only will this protect the mattress, it will also ensure that you can treat the accident as just that – an accident, not a disaster. Both you and your child will sleep better knowing that there isn't a major clean-up job to worry about.

Medical help

Some studies show that children who wet their beds may have an abnormally low level of antidiuretic hormone (ADH). This hormone helps the kidneys to retain water, and if there's a deficiency, more urine gets into the bladder. A doctor can prescribe a nasal spray containing a synthetic version of the hormone, to be used before bed. But behaviour modification (with the help of a bedwetting alarm) may be more effective.

Enlist your child's help

• Get your child to assist you with the **tasks that go along with bedwetting**, like laundering the sheets, making the bed or putting out a fresh nightie or pair of pyjamas. Make it clear that participation isn't a punishment, just a responsibility.

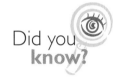

Did you know?

Research suggests that if both parents wet the bed when they were children, their child has a 70 per cent chance of having the same problem.

Bites and stings

If you live near a polar ice cap, you'll never have to worry about mosquitoes, bees, wasps or jellyfish. For the rest of us, confrontations with these irritating predators are as inevitable as a wet bank holiday. Insect repellent is an effective deterrent for many airborne pests. Others, however, seem ever bold and their bites are worse than their buzz. Here's how to recover from an assault and protect your skin from further attack.

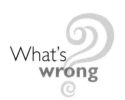

What's wrong

Some insects bite you because they're hungry and they see you as food. Mosquitoes, ticks and fleas fall into this category. Others sting you because they regard you as a threat. These include wasps and bees. Mosquitoes inject you with a little saliva that leaves a maddeningly itchy bump, while bees and wasps penetrate skin with a poison that makes you howl and run.

WASP AND BEE STINGS

Get out the credit card

● If you've been stung by a bee, **scrape away the sting** as soon as possible using the edge of a credit card, a knife blade or your fingernail. As long as the sting remains in your skin, the little sac of poison attached to it keeps pumping its contents into your body. Don't use tweezers or pinch the stinger with your fingertips, as you'll squeeze more venom into your skin.

Pamper the sting site

● As soon as you have got the sting out, soak the area in **vinegar** or a solution of **bicarbonate of soda** in water for a few minutes (1 teaspoon of bicarb into a glass of water). Make sure you use the right one: bee stings are acidic so need an alkaline neutraliser (remember 'bee for bicarb'), whereas wasp stings are alkaline so need acidic vinegar to neutralize. Dip a cotton wool ball in the liquid and tape it to the sting site. It will help to relieve redness and swelling.

● Treat the area with an enzyme based **meat tenderizer** straight away. It contains enzymes that break down the venom, reducing swelling and inflammation. Take a few spoonfuls of meat tenderizer powder, add enough water to form a paste, smear on the paste and leave it there for an hour.

● Apply an **aspirin paste** to stop the itching. Crush 1 or 2 aspirin tablets on a chopping board. Add just enough water to make a paste, then dab the paste onto the sting. Ingredients in aspirin help to neutralize the venom. (*Alert* Do not use this tip if you are allergic to aspirin or on a child under 16.)

Stingers in the sea

One doesn't tend to associate stinging jellyfish with the tame British coastline, but the Marine Conservation Society says that thousands of jellyfish now invade our coastal waters. Whether you holiday in Devon or Scotland, you could find yourself surrounded by a swarm of them. Most are completely harmless or inflict only mild stings, which should be rinsed with sea water, rather than fresh water, then bathed in vinegar over a 30-minute period. But there is always the risk of allergy to the sting – or the rare possibility of an encounter with a stranded lion's mane jellyfish. These creatures can be up to 2m (6ft 6in) wide. If you are unlucky enough to be stung, get to a doctor as soon as you can.

• Apply an **ice pack** to numb the area and slow down swelling. If you put a flannel between the ice pack and your skin, you can leave the ice pack in place for up to 20 minutes.

• **Papaya** contains enzymes that neutralize insect venom. If you happen to have papaya in your lunch box or fruit bowl, simply lay a slice on the sting for an hour.

• Rub on a slice of **onion** or **crushed garlic**. Both contain enzymes that seem to break down inflammatory compounds.

• **Sugar** works too. Just dip your forefinger in water, dip it in sugar and touch the sting site.

• To help reduce swelling, try **bromelain**, a protein-digesting enzyme derived from pineapple. Take three doses of 500mg in a single day. Stop taking it as soon as the swelling goes down.

• **Tea tree oil** will also help to reduce the swelling. Apply one drop several times a day.

• To stop the itching, dab on a drop or two of **lavender oil**. Wait about 15 minutes to allow the oil to take effect. If the area starts to itch again, apply more – but just one or two drops at a time. Or rub in **calendula cream** several times a day.

INSECT BITES

Instead of scratching...

• Rub an **ice cube** on the bite straight away. This helps to decrease the inflammation that causes itching.

• Essential oils can help to stop the itching from mosquito bites. Try **eucalyptus oil**, **clove oil** or **peppermint oil**. Put a small amount on a cotton wool ball and apply it to the site.

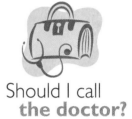

Should I call the doctor?

If someone has been stung by a bee or wasp and then has trouble breathing, feels faint, or has swelling in the mouth or throat, a rapid pulse or hives, dial 999 or get the victim to the nearest hospital or doctor. These are signs of a potentially fatal allergic reaction called anaphylaxis. Anyone who receives multiple insect bites or stings needs medical attention. This can be dangerous even for someone who is not allergic. If you develop a raised circular red rash or the area appears ulcerated or infected, you should also see a doctor.

Watch out in meadow, moor and woodland

Contrary to popular belief, tick-borne infections in the UK are countrywide – not limited to 'high risk' areas such as the New Forest or the Lake District. The incidence of Lyme disease is on the increase due to a growth in tick numbers. Ticks tend to be found in areas where deer and sheep graze, and in woods and moors.

• After a hike in the woods or a camping trip on the moors, it is advisable to check your body from head to toe when you undress. (You could ask your partner to check any parts you can't see.)

• If you find a tick that isn't attached to your skin, pick it up with a tissue and dispose of it.
• If a tick has latched onto your skin, clean the area with alcohol and use tweezers to grab it by the head, as close to your skin as possible. Slowly pull until it lets go. If you yank it off or twist or squeeze, the head can break off in your skin and remain there until infection sets in.
• Clean the area, apply an antiseptic and visit your GP. A course of antibiotics will deal with early-stage Lyme disease; later on it's much harder to treat.

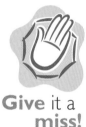

Give it a miss!

You may have heard that the best way to get rid of a tick that's latched onto your skin is to touch it with a glowing cigarette. Don't. The heat will probably make the insect burrow even deeper. Smearing the tick with petroleum jelly or oil won't cause it to come loose, either. Removing the head slowly with tweezers is the only effective way to get the job done.

• **Peppermint** has a cooling effect and can also increases circulation to the bite, speeding up the healing process. Use the essential oil if you have it, or check the ingredients of your **toothpaste**. If it contains peppermint oil, apply a blob.
• **Underarm deodorants** contain ingredients that reduce skin irritation. If you get an insect bite, try spraying or rolling on some deodorant and see if it works.
• Look for an anti-itch spray or gel that contains **menthol**, a classic skin-soother. Keep it in the fridge so it's always ready when you need it. The coolness will provide extra itch relief.
• Buy **anti-itch cream**. Various preparations are available over the counter. Lanacane cream contains topical anaesthetic; Anthisan and Wasp-Eze both contain antihistamines. And Eurax-HC contains hydrocortisone (a steroid) plus crotamiton, an anti-itch ingredient specifically for insect bites.

The power of prevention

• Use an insect repellent that contains **DEET**, the most effective insect repellent for use on the skin. Adults can safely use any DEET product (following directions on the label). Don't use any cream containing more than 10 per cent DEET on children and don't let a child handle insect repellents.
• Make your **clothes uninviting**. Permethrin is a synthetic version of an insect-repelling compound that is found in

chrysanthemums. You can buy it in spray form at specialized outdoor shops and online. Choose those clothes you are most likely to be wearing during times of high insect exposure, spray them lightly to dampen, turn them over and spray again. Then hang them to dry. The repellent lasts through several washes. **Bed nets** should be treated with permethrin every month.

- Mosi-Guard Insect Repellent is a range of natural, non-toxic insect repellents made from a blend of **eucalyptus oils**. Approved by the London School of Hygiene and Tropical Medicine, all these forms of insect repellent are safe for use with children and on sensitive skins. As well as being safe on skin they are also harmless to plastics and clothing.

- **Citronella**, a lemony scented oil that comes from a variety of grass, is found in insect-repelling candles as well as sprays. Follow label directions.

- Several days before you take a camping or hiking trip into insect territory, start eating **garlic**. Have a clove or two every day. The smell of garlic in sweat repels many insects.

- If you prefer to smell sweeter than garlic, try using Avon's **Skin-So-Soft** shower gel or bath oil – insects don't like it.

- If you don't want to attract **bees**, don't mimic a flower: avoid scented products and don't wear brightly coloured clothes.

What about animal bites?

The family pet is responsible for large numbers of hospital visits – especially children with dog bites. Cat bites are much less common, but four times as likely to cause infections.

If someone is bitten by an animal, clean the area thoroughly, no matter how small the injury: animals' mouths are full of germs and cleaning will reduce the chance of infection. Clean a small bite with plenty of plain tap water (antiseptics may damage skin tissue and delay healing). A large, deep or dirty bite should be cleaned and dressed by a nurse or doctor.

You may need a tetanus jab after a bite, but this is not necessary as long as you have had five tetanus injections during your lifetime. Most people born after 1961 – the start of routine immunizations – fall into this category. If you were born before 1961, or are in any doubt about your immunity, have a booster as soon as you can.

Blisters

What is the best thing to do with a blister? Drain it? Or leave it alone? In general, don't interfere with blisters that are small or those that probably won't pop on their own. They are less likely to become infected if you leave the natural covering of skin intact, and give the area time to form new skin under its protective cushion of fluid. Meanwhile, these tips will relieve the pain and itching and speed up healing. If your blister is large, or in an area where you can't avoid putting pressure on it, drain it the proper way. Never pop a burn blister, though, as there's a risk of infection if you do.

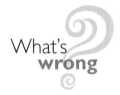

What's wrong

The most frequent cause of blisters is excessive friction on moist skin. As a blister forms, clear fluid accumulates in a pocket between the layers of the skin. Sometimes a small blood vessel in the area is damaged, and the fluid in the blister becomes tinged with blood. These types of blisters are generally found on the hands and feet, but can occur elsewhere too. Other potential blister causes include sunburn and other burns, eczema and other skin conditions.

Let it be

• Leave a blister intact if at all possible, and if it's going to pop, let it do so on its own – keep the blister clean with soap and water. You can dab on **petroleum jelly** such as **Vaseline** or some other emollient to minimize further friction.

• Whether and when to **cover a blister** depends very much on the site of the blister – if it's likely to get banged, it should be covered. Cover it with an adhesive **plaster** and change it at least once a day. If it is not likely to get knocked, it's best left open to the air.

• Protect the blister with a piece of **moleskin** – a soft, adhesive cushion available from pharmacies. Leave it on for two days, and remove it carefully so that it doesn't tear the fragile skin beneath.

• **At night**, remove all dressings from the blister to expose the area to the air. This will speed up healing. However, if the blister is in a vulnerable area and likely to rub on bedclothes, then keep it covered with a light dressing.

• Apply **calendula cream**, a product made from marigold. It's traditionally used as a soothing wound healer. To keep the cream clean, cover it with an adhesive plaster or a gauze pad.

• If you don't have any calendula cream, apply some **aloe vera gel** to the blister and cover it with a dressing. But be sure to use the pure gel of the plant – cut a leaf and squeeze the healing gel from the middle – as manufactured products may contain ingredients such as alcohol, which have a drying effect.

• Try **Preparation H**. This may not be the normal use for a haemorrhoid cream, but it contains ingredients that relieve itching and burning, and it also provides a coating that protects the skin.

• Relieve pain and itching with a **wet flannel**. Soak the cloth in cold water, wring it out and lay it over the blister.

If it pops by accident...

• Wash the blister with soap and water. Apply a healing cream or gel and cover with a clean dressing. Four times a day, remove the dressing and treat the raw area with a mixture made up of one part **tea tree oil** and three parts **vegetable oil**. The tea tree oil will help to kill bacteria and will also prevent infection.

Practise the art of careful draining

Do not drain a blister unless absolutely necessary – if it is especially large, for example, or in a spot where you can't avoid putting pressure on it.

• Sterilize a needle. Use a pair of pliers or tweezers to hold the needle over a naked flame for a few seconds until it glows red. Let it cool. Clean the blister with **surgical spirit** or an antiseptic cleanser such as **Betadine**.

• Open a **sterile gauze pad** and lay it gently on top of the blister. Pierce the edge of the blister, sliding the needle in sideways, and gently squeeze out the liquid by pressing down on the gauze pad. Make sure you don't tear or remove that top layer of skin – it's protecting an extremely sensitive circle of skin beneath.

• Apply an antiseptic cream such as **Savlon** and cover it with a clean dressing. Or cover it with **Second Skin**, a blister dressing made by Spenco. It's a moist, jelly-like covering that absorbs pressure and reduces friction. It can be cut to size and taped in place. Change it twice a day.

• If the blister refills again later, **drain it again** the same way.

• Apply a mixture of **vitamin E** and **calendula cream** to help your skin to heal faster. Vitamin E comes in capsules. Slice open a capsule, mix equal amounts of the vitamin and calendula oil, and apply the mixture to your blister. Reapply as needed for up to a week.

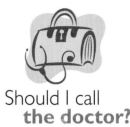

Should I call the doctor?

If your blister is extremely large – more than 5cm (2in) across – you should see a doctor. Any symptoms of infection should also be looked at by a doctor. These include pain that isn't lessening day by day, a raised temperature, redness that extends beyond the borders of the blister, or the fluid coming out of the blister is not watery but thick, or has an unpleasant smell. Some disorders that cause blisters, such as chicken pox, eczema and impetigo, may also require a doctor's care.

Felled by a blister

The power of prevention

• Don't assume you know your proper shoe size or that your feet haven't changed since you last bought shoes. **Have your feet measured** every time you buy. And when you try on shoes, be sure you're wearing the same kind of socks you will be wearing with the new shoes.

• Shop for shoes in the **afternoon**. Your feet swell during the day, and if you buy a pair in the morning, you might be getting half a size too small.

• Make sure new shoes are **roomy in the toe area**. When you're standing up, you should have a thumb width of space between your longest toe and the end of your shoe.

• For long walks or hikes, try wearing **two pairs of socks** to reduce friction. The inner pair should be made of a thin fabric like acrylic that draws out sweat, with an outer sock made of cotton.

• You may also want to **use an antiperspirant** on your feet to keep them dry. Dry feet are less likely to develop blisters.

• Cover blister-prone spots with a lubricant such as **petroleum jelly** such as Vaseline or a thick nappy ointment before you go for a run.

• Gardeners can prevent blisters on their hands by wearing **soft leather gardening gloves**. If you always get blisters when you hoe the garden, even if you wear gloves, look for a hoe with a larger handle or a cushioned grip.

• Anyone who plays racket sports will probably have to contend with hand blisters. But if they keep recurring, get advice from your local sports shop about **changing the grip** on your racket or wrapping it with an absorbent, soft covering.

Body odour

To tackle body odour, you have to stop the problem at its source. If antiperspirants (which block sweat glands) and deodorants (which neutralize or mask odours) don't do the trick or you prefer a natural approach, there are myriad paths to an agreeable essence. BO battles begin in the shower or bath and continue throughout the day.

Choose an effective soap

- Pick a **deodorant soap**, such as Wright's Coal Tar, tea tree oil soap (from Holland & Barrett) or anti-bacterial hand-washes, such as Boots, Carex or supermarket own brands. These leave ingredients on your skin that continue to kill bacteria even after you've finished washing. If the soap doesn't irritate your skin, use it every day. Some people find these soaps too drying, in which case their use should be restricted to the underarms and groin, where they are needed most.
- If deodorant soap doesn't do the trick, then bring out the big guns. **Antibacterial surgical scrubs**, such as Hibiscrub or Betadine, are available over-the-counter in most pharmacies. These are so effective that they are used to clean patients before surgery. But as these products can dry your skin, you should use them only in the shower, so you can rinse off quickly, and only on high-smell areas such as the armpits and groin. Squeeze out a little of the cleanser, wash the target areas, then rinse off and finish your shower with ordinary soap.

Beyond deodorant

- Use a cotton wool pad to wipe **vinegar** onto your armpits during the day to cut down the numbers of odour-causing bacteria. Don't use immediately after shaving, though, or it will sting badly. The same applies to witch hazel (below).
- Dab on **witch hazel.** You can splash it directly onto your skin or apply it as often as you like with a cotton wool pad. The refreshing, clean-smelling liquid is both drying and deodorizing.
- Dust **bicarbonate of soda** or **cornflour** on any problem part of your body. Both of these powders absorb moisture, and bicarb also kills odour-causing bacteria.

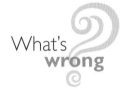

What's wrong?

Long ago, nature provided us with strong smells to entice the opposite sex. But BO won't get you far today. The problem starts with certain types of sweat. Eccrine glands produce clear, neutral-smelling sweat, which cools your body as it evaporates. Apocrine glands, concentrated in your armpits and groin, secrete a substance that bacteria feast upon, causing strong odours. Stress, ovulation, sexual excitement and anger can cause the apocrine glands to kick into overdrive. Some diseases cause the body to produce particular odours, and so do some drugs, such as the antidepressant, venlafaxine (Efexor) and bupropion (Zyban), a drug used to aid nicotine withdrawal.

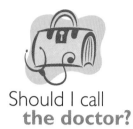

- **Shave regularly** under your arms. Armpit hair increases body odour because it traps sweat and bacteria.
- **Change your shirt** every day – and probably twice a day in hot weather.

Help from the garden

Any of the liquids mentioned below can be used in the underarm area, but not around the genitals.

- Apply **tea tree oil** to problem areas, as long as it doesn't irritate your skin. This oil, from an Australian tree, kills bacteria and also has a pleasant scent.
- Essential oils of **lavender, pine** and **peppermint** fight bacteria and smell pleasant. Some people have a skin reaction to certain oils, so test a small patch of skin before using.
- The fragrant kitchen herb **sage** can fight bacteria and reduce perspiration. You can buy sage tincture or diluted sage oil in health-food shops, or brew some sage tea from the fresh or dried leaves and store it in a bottle in the fridge. After using sage, be sure to wash your hands before touching your face.
- Citrus fruits such as **lemons** change the pH level of your skin, making it more acidic. All bacteria, including the odour-causing kinds, have a hard time surviving in a highly acidic environment. Just rub on some lemon juice and pat dry.

Eat green, smell clean

- Eat plenty of **spinach, chard** and **kale.** These and other leafy green vegetables are rich in chlorophyll, which has a powerful deodorizing effect in your body.
- Or buy tablets containing **chlorophyll.** Many brands are available, made from plants like kelp, barley grass, and blue-green algae. Check the label for the dosage recommendation.
- Chew a few sprigs of **parsley**, credited with anti-odour properties. Or prepare parsley tea by steeping a teaspoon of chopped fresh parsley in a cup of boiling water for 5 minutes. Let it cool a little before you drink it.
- **Lime tree tea** stimulates the excretion of waste products from the body, which may in turn make sweat sweeter. Also known as linden tea, it is made from lime tree blossom and is delicately fragrant, a little like jasmine tea.

Boils

There's only one thing to do with a boil: get rid of it fast. And you can, but not by squeezing it. Instead, use a combination of heat and moisture to bring it to a head, followed by safe and sterile methods to induce draining and provide pain relief. Alternatively, try drying treatments to shrink the offender to extinction.

Bring heat to the boil

- **Moist heat** will help to bring a boil to a head. Among the various folk remedies is a grocery list of items that seem to work when heated – including warm bread, milk, cabbage and even figs. But a simple flannel works, too. Soak a clean flannel or hand towel in very hot water – as hot as you can stand without burning yourself. Wring it out and apply it to the boil for 30 minutes at a time, several times a day.

- You can also use warm **thyme** or **camomile tea** instead of plain water when you prepare the compress. Thyme contains an antiseptic compound called thymol that may help to prevent infection. And camomile tea contains the chemical camazulene, which has anti-inflammatory properties.

- Also beneficial is a compress of the homeopathic tinctures of **calendula** (marigold) and **hypericum** (St John's wort). Put 1 teaspoon of each tincture in a cup of hot water and saturate a pad of cotton gauze. Apply this compress several times a day to decrease pain and inflammation.

- A warm, moist **tea bag** will act as a compress all on its own. Tea contains tannins, astringent compounds with antibacterial properties.

- If you like using folk remedies and have a **green cabbage** to hand, use a cooked outer cabbage leaf to draw the pus out of a boil. First, boil the cabbage leaf for a minute or so. Let it cool slightly and wrap it in gauze. Fix the gauze-covered leaf over the boil with adhesive tape such as Micropore and leave it in place for an hour. Use a fresh leaf and gauze each day.

- If the boil is in a hard-to-reach area, simply soak in a **hot bath**. While you're in the bath, keep the water as hot as possible without burning your skin.

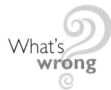

What's **wrong**

Sometimes called an abscess or a furuncle, a boil by any other name is still a boil. Highly infectious bacteria – usually staphylococci – work their way down a hair follicle into your skin. The boil fills with pus, swells and forms a white or yellow 'head' as the fluid forces its way upwards. Usually, boils occur where clothing rubs against your skin or where moist body parts are in constant contact: on the neck, under the arms, near the buttocks or around the inner thighs. Usually, a boil bursts on its own within about two weeks, and that starts the healing process. If you can bring the boil to a head and help pus to escape, you can often safely accelerate this process.

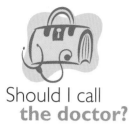

Should I call the doctor?

Seek a doctor's treatment for boils on the face as they might allow bacteria to get into your sinuses (leading to sinusitis), blood (septicaemia) or even brain (cerebral abscess). And if you frequently get boils of any size, you should have a medical examination to check that you are not developing diabetes or an immune-system problem. Also see your doctor if you develop boils in the armpits, in the groin or (if you're a breastfeeding mother) in your breasts. Otherwise, a boil needs attention if it's larger than 1 cm (½ in) across or if you detect signs of infection – intense redness, chills, a fever or swelling anywhere on your body.

Draining a boil

• To drain a boil after it comes to a head, **sterilize a needle** by holding it over a naked flame until the tip glows red, using tongs so you don't burn your fingers. When cool, gently prick the thin layer of skin on top of the boil. (*Alert* Do not attempt this procedure if you detect any signs of infection such as redness or inflamed-looking streaks around the boil.)

• Once the head is popped or has ruptured on its own, place a clean, **warm flannel** on top. First soak the flannel in a solution of **salt water** (mix a teaspoon of salt into a cup of hot water). Over the next three days, as the boil drains, replace the compress as frequently as possible.

• Each time you take off the flannel, use **liquid antibacterial soap** to clean the boil and the surrounding skin. Then apply magnesium sulphate paste BP, which is an over-the-counter preparation specifically for boils, or an antibacterial such as Betadine (povidone-iodine 10%), available in alcohol or aqueous solution, as a dry powder spray or as an ointment, on and around the boil to prevent the spread of infection.

All dried up

• Sometimes a boil will go away if it just dries out. To help kill the bacteria causing the boil – as well as dry it out – apply an acne medication containing **benzoyl peroxide** twice a day.

• Another way to make a boil clear up is by applying **tea tree oil**. This natural antiseptic kills germs and helps your skin to heal faster.

The power of prevention

• If you've had problems with boils in the past, consider switching to an **antibacterial cleanser**, such as Boots' ACT wash bar, Clearasil or Betadine skin cleanser or any alcohol-in-water-based cleansing gel.

• With heat and pressure, bacteria can get trapped in body hair. Avoid wearing tight trousers, a sweatband or any other clothing that rubs against your skin and traps perspiration. Instead, opt for **loose, comfortable clothing**.

• **Don't share clothes** with anyone who has a problem with boils. The infectious material can spread on contact. For the same reason, you shouldn't use anyone else's flannels or towels.

If someone in your household has boils, their laundry should be washed separately, and ideally in a hot wash – at a minimum temperature setting of 60°C.

• People who are overweight are at greater risk of getting boils because they tend to occur where moist skin is rubbing against itself. **Losing a few pounds** can help.

• In areas where skin friction leads to boils, **dust on some talc** to reduce moisture and chafing. (*Alert* Women should not use talc in the genital area. Talcum powder has been linked to ovarian cancer.)

• Pressure on the skin can also lead to boils, which is why they so often crop up on the part of your body you sit upon. If you sit in a car a lot, consider getting a **beaded seat pad**, which allows air to circulate behind and beneath you.

Breastfeeding solutions

For many new mothers, it's a shock to discover that breastfeeding, which seems so natural, is not necessarily easy. You'll probably be given much useful advice by your midwife, health visitor and friends, but every newborn gives birth to a brand new nursing experience. When your breasts start producing a regular milk supply a few days after birth, they may feel painfully tight and your baby may have trouble latching on. Many other factors affect your baby's feeds – and your own comfort. When problems arise, like nipple soreness or a blocked milk duct, it helps to know a few age-old tricks.

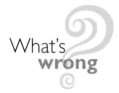

What's wrong

A number of problems can arise during breastfeeding that leave the mother sore and the baby irritable and sad. The most common problems are incorrect positioning of the baby and faulty latching on. Other issues include cracked or sore nipples, blocked milk ducts and breasts that are painfully engorged with milk (or, conversely, don't seem to be producing enough milk). Also, especially in the first few weeks, breastfeeding can be a physically tiring process, and it may take a while for mum and baby to learn how to work smoothly together.

Take the pressure off

- If you feel uncomfortably full, before starting a feed **express a little milk by hand.** Press repeatedly with your fingers above and below the areola (the dark area around the nipple). This will take off some pressure and allow your baby to attach more easily. The smell and taste of the milk will also encourage the baby to latch on.
- If your breasts are so full that no milk comes out, **apply a warm, damp compress** for several minutes. A wet flannel will work, or try a disposable nappy, which holds a lot of water and retains heat. Just soak the nappy in hot water and lay it over your breasts when you're in the bath.
- **Use a breast pump** if the baby falls asleep while feeding or finishes feeding and you still feel uncomfortably full – pumping a little milk may relieve the tension. But as this will encourage more milk next time, don't make it a routine thing or you're producing more than the baby requires.
- **Nurse often**, day and night. In fact, you should nurse about 8 to 12 times during every 24-hour period. This will keep your breasts from filling up with too much milk. Feed your baby every time he or she seems interested in eating.

Position yourself (and your baby) for success

- **Use a nursing pillow**; this is a horseshoe-shaped cushion which is specially designed for nursing mothers. It fits around your midriff, providing a convenient armrest when you're breastfeeding your baby. Nursing pillows are available from stores such as Mothercare, from catalogues such as Blooming Marvellous and online.

- Make sure your baby is **not too warm.** If infants are too warmly wrapped while nursing, they're more likely to doze off in the middle of feeding.
- Feed your baby in a **quiet, dimly lit** environment. Being relaxed makes the process easier for everyone.
- When you feed the baby, make sure **the entire body is facing yours.** Hold the buttocks in one hand, supporting the head in the crook of that elbow. Slide your other hand under your breast, fully supporting it. **Tickle your baby's lower lip.** This will prompt the mouth to open wide. Pull the baby straight in, quickly, so the mouth attaches to your areola (the dark area around the nipple). Be sure **the whole areola** is taken, or as much of it as possible.
- Sucking will stop when the baby is full. If you need to detach the baby from your nipple for any reason, such as to transfer to the other side (or to answer the door), gently insert your little finger between the corner of the baby's mouth and the skin of your nipple to **break the suction.** Babies have a natural survival reflex: they hold on tighter if they're suddenly interrupted while sucking. If you can gradually break the seal between your nipple and the baby's mouth before you pull the infant away, you'll reduce tugging, which can contribute to nipple soreness.

Left, right, left

- To make sure each breast is doing its share, start each feed with the breast you ended with at the previous feed. If you are so tired that you can't remember which breast that was, **fasten a safety pin** to your bra on the side you need to begin next time. By switching the breast you offer first, you give each one a chance to get completely emptied.

Become more productive

- If you feel you aren't producing enough milk, drink one glass of **alcohol-free beer** a day. There's a yeast derivative in the beer that increases levels of prolactin, a hormone that influences milk production. Just make sure it's alcohol-free and drink the beer 30 minutes before a feed.

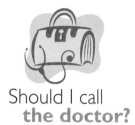

Should I call **the doctor?**

If you are worried that your baby isn't getting enough milk or if your baby fails to feed at least once during the day, get in touch with your midwife, health visitor or GP straight away. You also need to see your doctor if you have a red, tender area on a breast, accompanied by flu-like symptoms and a raised temperature. These are symptoms of a breast infection known as mastitis, which is caused by bacteria slipping into your breast through cracks in the nipple. It is treated with antibiotics. Drink plenty of water, go to bed if you can and continue to breastfeed your baby – even more frequently – while the infection heals.

● Apply **pressure** to your chest to stimulate milk flow. According to doctors who specialize in acupressure, the best pressure points are directly above your breasts. Place your thumbs between the third and fourth ribs straight down from your collarbone and in line with your nipples. Press steadily for a minute or so. If this procedure helps, you can repeat as often as you like.

● Drink **fennel tea** each morning. Herbalists have long recommended fennel to first-time mothers to help increase milk production. Some research indicates that fennel may have a mild oestrogen-like effect, which could encourage the production of breastmilk. Or perhaps babies just like fennel's mild liquorice-like taste. Put a teaspoon of fennel seeds into a cup of boiling water, leave to infuse for two or three minutes, strain and drink the tea.

Munch some healthy encouragement

● **Eat garlicky foods.** Apparently garlic affects the flavour of mother's milk in a way that appeals to babies. One US study showed that babies took more milk and stayed at the breast longer if their mothers ate some garlic a few hours before breastfeeding. It's also very good for you.

Nip soreness in the bud

● If one nipple is very painful, **offer the other one** first to your baby. Even if you used it during the previous feed, you'll want to favour the good nipple until the sore one feels better.

● Between feeds, place a **cold flannel** on each breast to relieve soreness.

● If your nipples are cracked or tender, let them dry naturally in the air after a feed. Speed up healing with **your own milk**: once the nipple is dry, express a drop and apply it to your nipples. Other healing salves include **vitamin E oil** – simply squeezed out of a pierced capsule (clean off any oil before the next feed), olive oil, sweet almond oil or lanolin cream.

Keep milk ducts clear

● For a blocked milk duct (which may present itself as a red, tender lump in your breast), soap the affected area while you're in the bath or shower and then gently run a **wide-toothed** comb over it to stimulate milk flow and help clear the blockage. (In general, however, avoid using soap on your nipples, as it can dry them out.)

- **Empty your breasts** as completely as possible during each feed. Offer your baby the affected breast first.
- Try to gently **massage the lumpy area** towards your nipple during feeding.
- Increase bloodflow to the area by placing **a warm flannel** on your breast, then gently massaging the breast.
- Make sure your **bra fits properly**. Specialist maternity stores and lingerie departments in larger stores often have advisers who can help you to choose the right bra. Ideally, choose a cotton bra with broad straps. The opening for feeding must not be too small or the fabric can press into the breast and cause a blockage.

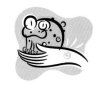

Old **wives' tale**

For a long time, it was believed to be 'common knowledge' that a mother's breasts would become too full of milk if she fed her baby very frequently. Actually, frequent nursing keeps them better drained – and your baby will be happier, too.

Breastfeeding support when you need it

When problems arise, you want instant answers. Several organisations have 24-hour helplines and helpful websites.

- **La Leche League** (www.laleche.org.uk) is highly recommended. It offers mother-to-mother support, encouragement, information and education. It also aims to promote a better understanding of breastfeeding as an important element in the healthy development of the baby and mother. Its 24-hour helpline number is 0845 120 2918

- **The National Childbirth Trust** (www.nctpregnancyandbabycare.com) offers free help and support with breastfeeding. Phone the NCT breastfeeding line on 0870 444 8708.
- **BabyCentre** (www.babycentre.co.uk/breastfeeding) is a parent-focused website with lots of friendly advice on all aspects of breastfeeding, from getting started to overcoming problems and weaning.

Breast tenderness

Just as the moon has phases, so breast discomfort waxes and wanes. Here are some suggestions for easing the discomfort created by your hormones. Vitamins, herbs and oils can work to keep fluid retention in check and coax your hormones into a breast-friendly balance (more progesterone, less oestrogen). And a few dietary changes may help to relieve some of that breast pain, too.

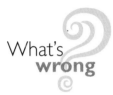

What's wrong

The uterus goes through a cycle of changes each month and so do the breasts. Shifting levels of hormones – mainly oestrogen and progesterone – trigger tissue growth and fluid retention in the breasts as the milk glands get ready for potential pregnancy. This can lead to pain and may also cause lumps to form. Cyclical breast tenderness was once called fibrocystic breast disease, but is now recognized as just a side-effect of menstruation. Almost half of women under 50 experience it. Breast tenderness tends to be most noticeable just before menstruation. It can also be related to the taking of certain drugs, such as the stomach acid suppressant, cimetidine (Tagamet).

A soothing soap

• When you're in the shower, soap your breasts and gently **massage** them from the centre of your chest out towards your armpits. This improves blood circulation and the drainage of lymphatic fluid, the clear fluid that carries infection-fighting substances around your body.

Take cold comfort

• Wrap a towel around a bag of **ice cubes** or frozen peas and apply it to each breast for about 10 minutes. The cold-pack treatment reduces swelling and dulls the pain.

Consider taking supplements

• **Dandelion** is a natural diuretic. Take the herb in capsule form, or make a tea using powdered dandelion root, available as sachets from health-food stores or online. Infuse a tea bag in a cup of boiling water for 10 minutes and drink 2 cups a day, an hour after main meals.

• Try **evening primrose oil**, a traditional herbal remedy for premenstrual symptoms. It contains an essential fatty acid called gamma-linolenic acid (GLA) that may help to balance a woman's hormones and appears to ease cyclical breast tenderness. Take 1000mg of the oil in soft capsule form three times a day during the last ten days of the menstrual cycle. Take it with meals to enhance absorption.

• **Vitamins E and B_6** may also work together to help prevent breast pain. Try 500mg (800 IU) of vitamin E a day, together with 50mg of B_6. While you won't be able to meet these goals with food alone, you can increase your dietary intake of these helpful vitamins by eating wheatgerm, vegetable oils, nuts, seeds and whole grains for more vitamin E, and avocados, fish, poultry, lean meats, bananas and spinach for B$_6$.

Get a new lift

- Consider wearing a **support bra** instead of an underwired bra when your breasts are tender. You may want to wear a soft support bra to bed to reduce night-time jostling. When you try on a new bra, make sure it cups your breasts without pinching. Once you buy new, more comfortable bras, throw away the old, out of shape ones that don't provide your breasts with proper support anymore.

Look at food solutions

- Eat more **soya beans** and other soya-based foods. Population studies have shown that in traditional Asian cultures where people consume a lot of soya, women have fewer oestrogen-related problems such as breast pain and menopause symptoms. Soya contains hormone-like compounds called phytoestrogens that can influence hormonal fluctuations related to menstruation and menopause. Try some soya-based meat substitutes, or add tofu to your meals. Soya milk is another excellent source; try it on breakfast cereals or in milkshakes.
- Consume plenty of **fibre**, such as fruit, vegetables, beans and pulses – kidney beans and lentils, for example – and whole grains. One US study found that women on a higher-fibre diet excreted more oestrogen.
- Aim to get fewer than 30 per cent of your calories from **fat**. Women who live in cultures where low-fat diets are the norm generally have a lower incidence of breast pain.
- Cut back your intake of **hydrogenated oils**, found in margarine, biscuits, manufactured pies and snack foods. When you eat these oils, your body loses some of its ability to convert the fatty acids in your diet (essential to your health) into GLA – a necessary link in a chain reaction that prevents breast tissue from becoming painful.
- Reduce your consumption of **methylxanthine**. 'Methyl what?', you may ask. Methylxanthine is the unfamiliar name of a group of stimulants that includes caffeine and

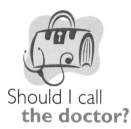

Should I call the doctor?

If you're taking any prescription medication, tell your doctor about any breast pain or tenderness, because it could be related to that drug. Other breast changes should be reported as well, especially any lump in your breast or under your arm. Soft lumps are usually the result of a build-up of fluid, but if a lump is more firm and round, your doctor may want to refer you for a biopsy to make sure it is noncancerous. Your doctor can help you to identify 'normal' lumpiness and distinguish this from lumps that should be tested. Even if you have come to expect breast pain associated with your period, tell your doctor if the pain becomes severe or if you notice discharge or blood from the nipple.

theobromine – found in coffee and chocolate respectively. It's present in many other common foods and drinks, too, including colas, tea, wine, beer, bananas, cheese, peanut butter, mushrooms and pickles. Most women who suffer from painful lumps on a cyclical basis will improve if they cut right down on, or eliminate, foods that are high in this compound.

● Go easy on the salt, and **watch your intake of sodium** from tinned soups and other processed and packaged foods. Sodium increases water retention, which causes your breasts to swell. Be especially careful to keep your salt consumption right down during the two weeks before your period.

Other ways to improve hormone harmony

● To help your hormones into a more breast-friendly balance, try a natural **progesterone cream** such as EquiGest (made by At Last Naturals). Although the cream is primarily recommended for PMS and menopause symptoms, you may find it helpful. Rub it into your skin every day, following the label directions.

● If you take contraceptive pills or hormone replacement therapy (HRT), then talk to your doctor about **altering your prescription**. A relatively minor dosage adjustment might help.

● **Exercise** vigorously for 30 minutes at least three times a week, especially during the week before your period. Exercise decreases the stress hormones in your body. And that is significant because those hormones play a role in causing breast pain. Exercise also helps to reduce fluids in your body while increasing levels of feel-good chemicals in your brain.

● Make regular, sacrosanct time for yourself and practise **meditation**, **breathing exercises** or other **relaxation techniques** that can reduce stress hormones.

Bronchitis

Your goal is to loosen the phlegm in your chest and get it moving, so that you can cough it up and out. The most direct approach to your lungs is the air you breathe; therefore inhalation treatments are the first step. Think of them as a steam cleaning for your airways. The right food and drink can also help to keep mucus on the move. At the same time, you'll want to get some germ-fighters into your system so as to discourage the bacteria adhering to the mucus. Here's what to do.

Dissolve the cough with steam

- **Breathe steam.** You can do that just by taking a hot shower, or pour steaming-hot water into a bowl and lean over it, draping a towel over your head to create a steam tent. If you use water from the kettle, wait for a minute or two before leaning over it, so as to avoid scalding your face. Inhaling the steam will help to loosen the secretions in your lungs. Many pharmacies sell a simple, cheap and safe steam inhaler – a two-handled beaker with a face mask attachment called Clearway.
- To make the steam treatment even more effective, add a few drops of **eucalyptus** or **pine oil** to the water. Eucalyptus helps to soften mucus in obstructed airways and has some antibacterial properties. (If you want to use eucalyptus leaves, simply boil them in a pot of water, then remove from the heat and inhale the steam.) Pine oil acts as an expectorant, so it will help you to 'bring up' phlegm from the bronchial tubes.
- Run a **humidifier** in your bedroom when you sleep to moisten the air you breathe. Make sure you follow the manufacturer's directions for cleaning the humidifier. Otherwise, bacteria and mould can accumulate in the works.
- If you have frequent bronchitis, consider an ultrasound, cool-mist humidifier (such as Bionaire, available for about £30 online). Let it run day and night when you are in the room.

Foods and drinks that help and hinder

- Eat **chilli peppers**, **hot spicy salsa** or dishes flavoured with **cayenne pepper**. Fiery foods thin the mucus in your lungs, helping you to cough more productively.

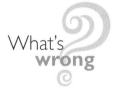

What's **wrong**

Short-lived cases of bronchitis are usually caused by a viral or bacterial infection, though they can also be brought on by allergies. The bronchial tubes swell up, and the cilia – tiny hairs lining the respiratory tract – become paralysed. Mucus accumulates, forcing you to cough heavily. You may also experience aching, shortness of breath, wheezing, sweating, chills, fatigue and a raised temperature. These symptoms generally go away after 10 days. Chronic bronchitis, on the other hand, can last a lifetime. Most chronic bronchitis is caused by smoking though it can arise from long-term exposure to dust.

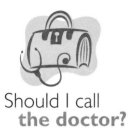

Should I call the doctor?

See your doctor if your cough is interfering with your sleep or your normal routine, or if breathing is difficult, or if you have a fever or if you are coughing up blood or yellow or green phlegm. Bronchitis can lead to pneumonia. You should also call the doctor if you think your child has bronchitis.

• To thin mucus and help you cough it up more easily, **drink plenty of water** – at least 8 large glasses a day. **Avoid alcohol** and caffeinated drinks, which dehydrate your system and make the mucus tougher to dislodge.

• Drink **mullein tea.** Mullein, also known as Aaron's rod, is a traditional remedy for respiratory ailments and is used to make expectorant cough syrups. It contains substances known as saponins, which help to loosen phlegm, along with a gelatinous mucilage that soothes raw mucous membranes. Boil a cup of water, remove from the heat, and drop in 2 teaspoons dried mullein flowers. Leave to steep for 10 minutes, then strain and drink the tea. You can drink up to 3 cups a day.

• To drink or not to drink milk? One school of thought claims that milk stimulates the production of mucus in the upper and lower respiratory tract and in the intestines. (The theory is that young calves, with four stomachs, need this extra mucus to help protect their intestinal tracts from strong stomach acids – but humans don't.) But other authorities say that there is almost no evidence of any **link between milk and mucus**, and that people actually do more harm than good by cutting out milk because they prejudice their calcium intake.

Supplement your efforts

• **N-acetylcysteine (NAC)**, a form of the amino acid cysteine, has been found to help thin and loosen mucus and reduce the recurrence of bronchitis. Interestingly, it is also the antidote for paracetamol poisoning. NAC is available from health-food shops in 600mg capsules. Take one a day on an empty stomach. If treating short-lived bronchitis, continue taking NAC for a few weeks after the cough has cleared up.

• **Echinacea** and **astragalus** are herbs that strengthen the immune system and help you to fight off bacteria and viruses. Take 200mg of either herb four times a day for acute bronchitis or twice a day for chronic bronchitis.

• For an acute attack of bronchitis, drink **thyme tea** to thin mucus secretions. Use 1 or 2 teaspoons per 240ml (8fl oz) boiling water and add honey to taste. Drink 3 or 4 cups a day. Other herbs that can be combined with thyme or used as alternatives are **elecampane, hyssop, plantain** and **angelica**. Use in the same way as thyme.

The power of prevention

- To prevent chronic bronchitis, the most essential advice is **don't smoke.** If you're a smoker, find out about programmes that will help you to give it up. Second-hand smoke is almost as bad, so avoid smoky pubs, and ask friends who smoke to do so away from you.
- If your job exposes you to lots of dust, fumes or pollutants – any of which can contribute to chronic bronchitis – be sure to wear an efficient **mask** or **respirator** to filter the impurities from the air you breathe.
- To reduce your risk of getting viral bronchitis, **wash your hands** frequently and keep them away from your face, especially when you've been near someone who has a cold.
- **Clean your nose and sinuses** with a saline solution (see Allergies, page 35) to help prevent allergens and infectious agents from getting into your lungs.
- **Vitamin C** helps you to fight off respiratory viruses. It works well in conjunction with supplementary flavonoids. Take up to 500mg of vitamin C and 250mg flavonoids twice a day.

Give it a miss!

When you're coughing, it can be very tempting to take a cough suppressant. But if you have a wet, productive cough, you shouldn't try to suppress it because your lungs are expelling bad mucus. You could try an expectorant cough syrup. These claim to loosen mucus, so the coughing clears out your bronchial passages. Expectorant cough mixtures contain the ingredient guaifenesin. They include Adult Meltus Expectorant with Decongestant and Beechams All-In-One. However, many doctors believe that the most effective way to loosen mucus is to drink plenty of fluids.

Bruises

There are several steps you can take to reduce the pain of a bump and encourage faster fading of the bruise. First, you want to reduce bloodflow to the area with ice and compression to minimize discoloration. Next, use heat to boost circulation and help to clear away the pooled blood. At the same time, as long as the skin isn't broken, a number of herbal ointments and compresses can help to erase the evidence of a careless moment that left its mark.

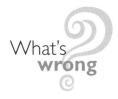

What's wrong

You've taken a bump, blow or knock that was hard enough to damage small blood vessels under your skin. Blood leaks out of these blood vessels, called capillaries, and seeps into the surrounding tissue. For a while you see the traditional black-and-blue colours, which are the trademark of most bruises. As the pooled blood gradually breaks down, the colours take on a full palette of hues, from purple to green and yellow. Normally, bruises fade in 10 to 14 days without any treatment.

Speed up the fading process

● Apply **ice** as soon as possible. If you cool the blood vessels around the bruised area, less blood leaks into the surrounding tissue. Flexible gel-filled ice packs, specifically designed for injuries, are available from sports shops and athletes will usually keep a couple of them in the freezer. For most of us, a bag of **frozen peas** wrapped in a towel is perfectly adequate. Or soak a flannel in ice-cold water and lay it over the bruise for 10 minutes. Whatever chilling agent you use, take it off after 10 minutes and wait for 20 minutes or so before you re-apply it so you don't overchill the skin underneath.

● If you've bruised your arm or leg, immediately wrap an **elastic bandage** around the bruised part. By squeezing the tissues underneath, the bandage helps to prevent blood vessels from leaking. The bruise won't be quite as severe.

● **Reduce bloodflow** to the bruise to minimize discoloration. If you bruise your leg, for instance, and you can take a break, settle into a sofa or armchair with your leg up on a pillow, above heart level. If your arm is bruised, try to keep it propped up above heart level whenever you're sitting.

Apply some heat

● After cooling the bruise for 24 hours, start applying heat to bring more circulation to the area and help to clear away the pooled blood. Use an **electric heating pad** for 20 minutes several times a day. Be sure to follow the instructions on the heating pad: in order to avoid burns, the pad should be placed so that it lies on top of – not under – the bruised limb.

- Alternatively, you can apply a **warm compress** either under or over the bruised area. A hot-water bottle will work. Or use a **microwavable heat pack**, available from medical supply stores or online.
- A warm compress of **comfrey** can also offer comfort. Comfrey contains compounds that reduce swelling and promote the rapid growth of new cells. Make a warm herbal solution by pouring a pint of boiling water over 30g dried comfrey leaves or 60g fresh leaves. Steep for 10 minutes, then strain. This is for external use only – do *not* drink. Soak a gauze pad or a flannel in the solution and apply it to the bruise for an hour. (*Alert* Do not use on broken skin or if you have an open wound.)
- **Vinegar** mixed with warm water will help the healing process. Vinegar increases bloodflow near the skin's surface, so it may help to dissipate the blood that has pooled in the bruise area. **Witch hazel** will also do the trick.

Here's the rub

- **Arnica** is a herb that has long been recommended for bruises. It contains a compound that reduces inflammation and swelling. Apply arnica ointment or gel to the bruise daily.
- Take a handful of fresh **parsley** leaves, crush them and spread them over the bruise. Wrap the area with an elastic bandage. Some experts claim that parsley decreases inflammation, reduces pain and can make a bruise fade more quickly.
- Gently rub **St John's wort** oil into the bruise. St John's wort is often taken as a capsule or tea for mild depression but the oil has long been known as a wound healer. It's rich in tannins, astringents that help shrink tissue and control capillary bleeding. For the best effect, start this treatment soon after the bruise occurs, and repeat it three times a day.

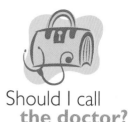

Should I call the doctor?

If your bruises appear mysteriously – that is, in places that you haven't even injured – see your doctor. Sometimes bruises are a warning sign of serious conditions. Consult your doctor if you bruise a joint and it leads to swelling, if a bruise doesn't fade after a week, if it's accompanied by severe pain or fever, or if you sustain a bruise on the side of your head over your ear (this area fractures easily).

A do-it-yourself flexible ice pack

If you tend to like active sports – or you bump your shins at regular intervals – it helps to have an ice pack handy. To prepare one in advance, fill a resealable plastic bag with 2 cups water and ⅓ cup surgical spirit. Zip it shut and put it in a container in the freezer. Overnight it forms a slushy ice that will conform to any body part that gets damaged in the course of daily activities. Keep zip side up to minimize risk of leaks.

Choose painkillers with care

Don't take aspirin when you've just sustained a bruise – it can make things worse. Aspirin thins the blood, which means it can pool more easily under the skin and intensify the characteristic black-and-blue effect. The same applies to ibuprofen. Instead, take paracetamol as pain relief for a bruise. If you think you bruise too easily, and you take aspirin regularly (to reduce your risk of heart attack, for example), then discuss the problem with your doctor, but don't stop taking the aspirin unless advised to.

Swallow, please

- **Bromelain**, an enzyme found in pineapples, actually 'digests' proteins involved in causing inflammation and inducing pain. Take up to 500mg of bromelain daily between meals until the bruise has faded.
- Try a **homeopathic version of arnica.** As soon as you get the bruise, start taking 1 dose every 4 hours. Take 4 doses the first day, then reduce your dosage to 2 or 3 pills daily as the bruise fades.

The power of prevention

- If you feel that you bruise too easily, you may be deficient in **vitamin C.** It strengthens capillary walls so they're less likely to leak blood and create a bruise. Get additional vitamin C by eating more peppers and citrus fruit or take supplements of up to 1000mg a day in divided doses.
- Increase your intake of **flavonoids** by eating more **carrots, apricots** and **citrus fruits.** These help vitamin C to work more efficiently in the body. Grape seed extract is also a rich supplier of flavonoids. Take up to 100mg a day.
- People who are susceptible to bruising may be deficient in **vitamin K,** which you can get from kale, broccoli, Brussels sprouts and leafy green vegetables, as well as from multivitamin supplements, which you should take with meals to enhance absorption.

Burns and Scalds

Prompt first aid is all that is needed for most minor burns and scalds. The first healing step is to immerse the burnt area in cold water for at least 20 minutes. This cools the skin, stops burning and relieves pain. Follow up by keeping the area clean and applying soothing compresses and boosting your body's ability to heal itself by taking one of the remedies recommended here.

First things first

- **Act fast.** You can safely treat burns that affect only the top layer of skin, depending on size: even first degree burns require medical attention if they cover a large area (bigger than hand-size). Deeper burns and those caused by electricity need emergency medical attention.
- As soon as you can, get the burnt skin under **cold running water** if possible (running water stays cold), for at least 20 minutes. If there's no water available, use any other cold, non-irritating liquid such as **milk** or iced tea.
- Remove **jewellery or clothes** that may constrict the area if swelling occurs.
- Cover the burn loosely with a temporary dressing of **cling film** or a **plastic bag**. A wet cloth can be put on top to provide cooling after the initial 20 minutes cold water treatment.
- Take care not to break any **blisters**. They are nature's protective coating.
- **Leave the burn alone** for at least 24 hours so it can begin to heal on its own. If a blister bursts, clean the area and apply some antiseptic cream before covering with a loose dressing.

Look to nature's healers

Once your burn has had two or three days to heal, you can try applying any of the following remedies.
- Squeeze or scrape some **aloe vera gel** from a freshly cut leaf and apply it to the burn. The cooling gel reduces pain, moistens the skin and keeps bacteria and air out of the burn. If you don't have a plant, apply an aloe vera based cream or gel two to three times a day.

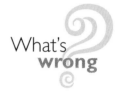

What's **wrong**

A burn is damage to the skin caused by wet or dry heat, chemicals or electricity. Most burns happen at home, and are caused by scalding water, hot oil or grease or hot foods. The mildest burns are known as 'first degree'. They may be red and tender with some swelling. You can treat these yourself provided they cover an area no larger than your hand. More serious injuries may result from fire, steam or chemicals. Moderate (second degree) burns are red and painful with blistering and swelling. Severe (third degree) burns don't hurt to begin with due to nerve damage; the skin is charred or black, white or red. There is no blistering but serious swelling. Severe burns require urgent hospital treatment.

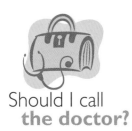

Should I call the doctor?

If someone suffers a severe burn, including a chemical or an electrical burn, he or she needs urgent medical attention. Dial 999 or get the person to the nearest hospital A&E department as soon as possible. A mild burn needs medical treatment if it covers a large area of skin or is very painful. Seek medical advice for a burn on the face or hands, or if the burn covers an area larger than the hand of the person affected (thus a smaller burned area for a baby than for an adult). Also see a doctor if the victim has a fever, chills, vomiting or swollen glands; or if the site of the burn smells unpleasant or oozes pus.

• The daisy-like flowers of **camomile** have long been used in burns remedies. To help a burn heal more quickly, apply camomile cream (from health-food shops) or **make a compress** using a cotton cloth soaked in a strong infusion of camomile.

• Another gentle healer is **calendula ointment**, made from the flowers of garden marigolds. Apply as often as needed.

• You can make a soothing compress by soaking a cloth in diluted distilled **witch hazel** or cooled tea made from **marigold**, **chickweed** or **elderflowers**. Apply the compress three or four times a day.

• The yellow flowers of **St John's wort** contain hypericin, a substance renowned for its ability to heal wounds and burns. It is the active constituent in **hypericum ointment**, which can be applied to a burn three times a day. The flowers are also dried and can be used to make a healing compress. Put one teaspoon of the dried herb into a cup of boiling water, steep for five minutes and strain. Soak a cloth in the cooled tea and apply to the burnt area twice a day.

Comfort foods

• Slap on some **honey**. Researchers in India found that honey was more effective on burns than silver sulphadiazine – the effective ingredient in conventional burns treatment creams. The study observed that burns dressed with honey healed faster and with less pain and scarring.

• Soak a flannel in ice-cold **whole milk** and apply to the burn for ten minutes at a time.

Homeopathic remedies

• Apply **Urtica** or **Hypercal** – available as ointments or tinctures – to any burns that have not blistered.

• For burns that blister, take **Cantharis** by mouth every hour.

Heal from the inside out

• Immune system boosting **echinacea** can help your skin to repair itself and fight off infection. Buy the tincture (1:5 in 45% alcohol) and take 15 drops in water three times a day.

• **Gotu kola** (or Indian pennywort) is a small tropical plant whose leaves have valuable wound healing properties. They are

Children at risk

Pre-school children are at greatest risk of accidental burns. Domestic fires are the most obvious danger zone. If you have a fireplace, don't put anything on the mantelpiece that might tempt your child to climb up to reach it. If you have an open fire, you must have a fireguard *by law* if you have children in the house. Choose a large 'childproof' guard and anchor it to the wall to protect your child from danger.

Kitchens pose lots of dangers. If possible, keep your child out of the kitchen while you're cooking. Keep the kettle flex away from the edge of the worktop; turn saucepan handles in – and always use the back rings if you can – and never throw water over oil fires, such as in a chip pan, because this will cause a fire explosion. Instead, cover the pan with a damp towel to smother the fire.

Barbecues are a major cause of serious burns: they can suddenly shoot flames when inflammable liquids drip onto the coals. Young children are also more likely than older children or adults to be scalded. Most scalds are caused by hot drinks being spilt – a cup of tea or coffee is still hot enough to scald a child 15 minutes after being made. Keep all hot drinks well out of children's reach and use placemats instead of a tablecloth that a child could pull.

Even bathtime is hazardous, especially once your child has learnt how to turn on the taps. Always turn on the cold tap first when running a bath, and set hot water thermostats no higher than 54°C (120°F) so as to reduce the chance of scalding. It takes just three seconds for a child to get burnt.

used in capsules as well as external ointments. For burns, take one or two 300mg capsules with food, up to three times a day.

COOL A SCALDED MOUTH

Gulping a hot drink, taking a mouthful of microwaved mince pie, biting into a cheesy pizza – all these can cause excruciating burns inside your mouth. The tissue on the roof of your mouth is very thin and burns easily. Like an injury to any other part of your body, a burn inside your mouth will take time to heal. Left to its own devices, your mouth should heal completely in a week or so, and you may be able to reduce healing time if you act quickly to cool down the burn.

Water, water everywhere

• Just like a burn to the skin, the best thing you can do with a scalded mouth is to cool it down. And the easiest way to do that is with **cold water**. Spend 5 or 10 minutes simply rinsing, spitting and gargling with cold water until the pain in your mouth eases.

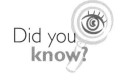

Did you know?

The ancient Egyptians used leeks to heal burns. Although this remedy is not used today, there was in fact some benefit to using leeks as they have significant antibiotic properties and would have helped to ward off infection.

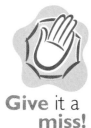

Give it a miss!

An old-fashioned remedy for a burn was to smear it with butter. This is probably as sensible as trying to put out a fire with petrol. Applying fat to a burn will simply hold in the heat and worsen the burn. Stick with lots of cold water instead.

- An even faster method is to use ice if you can get hold of some quickly. **Suck ice cubes** until the stinging stops.
- Once you've finished the initial cooling off, rinse and gargle with a **salt water solution**. Stir half a teaspoon of salt into a glass of warm water and use it to wash your mouth out. (Don't swallow it.) The salt is antiseptic and will help to clean and disinfect the burn.

Cool and sweet
- The fastest and most enjoyable way to cool down a pizza-scalded mouth – especially if you're eight years old – is with a scoop, or three, of **ice cream**.

Don't slow down the healing process
- For a few days after burning your mouth, **steer clear of hot drinks**. Let tea and coffee cool to lukewarm before inflicting them on your mouth, or stick to cold drinks for a while.
- Temporarily take **crusty baguettes off** the lunch menu. The same applies to crisps, raw carrots and crunchy apples. Any of these foods can scratch a healing burn.
- You may want to **avoid hot spices**, too, as these will irritate the damaged skin.

Try a healing herbal mouthwash
- **Blackberry leaves** have antibacterial and anti-inflammatory properties. Make a decoction by putting 10g dried leaves into 100ml (3½fl oz) cold water. Bring to the boil and leave to infuse for 15 minutes. Strain, sweeten with honey if you wish, and use as a mouthwash and gargle as often as you like.

Bursitis and tendinitis

There's nothing worse than having an arm or leg out of action as a result of pain caused by bursitis. Because the condition arises when repeated movement puts a strain on a specific joint, bursitis often affects the elbows of gardeners and golfers' shoulders. Tendinitis, too, is a repetitive strain injury. Runners can suffer from Achilles tendinitis; typists often experience the pain in their wrists. Healing for both conditions begins with acknowledging the need for a break from the activity that triggered the flare-up. Remedies designed to reduce the inflammation will help to ease the soreness.

Have a rest

- **Take a break** before you repeat the activity that triggered the pain. Be patient, as the problem may take several weeks to resolve.
- To hold down swelling, wrap an **elastic bandage** around the joint – but not too snugly. Then elevate the joint above the level of your heart. If it's your elbow that hurts, keep it on a high armrest, or sit in a low chair with your elbow propped up on the table. If you're treating your knee, lie on your back with the knee propped up on pillows.

Run cold and hot

- **Ice your sore joint** to ease pain and inflammation. Wrap up an ice pack in a towel and apply it for 10 to 20 minutes every four hours. Or freeze a paper cup full of ice, tear off the top edge, and rub the ice where it hurts. Repeat the treatment three or four times a day, allowing 2 to 5 minutes for each ice application.
- After about three days of giving joints the cold treatment – or until the joint no longer feels warm to the touch – start **alternating cold with heat.** Heat increases bloodflow to the injury, helping it to heal faster. Use a microwavable heat pack or an electric heating pad. Or, for contour-hugging warmth, place 2 to 3 cups of rice in a large sock, tie up the top and microwave it for 60 to 90 seconds. The rice will mould itself snugly to a knee, elbow or ankle.

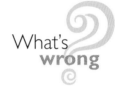

What's **wrong**

These somewhat related conditions are often the price you pay for too much repeated motion, whether doing something fun like playing tennis, or less fun, like shovelling snow. Bursitis is inflammation of the bursae – tiny, fluid-filled sacs that provide cushioning where muscle touches bone or rubs up against another muscle. Tendinitis is inflammation of the tendons, the tough cords that attach muscles to bones. Where bursitis often feels like a dull ache in a joint, tendinitis tends to produce sharp pain. These conditions crop up most often in the shoulders, hips, elbows, knees and ankles.

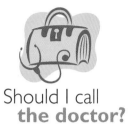

Should I call **the doctor?**

Reach for painkillers

● **Ibuprofen** is an effective anti-inflammatory that will help to relieve the swelling. It is very effective for short-term relief of this kind of pain.

● Try **Indian frankincense (boswellia)**. The body produces certain chemicals that actually increase pain. But this extract from the resin of the frankincense tree reduces production of those chemicals. Take one to two 150mg tablets three times a day. As the pain fades, reduce the dosage.

● Consider a **homeopathic remedy**. If your joint is stiff and painful when you move it but feels better with more use, take a dose of *Rhus toxicodendron* at the 6c or 12c dilution every 3 to 4 hours until you feel relief. (The 'c' stands for 'centesimal' – a dilution of 1:100. The more dilutions carried out, the more potent the remedy is considered to be.) If the joint pain becomes worse as you move, take **bryonia** at the 6c or 12c dilution every 3 to 4 hours until the pain diminishes. For pain that comes on suddenly and acutely, homeopathic physicians recommend **ruta** and **arnica**; the suggested dose is the 6c or 12c dilution every 3 to 4 hours.

Soothe with a rub or a poultice

● To soothe the aching area, rub on **arnica** cream or gel – a remedy derived from the flowers of a mountain daisy – two or three times a day. Arnica reduces swelling and inflammation, and is therefore also recommended for treating bruises and sprains. For even greater relief, press a **hot-water bottle** or heating pad against the joint after you've applied the arnica.

● **Tiger Balm**, a menthol-laced cream imported from China, can melt away pain. Rub it into the sore area once or twice a day. But it's a good idea to test a small patch of skin first. This is hot stuff, and some people develop a rash or redness if they use it too often. (*Alert* Do not get Tiger Balm near your eyes or mouth, and wash your hands after using.)

● Use a soothing **ginger compress** to help stop the hurt from the outside in. Chop 2 tablespoons of fresh root ginger, mix into 500ml (18fl oz) boiling water and leave to steep for 20 minutes. Immerse a folded piece of cloth in the warm tea and wring it out. Lay the damp cloth over your sore joint for 5 minutes. Repeat three or four times a day.

- **Vinegar**, applied topically, also eases aches and pains. Soak a flannel or tea-towel in equal parts hot water and vinegar. Wring it out and apply.

Swallow some soothers

- **Ginger** isn't just for compresses. Supplements of this natural anti-inflammatory can also help. For acute pain, take one 250mg ginger root capsule twice a day. (*Alert* Do not take ginger if you take blood thinning drugs such as warfarin or aspirin as it may interfere with blood clotting mechanisms.)
- Give the 'curry cure' a go. **Curcumin** is the active constituent in turmeric, the yellow Indian spice that's a key ingredient in many curry recipes. Turmeric has an age-old reputation as an anti-inflammatory and pain-relieving agent, but it seems to be curcumin that does the real work: it has been found to inhibit the synthesis of prostaglandins – hormone-like compounds in the body involved in the transmission of pain signals. Take 400 to 500mg of the dried standardized root extract three times a day.
- **Bromelain**, an enzyme found in pineapple, reduces inflammation. The strength of the standardized extract is measured in milk-clotting units (MCU). To achieve a strong therapeutic effect, a product must contain at least 2,000 MCU. Take 500mg on an empty stomach three times a day.
- **A bowl of cherries** is reputed to ease arthritic pain; eat at least 20 cherries a day for pain relief equivalent to one aspirin.
- Supplemental antioxidants can help to strengthen and repair connective tissue in your joints. **Grape seed extract** contains powerful antioxidant flavonoids called OPCs (oligomeric proanthocyanidins). It is available in capsules: take 200mg at the same time each day.

Choose fats that care for your joints

- **Omega-3 fatty acids** help to reduce inflammation. Increase the amounts in your diet by eating more oily fish, such as salmon, fresh tuna and mackerel. And consider taking fish oil supplements, in a dose of 1000–2000mg a day. Omega-3s are also found in flax seeds (linseed). Take 1 or 2 tablespoons of ground flax seeds with a glass of water up to three times a day, or 1 tablespoon of flax seed oil once or twice a day.

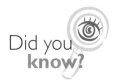

Did you know?

Flare-ups of bursitis and tendinitis have been called a lot of different names. Tennis elbow, for instance, is one of the most common forms of tendinitis. Heel pain may be caused by bursitis, tendinitis or both. Rotator cuff pain in the shoulder – a common complaint among bowlers – is also related to bursitis and tendinitis.

DO-IT-YOURSELF HEALING

DO-IT-YOURSELF HEALING
TREATING AN ACHING SHOULDER

If your shoulder is hurting, you might be tempted to rest your arm to ease the pain. But don't wait too long before you start using it again or you might develop a condition that is commonly called 'frozen shoulder'. Once you've treated the shoulder to the point where it is no longer excessively sore, do some daily exercises to make sure the joint remains flexible.

Lie on a bed or firm sofa face down, with your sore shoulder just slightly over the side of the bed and your arm hanging down. Swing your arm gently back and forth. Do this for 15 to 30 minutes, three to five times a week. (That's a long time to swing your arm, but fortunately it's easy to watch television from that position.)

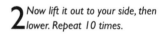

2 *Now lift it out to your side, then lower. Repeat 10 times.*

1 *Stand with your arms at your sides. Raise your affected arm in front of you until it's pointing at the ceiling, then lower it back down. Repeat 10 times.*

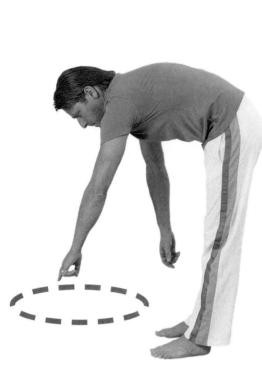

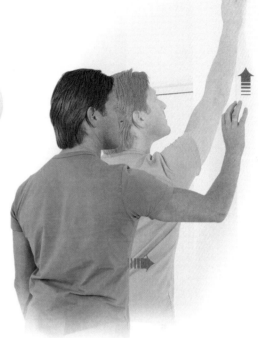

Bend over with your arms hanging loosely in front of you and swing one hand around as if you were drawing circles on the floor. After you've 'drawn' 10 circles with one hand, repeat with the other.

I Stand facing a corner and place the fingertips of one hand against the wall. Use your fingertips to 'crawl' up the corner, stepping closer as your hand moves higher.

2 When your arm is fully extended, hold the position for a few seconds, then lower your arm. Repeat 3 times, then do the same exercise with the other arm.

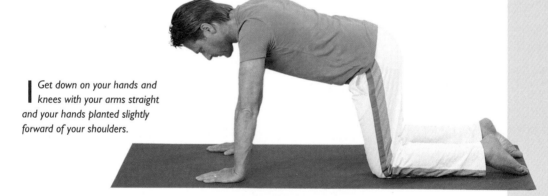

I Get down on your hands and knees with your arms straight and your hands planted slightly forward of your shoulders.

2 Gradually sit back on your heels until you can feel the stretch in your shoulders. Then return to the starting position. Do 5 repetitions.

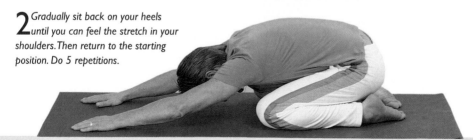

• **Avoid** chips and other packaged and processed foods that contain **hydrogenated oils**, and forgo fried foods, which are often cooked in those oils. These substances increase the inflammation in your body.

Warm up properly before exercise

• As you resume sports or other normal activities, the joint that's been giving you pain will need some extra attention. Give the muscles near the joint a good **massage** – either on your own or with the help of a professional masseur – for additional pain relief and relaxation.

• Always **stretch** properly before and after you exercise.

• If you have experienced knee pain, make sure that you're using the **correct shoes** for your sport. This is especially important before you resume a sport like tennis or running, where it's critical to have shoes that fit properly and are in excellent condition. Get rid of those worn-out pairs that have simply seen too many miles.

The power of prevention

• Start a **strength-training** programme using light weights to improve the muscles around the injured joint.

• Avoid going to sleep with **your arm bent over your head** – that is a classic trigger for bursitis.

• Be sure to interrupt long, repetitive chores with regular **stretch** breaks.

• If you're a tennis player, avoid tennis elbow by making sure your racquet has a large-handled grip and decreased string tension. Also, tennis elbow can develop if the racket head is too big or too small. Have the **grip**, **tension** and **racket size** checked by a tennis instructor.

• When working on your knees – pulling weeds, for example – kneel on a specially-designed **foam-rubber pad**.

Calluses and corns

In every pharmacy there is shelf space devoted to the tender care of calluses and corns. This is a good place to start in your search for relief. But the quest for treatment ingredients can take you much farther afield. If your feet are affected, you need the right oil to soften hard skin, customized patches for day-long protection, along with socks, shoes and insoles to protect you from pain. For hands, the right gloves can help a lot. Here are some ways to ease the irritation of calluses and corns.

Scrape and sand down

• If a callus is causing pain or irritation, you need to scrape away some of those dead cells so the callus won't put so much pressure on your nerves. Immediately after a warm shower or bath, when your skin is wet and softened, rub a **pumice stone** on the callus to remove dead cells. A pumice stone, available from pharmacies, is simply a rough piece of volcanic mineral. Don't try to grind the whole callus away in one sitting, as you will rub your skin raw. Instead, sand it down a little every day and be patient. If the callus is very thick or hard, the sanding project might take a few weeks.

• Soft corns occur between your toes when the bones in adjacent toes rub until the skin thickens. They're called 'soft' because the skin between the toes is generally more moist. A pumice stone won't fit the tight space between the toes, so buy a **callus file** instead and remove the thickened skin a little at a time, or relieve pressure between the toes with a foam wedge. If your feet need further attention, see a registered podiatrist or chiropodist who can remove corns painlessly, apply padding or insoles to relieve pressure, or fit corrective appliances for long term relief.

Soften up the opposition

• Instead of filing corns and calluses, you can soak and moisturize them until they become soft. For corns on your toes, use **olive oil** as a softener with a **corn pad** as protector. To protect the corn, you want non-medicated, doughnut-shaped pads, available from pharmacies. Place one of these pads around the

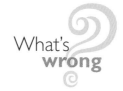

What's wrong

When your body tries to defend itself from injury, it sometimes creates strange armour. The outermost layer of skin piles up a thick fortress of dead cells whenever it is rubbed too much or too often. That is what happens when a badly-fitting shoe keeps rubbing the same toe or a metal-handled rake creates friction on the inside of your thumb. The epidermis gradually builds up a callus. That can evolve into a corn, which is simply a callus with a hard core. Calluses on the hands and feet can be painless and protective. But if a callus or corn presses on a bone or nerve beneath the skin, it can be as painful as a pebble between the toes.

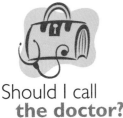

Should I call the doctor?

corn, apply a few drops of castor oil onto the corn with a cotton bud, then put adhesive tape over the pad to hold it in place. The little padded doughnut encircles the corn and shields it from pressure while also holding in the moisturizing castor oil. (Castor oil can leak through the bandage, causing stains, so wear some old socks when trying this treatment.)

• Another good way to soften calluses and corns is to soak them in water containing **Epsom salts**. Follow the directions on the packet.

Attack the corn with acid

• Look for medicated corn-removing patches that contain **salicylic acid.** Apply the patch after a bath or shower, and make sure you are treating only the hard callused area, not the soft skin around it – salicylic acid could cause burning or ulceration on normal skin.

• Another source of salicylic acid is **aspirin.** To create your own corn-softening compound, crush 5 aspirin tablets to a fine powder. Mix the powder thoroughly with ½ teaspoon of lemon juice and ½ teaspoon of water. Dab the paste onto the thickened skin, wrap the foot in cling film, then cover the film with a heated towel. Remove the wrap after 10 minutes and gently scrub the loosened skin with a pumice stone. (*Alert* This tip is not suitable for those allergic to aspirin.)

Relieve the friction

• To help protect a callus or corn on your foot from pressure, custom-design your own 'doughnut' pad using a piece of adhesive **moleskin.** Cut a circle larger than your callus or corn, fold it in half, and cut a half-circle in the centre. When you open it up, you'll have a padded ring. Stick it over your callus or corn.

• If you have a soft corn between two toes, stick a **foam toe separator** between them to keep them from rubbing each other. Look for these in the foot-care section at the pharmacy.

• Try socks that have very **thick, cushioned soles.** They could stop your calluses from getting worse.

• Sometimes, adding an over-the-counter **insole** to your shoes can decrease the pressure on the area with the callus and help it to recover more quickly.

The power of prevention

- Apply a lotion containing **urea**, such as Aquadrate, to rough spots before they turn into troublesome calluses. Start with a small amount, as urea-based lotions can sting.
- Another way to prevent skin from toughening up is by soaking your feet in a bowl of **warm water** once a week. Afterwards, apply a **moisturizing lotion**.
- **Choose shoes that fit well.** You should have a thumb's width between your longest toe and the end of the shoe. Shoes should be wide enough so that your toes and the balls of your feet aren't cramped from side to side. But if shoes are too roomy, your feet slide around and rub against the sides.
- Since feet naturally swell during the day, **shop for shoes late in the afternoon** when your feet are plumpest. If you shop in the early morning, you might end up with a pair of shoes that are too small.
- For women, it's advisable to **save the high heels for special occasions.** Even for the big night out, however, you should choose high heels that have a lot of cushioning in the front to reduce pressure on your toes.
- Don't play tennis in your running shoes. For each sport, select the **appropriate type of shoe**. A lot of research and engineering has gone into the development of shoes that are perfect for particular foot movements.
- To prevent calluses on your hands, wear thickly cushioned **gloves** when you're doing work such as raking, painting or pruning.

Give it a miss!

Some people may advise you to trim calluses and corns yourself, using a callus knife, a razor blade or scissors. Don't try it. No matter how awesome your surgical skills, you have better things to do than practise on your own flesh. There is real danger of infection from mishandling sharp instruments.

Carpal tunnel syndrome

The last time you needed a signed sick note from your doctor, you probably had an infection that made you feel lousy. This time, you don't even feel ill. But if you are suffering from carpal tunnel syndrome (CTS), you may well need some time off work because you must take a break from whatever has inflamed the tendons inside your carpal tunnel. Once you've got permission to give your wrists respite, you can use splints, supplements and exercises to help them to recover. But as you get back to normal, take some preventive steps and keep up the strengthening exercises.

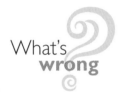

What's wrong

Inside each wrist is a narrow passageway called the carpal tunnel. Running through this tunnel are nine tendons that move your fingers, along with the median nerve. These tendons can become inflamed and swell up, compressing the nerve. Repetitive hand motion is a well-known cause of carpal tunnel syndrome, but other trigger factors include pregnancy, contraceptive pills, rheumatoid arthritis, hypothyroidism, diabetes and being overweight. The most common symptom is pins and needles; others are numbness in your fingers and thumb, pains that shoot up your wrist and forearm, soreness in the neck and shoulders and hand weakness.

Get to grips with the pain

- To quickly ease the pain and inflammation, cool your wrists with an **ice pack** wrapped in a thin towel. Leave it on for about 10 minutes. Repeat the treatment every hour or so.
- **Heat** can also ease pain by relaxing muscles. Soak your hands and wrists in warm to hot water for 12 to 15 minutes before you go to bed each night. However, because heat could also increase the pressure in the area, don't do this if it makes your symptoms worse.
- Twice a day, rub your wrists with an ointment containing **arnica**. This herbal remedy, renowned for its anti-inflammatory properties, helps to ease aches and pains. Apply a pea-sized blob of cream to the inside of each wrist, then massage the area with the thumb of the other hand all the way to the base of your palm. Repeat every morning and night until your symptoms ease.
- Many people find that **rapid wrist flicks** help to ease their symptoms, especially at night.
- **Wear a splint at night**. While asleep, you may be bending your hand and wrist under your pillow and this puts pressure on your wrist. In fact, people with CTS are often woken by the pain. A splint holds your fingers in a neutral position and relieves pressure on the median nerve. You can buy a splint from some chemists, but it's important to get the right size and make sure you know how to wear it properly – ask your pharmacist for advice.
- You may also want to **wear a splint during the day**, especially if you're doing jobs that require a lot of hand motion.

Beneficial supplements

- **Bromelain**, an enzyme derived from pineapples, digests inflammatory proteins, so it can reduce inflammation in your sore wrists. Along with reducing the pain, it may help you to heal faster. Bromelain's potency is measured in MCU (milk-clotting units). Look for supplements rated at least 2,000 MCU and take 1,000mg twice a day during a CTS flare-up. You can cut down to 500mg twice a day once your symptoms start improving. Make sure you take bromelain between meals. If you take it near mealtimes, much of its potency will be wasted digesting your food.

- The herb **St John's wort**, best known as an antidepressant, can also help to repair nerve damage and reduce pain and inflammation. Take up to 250mg of extract standardized to contain 0.3 per cent hypericin three times a day. If that's not working after two weeks, take 300 to 400mg three times a day.

- Take 1 tablespoon of **flax seed (linseed) oil** every day, and give it at least two weeks to have an effect. Flax seed oil is rich in omega-3 fatty acids, which reduce inflammation. Take it with food for better absorption. If you like, you can stir it into orange juice or add it to salad dressing.

- **Curcumin** is an anti-inflammatory component found in the spice turmeric. In Ayurvedic medicine – which originated in India – turmeric has a long history of use as a medicine for pain and inflammation. But the spice alone doesn't really pack the

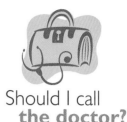

Should I call the doctor?

Seek a doctor's advice if symptoms interfere with your daily activities. If carpal tunnel syndrome goes untreated, you could be left with a weakened grip in your hands and significant pain in your forearms or shoulders. Also, because the condition is associated with arthritis, diabetes and an under-active thyroid gland, a doctor should evaluate you to ensure you don't have any of those conditions in addition to CTS.

B for benefit?

Vitamin B_6 is probably the most well-known supplement when it comes to treating carpal tunnel syndrome, but it is also controversial. Many experts claim it works but there are also many who claim it doesn't. On top of that, excessive vitamin B_6 (anything over 50mg a day) taken for a long period can even cause nerve problems.

Supplementation with B_6 might be helpful because the vitamin is important in maintaining healthy nerves, and it may speed up nerve impulses to your hands. Some people claim CTS is actually caused by

vitamin B_6 deficiency. What we know for sure is that some people require more of the vitamin than others and stress can increase your need for it.

To err on the side of caution, eat plenty of foods rich in the vitamin, including chicken breast, wholegrain cereals, brown rice, salmon, green vegetables and egg yolks. If you want to try a supplement, take up to 50mg of B_6 a day, in divided doses, until your symptoms improve. If you then wish to continue supplementation, reduce the daily dose of B_6 to 10mg a day.

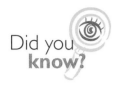

Did you know?

punch of supplements. Look for a supplement standardized to contain 95 per cent curcumin and take 300mg three times a day, with meals.

● Try taking 300mg of **magnesium** two or three times a day. This mineral is involved in nerve function and muscle relaxation. A supplement may help, especially if you don't eat a lot of magnesium-rich whole grains, nuts, legumes, dark green leafy vegetables or shellfish. The most absorbable form is magnesium citrate. The only side effect might be loose bowel movements. If you have that problem, reduce the dose or try magnesium gluconate, which has a gentler effect on the digestive tract.

Take precautions at the keyboard

● If you spend a lot of time in front of the computer, **adjust your chair and keyboard**. Your arms should be bent at a 90 degree angle when you type so that your wrists are parallel with the ground. Your knees should also obey the 90 degree rule. And sit up straight, making sure your shoulders are not slumped forward.

● If the keyboard can be lowered, bring it down to a position where the **keys are slightly lower than your wrists** so that your fingertips drop down to rest lightly on the keys.

● **Tap the computer keys** rather than pounding them. The less pressure you apply, the better.

● Use ergonomic, hand-friendly products whenever possible. Especially helpful is **a wrist rest**, sold at most office equipment suppliers.

● Get a **contoured keyboard** or **split keyboard.** These are specially designed so your hands can rest in a natural position while your fingers tap lightly on the keys. (The pressure required to depress a key is much lighter than on regular keyboards.) In contour models, two sets of keys are held in a single, moulded frame, with comfortable areas to support each of your wrists. Split keyboards have separate frames that can be angled in different ways for maximum wrist comfort.

DO-IT-YOURSELF HEALING
CARPAL TUNNEL SYNDROME

When using a computer or doing any job that involves repetitive hand motion, it's essential to take regular breaks and do stretching exercises. Try to take a 15-minute break every few hours. Stand up, relax your shoulders and shake your arms to relax your wrists and restore circulation. Make a fist with each hand, hold for a few seconds, then open it, separating your fingers and spreading them as wide as possible. Repeat 4 times. Whenever possible, do the following exercises.

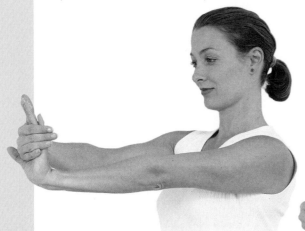

Extend your left arm straight in front of you and bend the wrist upwards. Place the fingers of your right hand against the palm of your left and pull back gently. Hold for a count of 10. Switch hands.

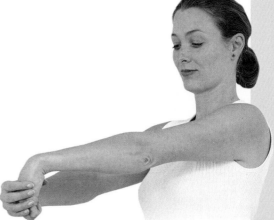

Extend your left arm and make a fist. Fold your right hand over the top of the fist and pull gently, holding for a count of 10. Switch hands.

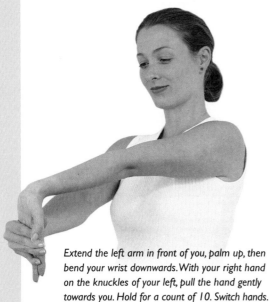

Extend the left arm in front of you, palm up, then bend your wrist downwards. With your right hand on the knuckles of your left, pull the hand gently towards you. Hold for a count of 10. Switch hands.

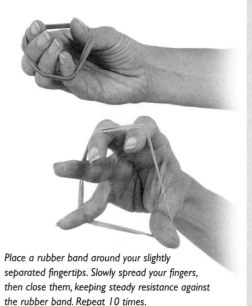

Place a rubber band around your slightly separated fingertips. Slowly spread your fingers, then close them, keeping steady resistance against the rubber band. Repeat 10 times.

Chapped lips

It is one of the few flaws in an almost-perfect design: our lips, so exposed to sun, wind and other irritants, don't have oil glands to keep them soft and moist. Nor do they contain much melanin, the pigment in our skin that allows us to tan and offers some protection from the sun. No wonder lips can become as parched and cracked as old shoe leather. If you want to keep lips kissable, give them some protection.

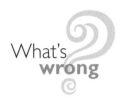

What's wrong

Your lips are dry, irritated and cracked. They may be sore or they may itch. Dry lips can be triggered by dry, cold winter weather, sunburn, allergic reactions, having a raised temperature or simply licking your lips too often.

Bring out the lip balm

- One all-natural salve is **beeswax**, such as Burts Beeswax lip balm, sold in pharmacies. Always coat your lips with balm **before you go out** to keep the elements at bay.
- Some people swear by **cocoa butter** to relieve chapped lips. (It also works on chapped hands.) Apply four or five times a day, or more often if your lips are very dry.
- A handy home remedy is **olive oil** or **vegetable shortening** which can effectively soften and moisturize chapped lips.
- If you have **vitamin E** capsules to hand, puncture one and apply the oil to your lips.
- **Petroleum jelly**, such as Vaseline, is an old-fashioned and effective chapped lips remedy.
- The label on one US brand of **udder cream** says that it's for cows but that most of its users have two legs. That's because it's so effective for chapped lips. Various products are available here but look for any formulated with lanolin and petrolatum (the stuff in petroleum jelly). You may find them in some country stores or you can order them online.

Moisturize from the inside out

- If your lips are continually chapped, drink eight 250ml glasses of **water** a day – more, if you can. While this won't prevent dryness, it will keep it from getting worse.

The power of prevention

- Apply a balm with a **sun protection factor (SPF) of at least 15** before you go out into the sun. Lips need just as much sun protection as the rest of your skin. (*Alert* Stop using

Get rid of the yeast

If you have whitish patches in your mouth and the corners of your mouth are cracked or chapped, you may have oral thrush, caused by a yeast overgrowth. To help clear the yeast, use over-the-counter miconazole gel (Daktarin oral gel). If you wear dentures and have this condition, be sure to clean your dentures thoroughly and frequently. Yeast can grow on them and spread by contact to your lips. Babies and toddlers can be affected, too. Sterilize dummies and teats frequently to get rid of the fungus.

the balm if your lips turn red and itchy. Some people have an allergic reaction to lip balms that contain sunscreen.)

● A dark, creamy **lipstick** helps to protect lips from the sun and keep moisture in.

● When indoor air is very dry, prevent chapped lips by running a **humidifier** in your bedroom while you sleep.

● Try eating more foods that are rich in **B vitamins**, such as meat, fish, whole grains, nuts and leafy green vegetables. Lack of B vitamins contributes to chapped lips in some people.

● **Avoid licking your lips.** Your saliva may momentarily provide a coating of moisture, but it evaporates quickly, leaving lips drier than before. And the saliva contains digestive enzymes that dry out tissue.

● Stay away from balms that contain **phenol** or **camphor**. These antiseptics can be very drying.

● **Don't give a child flavoured lip balms**. Children tend to lick the flavoured varieties straight off their lips, which further aggravates the chapping.

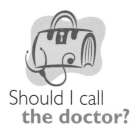

Should I call the doctor?

Usually, a little TLC takes care of chapped lips. But if they remain chapped after you've soothed them for two or three weeks, then see your doctor. You should also see a doctor if your lips are often cracked; you may have a yeast infection (oral thrush). An allergic sensitivity to ingredients in toothpaste, lipstick or lip balms can also cause dry lips. Occasionally, lips that are persistently red, dry or scaly can suggest a precancerous condition.

Chickenpox

Chickenpox lasts only a week or two, but generally the end can't come soon enough. If pain is the problem, ease it with paracetamol – never aspirin. If the itching is too much to bear, try cool baths and a children's antihistamine. And have a few other tricks to keep up your sleeve to minimize the misery.

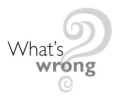

What's wrong

Your child has a common childhood illness, caused by the varicella zoster virus. The virus first appears as a rash or red spots on the trunk, which spread to other areas within a few days. There may be just a few spots or hundreds. Over a period of about a week, many of the spots turn into small blisters, which break and scab over. Your child may also have a fever and develop itching, which can be mild or intense. After the blisters heal, the virus goes into a latent stage and lives in sensory nerves in the body. It may surface years later in the form of the painful ailment, shingles.

Stay cool

- If it is winter, **turn down the heating** to the lowest comfortable temperature. In summer, **use a fan**. Heat brings more blood to the surface of the skin, exacerbating the itching.
- Let your child soak in a lukewarm bath for 15 to 20 minutes every few hours. Don't use soap. Instead, add half a cup of **bicarbonate of soda** to a shallow bath or a full cup to a deep bath to provide extra relief. **Colloidal oatmeal** (such as Aveeno) added to a bath also counteracts itching. If you don't have colloidal oatmeal (oatmeal that is so finely ground that it remains suspended in the water), place ordinary oats in a stocking, tie up the end and swish the stocking in the water.
- When your child feels like scratching, offer a **cool, wet flannel** to press against the itchy skin. Scratching can lead to infection and scarring. By using the flannel, the scratching urge is satisfied without doing any damage. As insurance against scratching, keep nails trimmed and put gloves on the child's hands at bedtime.

Attack the itching

- Should you slap on the **calamine?** Calamine lotion is a traditional remedy, long used to soothe the itching of chickenpox. However, doctors are now less keen to recommend it and dermatologists think it may even worsen itching.
- Apply an **antihistamine cream** to help calm the itching.
- Give **paracetamol** or **ibuprofen** syrup to make a child with a fever or headache more comfortable. Choose the right strength for your child's age and follow label instructions.
- If the itching is bad, give your child an **oral antihistamine** such as cetirizine if he or she is at least two years old. (And

Shun the blistering sun

If your child has recently been exposed to someone who has the chickenpox virus, keep him or her out of the sun. A dose of sunshine may make the blisters worse when they finally appear. Once the chickenpox is over, your child's skin will remain sensitive to the sun for as long as a year. You don't have to barricade your child in the house, but it is helpful to apply sunscreen every day – particularly in summertime.

always be sure to check the label first). This medicine can be especially useful at bedtime if itching interferes with sleep, because it causes drowsiness.

Calm the skin with cool cotton

• Keep your child in fresh **cotton pyjamas**. Cotton is less irritating than other fabrics. Choose pyjamas with long sleeves and long trousers to discourage scratching.

Mind that mouth

• If your child has chickenpox in the mouth (yes, it can happen), the best treatment is rinsing out or gargling with **salt water**. This will probably be harder than persuading your child that Brussels sprouts are delicious, but it's worth a try.
• Administer **ice lollies**. They can be soothing.
• Feed **bland food** like porridge, rice pudding, jelly, soups and bananas while the blisters are sore.

The power of prevention

• If your child hasn't had chickenpox, you can try to keep him or her away from children who have it. But it is **far better to get chickenpox as a child** than have to endure it as an adult.
• There is a **vaccine for chickenpox** but it is not given routinely to children in the UK. It may, however, be given to people who have not had chickenpox and who work or live with people who would be at high risk if they contracted the virus, such as those with weak immune systems (anyone with HIV or AIDS, or leukaemia, or on immune-suppressing medication such as chemotherapy).

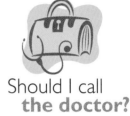

Should I call the doctor?

Chickenpox is usually more of an annoyance than a danger; most cases clear up in 10 to 14 days without problems. Call your doctor if your child develops a high fever accompanied by severe headache; or has a fever that lasts more than a few days; or feels severe pain in the limbs; or repeatedly vomits; or develops a cough; or has a large area of redness surrounding one or more blisters – a sign of infection. Also call your doctor if your child has convulsions, becomes disorientated or complains of neck pain. In very rare cases, chickenpox can result in meningitis.

HEALING SOUPS FROM AROUND THE WORLD

Soups have a lot to recommend them. They're comforting, easy to digest – and they provide nutrients that your body needs in order to recover. Chicken soup is the ultimate home remedy for colds. In China, hot-and-sour soup, with its rice vinegar, ginger and garlic, is used to break up congestion. Cabbage soup, popular in Eastern Europe, is now recommended as a home remedy for ulcers. Elsewhere in the world, other soup recipes are revered for their health benefits. Here are just a few.

India: horse gram soup for high blood pressure

In the farming communities of central India, an indigenous crop called horse gram is often prescribed to control high blood pressure. Horse gram is a small oval seed resembling lentils, with the aroma of freshly cut hay. When the seed-bearing pods of horse gram mature, they are picked, dried and beaten with wooden poles. The seeds are cleaned and sorted.

Kuluth saar, or horse gram soup, is a light dish with a slightly musty taste. It's often mixed with yoghurt and served with rice. Horse gram seeds are soaked for eight hours, then left to sprout for another eight hours before they're simmered in water. Other ingredients include kokum (a small, dark purple fruit from an evergreen tree) and many cloves of crushed garlic. A tablespoon of pomegranate seeds, ground into a fine paste, is sometimes added to a cup of horse gram soup to help dissolve kidney and bladder stones.

Horse gram may be available in specialist Indian food stores. But if you can't find horse gram, a bag of lentils will make a fine high fibre soup.

China: Ginkgo nut porridge for jet lag

Grace Young is a Chinese cook who flies thousands of miles every year. Whenever she returns to her family , there's a big pot of ginkgo nut porridge on the stove. It's a late-night snack (siu ye) that helps to heal the body from the damaging effects of flying. The ginkgo nuts in this recipe, according to traditional Chinese medicine, are beneficial for relieving coughs and reducing phlegm.

Key ingredients are dried bean curd (foo jook), unshelled ginkgo nuts (bock guo), and Chinese dried scallops (gawn yu chee) plus a generous helping of finely shredded ginger. Some cooks include rump steak as well.

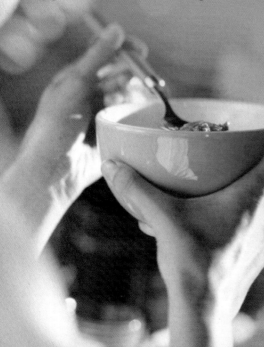

Philippines: ginger chicken soup for joint pain

Drugs such as aspirin and ibuprofen can ease painful arthritis flare-ups, but why not try this warming alternative: ginger soup. Ginger contains gingerol, a compound that blocks the action of prostaglandins, hormone-like chemicals that contribute to inflammation. Ginger can also help to combat the virus that causes flu. In the Philippines, ginger chicken soup (chicken tinola) is usually made with green papaya, but you can substitute fresh spinach instead.

Chicken tinola

The following classic recipe comes from the Maya Culinary Arts Centre in Manila.

6 tablespoons vegetable oil
3 cloves chopped garlic
2 tablespoons minced fresh ginger
1 large onion
1.5kg (3¼lb) boneless chicken,
    sliced for sautéing
1.75 litres (3 pints) water
2 large handfuls fresh spinach
fish sauce to taste
pepper to taste

In a heavy saucepan, heat half the oil and sauté the garlic, ginger and onion. When the onions turn clear (not brown), remove all the ingredients and set aside. In the same pan, add the remaining oil and stir-fry the chicken until it is cooked through. Return the garlic, ginger and onion to the casserole, add the water and bring to the boil. Reduce heat and simmer, partly covered, for 30 minutes. Add the spinach and stir. Just before serving, add the fish sauce and pepper.
Serves 8

United States of America: Mom's favourite chicken soup

This may well be one of the most popular home remedies ever invented. Recent research shows that there's even scientific fact behind the folklore: chicken soup can, apparently, help to prevent white blood cells from triggering inflammation and congestion in the upper airways.

There are many reasons to keep a pot simmering when you have a cold or flu. The rich, steamy broth breaks up congestion, and spicy ingredients such as garlic and onion have mild antiviral properties. To give the soup an extra cold-beating boost, slice a few cloves of garlic and add them to the pot when the soup is almost cooked.

Mom's favourite chicken soup

For extra congestion-busting power, add a few shakes of cayenne pepper and a tablespoon of chopped fresh ginger to this recipe.

1 whole chicken, cut into 8 pieces
1kg (2lb 3oz) chopped carrots
1kg (2lb 3oz) onions
4 cloves garlic, crushed
salt, pepper, parsley and dill to taste

Place the chicken pieces in a large pan, cover with water, and bring to a full boil. Reduce the heat to a simmer and skim off any foam that rises. Add the chopped carrots and onions, and simmer for 2 to 3 hours, topping up with water as necessary. Crush the garlic and add, then season to taste with salt, pepper, parsley and dill. For a thicker soup, scoop out a ladle or two of the vegetables, purée them in a food processor and stir back into the soup.
Serves 10

Colds and flu

It may be 'just a cold', but it's nothing to sneeze at. And flu makes you feel really ill. Fortunately, fast action on your part can mitigate some of the misery. Herbs, chicken soup, zinc – and even your hair dryer – are part of the healing arsenal. At the first sign of a sniffle, turn to these remedies, which can unstuff your head, boost your immune system and speed your illness on its way – unlike typical cold medicines, which can dry you out, put you to sleep, keep you up at night, do nothing at all to make you better faster – and may even prolong your illness.

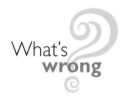

What's wrong

If your symptoms are above the neck – congestion, sore throat, sneezing, coughing – you probably have a cold, caused by any one of 200 viruses that other people's sneezes or coughs have placed in the air or on something you've touched. If you have all those symptoms plus a fever of 38.5°C (102°F) or more, headache, muscle aches, extreme fatigue, diarrhoea, nausea or vomiting, you're more likely to have flu. It usually lasts for a week or more and can leave you feeling weak and down-in-the-dumps for days or even weeks afterwards.

Nip it in the bud

- At the first hint of a cold, drink **elderflower tea**. Put 2 to 5g dried flowers into a cup of boiling water to make an infusion. Leave to infuse for 5 to 10 minutes and strain. Drink at least 3 cups a day. Elderflowers are only available from May to July so it's a good idea to make your own **elderflower cordial** – or make elderberry wine (the flowers and berries seem to be equally effective) – and keep it in the larder year round both as a pleasant drink and as a treatment for colds.
- **Sniff vitamin C powder** (available from pharmacies) at the first sign of a sniffle. Targeting the vitamin directly at the nasal mucosa can stop the virus in its tracks before the cold has a chance to take hold. This particular strategy is most effective for those who are subject to exceptionally high levels of physical stress, such as marathon runners. Be warned that sniffing vitamin C powder can sting a bit.
- **Zinc nasal gel** has been shown by one study to be effective in reducing symptoms of a cold and its duration. Zinc plays a key role in immune system activity and it is thought that delivering treatment via the nose works more effectively than an oral dosage. Do not take zinc for longer than a week, because long-term use of zinc can actually weaken immunity.

Head off a head cold

- As soon as you notice cold or flu symptoms, start taking 200mg of **vitamin C** five times a day, with food. Buy a brand with **added bioflavonoids**, which have been shown to enhance the effectiveness of vitamin C by as much as 35 per cent. If you develop diarrhoea, cut down on the dose.

• Take one 200mg **astragalus** capsule twice a day until you recover. This ancient Chinese herb stimulates the immune system and seems to be highly effective at fighting colds and flu. To prevent a relapse, continue taking 1 capsule twice a day for a further week once your symptoms have gone.

• **Goldenseal** stimulates the immune system and has germ-fighting compounds that can kill viruses. As soon as you begin to feel ill, take 125mg goldenseal extract (on its own or in combination with 200mg immune-boosting **echinacea**) four times a day for five days.

Bring on the flu fighters

• At the first sign of flu, take 20 to 30 drops of **elderberry** tincture three or four times a day for three days. Elderberry has been used in Europe for centuries to fight viruses, and one research study found that people who took it recovered from flu significantly faster than those who didn't. You can also buy elderberry lozenges (take six a day until symptoms subside).

• Naturopaths recommend **Oscillococcinum,** a homeopathic remedy for reducing the severity of flu symptoms. It is sold online and in some pharmacies and health-food shops. Be sure to use it within 12 to 48 hours of the first appearance of your symptoms. It comes in vials: take one vial every 6 hours.

• Try **N-acetylcysteine (NAC)**, a form of the amino acid cysteine. It helps to thin and loosen mucus and reduce flu symptoms. Take one 600mg dose three times daily.

Soothe a sore throat

• For a sore throat, fill a 250ml glass with warm water, mix in a teaspoon of **salt** and gargle. The salt will soothe the pain.

• The traditional sore-throat gargle – a squeeze of **lemon juice** in a glass of warm water – is ideal because it creates an acidic environment hostile to bacteria and viruses.

Sup chicken soup to combat a cold

• **Chicken soup,** *the* natural remedy of natural remedies, offers more than comfort for colds and flu. Modern scientists have

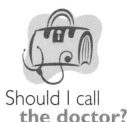

Should I call the doctor?

Colds are miserable but generally go away on their own, helped along by rest and home remedies. The same goes for less severe cases of flu; more severe cases may require a doctor's care. If you don't know whether it's a cold or flu, let the symptoms be your guide. Contact your doctor if you've had a fever above 38°C (101°F) for more than three days, or any fever above 39.5°C (103°F). Call, too, if you start to wheeze, find it hard to breathe, feel severe pain in your lungs, chest, throat or ear, or cough up copious amounts of phlegm, especially if it is bloody or has a greenish tinge. In children, a fever can quickly lead to dehydration, so it's important to keep pushing fluids and to talk to your doctor if you are worried.

Old **wives' tale**

Getting chilled does not cause a cold – at least not under laboratory conditions. In one study reported in *The New England Journal of Medicine,* two groups of people were exposed to viruses that cause the common cold. One group was exposed to the germs in a chilly 5°C (41°F) room; the other group, in a balmy 30°C (86°F) room. The result? Both groups caught colds at about the same rate.

confirmed that chicken soup stops certain white blood cells – neutrophils – from congregating and causing inflammation, which in turn triggers the body to produce copious amounts of mucus. It also thins mucus more effectively than plain hot water. Homemade soup is best – especially if it's made by someone you love (*see* Healing soups, page 114).

- Add fresh chopped **garlic** to chicken soup. The Egyptian pharaohs used garlic to fight infection and its healing powers are legendary. Among its active compounds are allicin and allin, shown in test-tube studies to kill germs outright. Garlic also appears to stimulate the release of natural killer cells, part of the human immune system's arsenal of germ-fighters.

Wet your whistle – and everything else

- Fighting off colds and flu can rob your body of moisture. Drink as much **water** as you can – eight or more 250ml glasses – to keep your mucous membranes moist and to help relieve dry eyes and other flu symptoms. Fluids also help to thin mucus making it easier to blow out.
- To help keep mucus loose, stay in a **moist, warm, well-ventilated room.** To keep the air in your bedroom moist, place bowls of water near the radiator (in winter) or run a humidifier. Or open the lid of an **electric kettle** and let the water boil, which will fill the room with steam.

A reeking remedy

- A dose of neat **garlic** – a natural antiseptic – will fight those viruses. If you're feeling brave, hold a small clove of garlic in your mouth and breathe the fumes into your throat and lungs. If the flavour gets too strong as the clove softens, just chew it up quickly into smaller pieces and swallow with water.

Get yourself vaccinated

Consider having a yearly flu jab. Health authorities advise it, especially for people with chronic heart or kidney disease; chronic lung diseases like asthma, bronchitis and emphysema; or those with diabetes or who have depressed immunity for any reason. It is also recommended for people over 65. The vaccine is usually available at your GP's surgery from early October. Have the jab early, as it takes at least two weeks for it to work, and you want to be protected before the flu season starts.

• You can also get a therapeutic dose of **garlic in capsule form**. The usual dose is 400 to 600mg concentrate four times a day, with food. Look for pills standardized to 4000mcg of allicin potential. If you develop indigestion, wind or diarrhoea when taking garlic, then you may find that enteric-coated capsules help to reduce these side-effects.

Blow that virus away

• You can cut short a cold with your … **hair dryer?** As outlandish as it sounds, inhaling heated air may help to kill a virus working its way up your nose. In one UK study, people who breathed heated air had half the cold symptoms of people who inhaled air at room temperature. Set your hair-dryer on warm (not hot), hold it an arm's length from your face and breathe in the air through your nose for as long as you can – at least two or three minutes and ideally 20 minutes.

Clear out congestion

• For a congestion-busting blast, buy fresh **root ginger** or **horseradish**, grate it and eat a small amount. (Or buy horseradish in a jar and eat as much as half a tablespoon.) To avoid the risk of a sore tummy, try these remedies after a meal.

• Drink a cup of **ginger tea**. Make it with a ginger tea bag or with ½ teaspoon of grated root ginger. Ginger helps to block the production of substances that cause bronchial congestion and stuffiness and it contains compounds called gingerols, which are natural cough suppressants.

• Spike stock or soup with a dash of **Tabasco sauce, chilli pepper flakes** or **wasabi**, the hot condiment (usually made from horseradish) eaten with sushi. All of these hot seasonings can increase a broth's decongestant power. In fact, adding any of them to any food can help you to breathe more freely.

• Wear **wet socks** to bed. Believe it or not, this soggy strategy is a recognized naturopathic remedy that can help to ease a fever and clear congestion. It works by drawing blood to the feet, which dramatically increases blood circulation. (Blood stagnates in the areas of greatest congestion.) First warm your feet in hot water. Then soak a thin pair of cotton socks in cold water, wring them out, and slip them on just before going to bed. Put a pair of dry wool socks over the wet ones. The wet

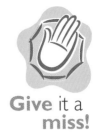

Give it a miss!

Some cold medicines contain an antihistamine, which works well for allergies, but does nothing for congestion caused by colds. In fact, antihistamines can make mucus thicker and therefore harder to blow out or cough up. If you're stuffed up, choose a simple decongestant. Otrivine and ephedrine are effective decongestant nasal sprays, but don't use them for longer than three days; over-exposure can cause a rebound effect that makes your nose even stuffier.

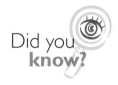

socks should be warm and dry in the morning, and you should feel markedly better. Only try this remedy in a reasonably well-heated room: wearing wet socks to bed would be unwise if the room was uncomfortably cold.

- Soak your feet in a **mustard footbath**. Add 1 tablespoon of mustard powder per litre of hot water in a large bowl – a washing-up bowl is ideal. The mustard draws blood to your feet, which helps to relieve congestion.

- An old-fashioned remedy for chest congestion is a **mustard poultice**. Grind 3 tablespoons of mustard seeds to a powder (or use ⅓ cup of mustard powder), add this to a cup of flour or fine oatmeal, then stir in just enough water to make a paste. Smooth a layer of petroleum jelly over your chest to protect the skin, then slap on the paste. The pungent aroma helps to unblock stuffy sinuses, and the heat improves blood circulation and eases congestion. Don't leave the poultice on for more than 15 minutes, however, or it may burn your skin.

Steam clean your nasal passages

- Pour boiling water into a large bowl, lean over the bowl and drape a towel over your head to create a **steam tent**. Breathe in through your nose and out through your mouth for 5 to 10 minutes. Don't put your face too close to the water or you risk scalding your skin or inhaling vapours that are too hot. Set the bowl on a steady table – don't attempt this remedy in bed.

- To make steam inhalations even more effective, add a few drops of **thyme oil** or **eucalyptus oil** to the water. Keep your eyes closed as you breathe the steam, as the combination of essential oil and steam can irritate your eyes.

- Add a few drops of **eucalyptus oil** or **Olbas oil** to a hanky. Whenever you feel congested, hold it to your nose and inhale.

Warm a stiff neck

- Flu can give you a horrible stiff neck. To ease the ache, wet a hand towel, wring it out, put it in a plastic bag and **microwave it for 60 seconds**. Or simply dip a towel in very hot water and squeeze it out. Check that it's not too hot, then wrap the towel around your shoulders and neck and lie down. (Put a beach or bath towel under you to keep the bed dry.) To **lock in the heat**, wrap a dry towel around the wet one.

The power of prevention

- During the colds and flu season, take 200mg **echinacea** up to three times a day. Alternate it every three weeks with other herbs that boost the immune system – such as **astragalus**, **goldenseal** and **pau d'arco**.
- **Wash your hands often** with soap and water, especially after you use a public toilet or if you work with people who are unwell. In 1998, a large US study ordered 40,000 naval recruits to wash their hands five times a day. The recruits cut their incidence of respiratory disease by a huge 45 per cent.
- Don't touch your face with unwashed hands. Carry a small bottle of **hand sanitizer gel** to use when you can't reach a washbasin.
- It may seem rude, but **avoid shaking hands** with anyone who has a cold.
- In winter, use a **cool-mist humidifier** to counteract the drying effect of central heating and keep indoor air moist.
- Practise **relaxation techniques** all year round, but especially during the colds and flu season. Research suggests that the more stress you're under, the more likely you are to become ill.
- **Get some rest.** Most people get colds or flu when they're run down. So phone in sick and sleep. Research shows that even if you are marginally sleep-deprived, your resistance to viruses declines dramatically. In one study, certain immune cells that stalk viral infections dropped by 30 per cent in people who got just slightly less sleep than usual in a single night.
- **Widen your circle of friends.** In a study of more than 200 men and women, people who had strong social ties developed fewer colds. Researchers gave the subjects nasal drops containing rhinovirus, the bug that causes most colds, and they found that those with only one to three social relationships were four times more likely to come down with a cold than those who had six or more friends.

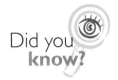

Did you know?

Making love keeps you well. To keep colds and flu at bay, make love at least once a week. One study found that men and women who were sexually active at least that often had higher levels of immune-system molecules called immunoglobulin A – which play an important role in shielding the mucous membranes from invaders – than people who weren't.

Cold sores

The goal of every cold-sore victim is to make sure that those sore and unsightly blisters are absent a lot more than they're present. Once you have the virus, you need to mount a consistent campaign to discourage flare-ups. Once you have learnt to recognize the telltale tingling or burning sensation that notifies you of a sore's imminent arrival, you can pepper it with your defensive home remedies.

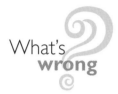

What's wrong

Cold sores are usually caused by the herpes simplex type 1 virus. The painful, fluid-filled blisters might appear on your lip, or you may have painful ulcers in your mouth and throat. If you get a sore once, you'll likely have a recurrence. A tingling sensation around your mouth heralds the sore's imminent arrival, usually within a day or two. The blister swells, bursts, oozes fluid, crusts over and fades, often in 7 to 10 days. Painful sores on your tongue and inside your lips and cheeks may accompany an initial outbreak. Common triggers of a new outbreak include sunlight, stress, menstruation and fatigue.

First aid for cold sores

- Apply **ice** directly to the sore. It will bring down the swelling and ease the pain temporarily. If you use this tactic early enough in the game – at the first sign of tingling – you may end up with a smaller sore than you otherwise would have.
- You can also use **aspirin** for pain relief, and it may have an added benefit. The results of one study (published in the US journal, *Annals of Internal Medicine*) suggested that taking 150mg of aspirin a day (two 75mg tablets) can cut the time a herpes infection remains active by 50 per cent.

Vanquish the virus

- Some studies have found the amino acid **lysine** helpful as a healer for cold sores. When you're having an outbreak, take 3000mg a day until the sore goes away. Research has shown that it thwarts the replication (copying) of the herpes virus.
- Herbal healers commonly recommend **lemon balm** (also called melissa) to treat herpes simplex type 1. Its essential oils contain substances that have been shown to inhibit the virus. In German studies, people with recurrent cold sores who used a lemon balm ointment regularly had less frequent outbreaks, or stopped developing the sores altogether. Lemon balm ointment may be available in health-food shops; if not, you can buy it online. Use it as often as needed.
- Dab the sore with a tincture of **myrrh** on a cotton bud up to 10 times a day. Myrrh directly attacks the virus that causes herpes. You'll find myrrh in health-food shops.
- Blend **tea tree oil** with an equal amount of **olive oil** and apply it to the sore two or three times a day. Tea tree oil is a

powerful natural antiseptic. Research conducted in the 1920s showed it had up to 13 times the antiseptic power of carbolic acid, which was then a common germicide.

- Eat **yoghurt** that contains live acidophilus bacteria. Some studies have shown that the acidophilus bacteria found in some brands of yoghurt actually hinder the growth of the virus.

- Buy an over-the-counter antiviral cream – **aciclovir** (Zovirax) or **penciclovir** (Fenistil) are both very effective – and keep it in the medicine cupboard. **As soon as you feel the telltale tingle** of an oncoming cold sore, you should start using the cream. Apply the cream five times a day for five days. At best, the medication can stop the eruption; in any case it will shorten the duration of the blister and lessen the pain.

Bolster your defences

- During an outbreak, take one 300mg capsule of **echinacea** four times a day. Studies have shown that the herb can boost your immune system's ability to fight off the virus.

- Take 1000mg of the immune-boosting flavonoid (plant pigment) **quercetin** each day in divided doses. Research published in the US *Journal of Medical Virology* has shown that this supplement can speed up the healing of cold sore blisters. It is available in pharmacies or health-food shops.

Don't crack up

- After the sore has crusted over, coat it with some **petroleum jelly** to prevent it from cracking and bleeding. When you do this, however, make sure you don't transmit the virus to the stuff in the jar. Instead of using your finger, apply the petroleum jelly with a cotton bud. Use a clean bud every time.

The power of prevention

- If you get more than three cold sores a year, you might benefit from taking a daily **lysine** supplement as a preventative. The recommended dose is 500mg a day.

- **Stay away from** foods rich in **arginine**, an essential amino acid that the herpes virus needs in order to thrive. If you want to take maximum precautions to avoid an outbreak, **avoid chocolate, cola, beer, peas, nuts** (peanuts, cashews, almonds and walnuts), **gelatin** and **whole grain cereals.**

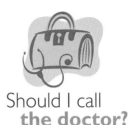

Should I call the doctor?

Yes, if this is your first outbreak, if your sores last longer than two weeks or if you get four or more cold sores a year. You may need the prescription-only form of aciclovir (Zovirax), an oral antiviral drug. Your doctor will also want to see you if your sore is accompanied by fever, swollen glands or flu-like symptoms, or if it is so painful that you avoid eating or brushing your teeth. Finally, if you develop eye pain or become sensitive to light, it may mean the virus has spread to your eyes. Get to a doctor quickly: your vision may be in jeopardy.

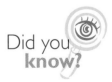

Did you know?

Nearly all of us carry the cold sore virus even when it's not causing symptoms. An estimated 80 per cent of adults in the UK are carriers of herpes simplex type 1, which causes most cold sores.

Give cold sores the brush-off

As the virus that causes herpes is carried in saliva, some extra dental hygiene precautions may be vital to avoid reinfecting yourself after an outbreak.

• Keep your toothbrush in a dry place, preferably on an open shelf where it's exposed to circulating air and sunlight.

If that means keeping it outside the bathroom, so be it. A damp toothbrush in a moist bathroom is an invitation for viral breeding.

• Buy a small tube of toothpaste, use it during the outbreak, then throw it away.

• Replace your toothbrush after an outbreak.

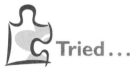

Tried...

When nothing else was available, people used a dab of vinegar to fend off a cold sore.

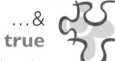

...& true

Vinegar is acidic and viruses don't do well in an acidic environment. Use a cotton wool ball dipped in any kind of vinegar and apply to the affected area, repeating several times a day at the first suggestion of the telltale tingle. Throw the cotton wool balls away after use.

• Take 15mg of **zinc** each day. In test-tube studies, this nutrient has been shown to block the replication of the virus. Zinc also boosts the immune system and fortifies the surface tissue on your lips and on the inside of your mouth, making it difficult for the virus to take hold.

• Try to **avoid whatever seems to trigger outbreaks**. Do cold sores appear after you've spent time in the sun or during periods of stress? Once you have identified potential triggers, you can begin to avoid situations likely to cause a sore.

• Use a **lip balm** that contains a sun protection factor (SPF) of at least 15. In one study of people with recurrent sores, those who didn't shield their lips were much more likely to develop blisters during extended exposure to sunlight.

• Like laughter and yawns, cold sores are contagious. **Don't kiss your partner** if either of you has a cold sore. Direct contact with the saliva of an infected person is usually necessary to pass the virus on, but if anyone in your house has cold sores, **don't mix up flannels**, towels, drinking glasses or toothbrushes.

• When you have a cold sore, **avoid touching your eyes**. Transmitting the virus to your eyes can cause a nasty infection that could damage your eyesight.

Conjunctivitis

Conjunctivitis, or pink-eye, can itch. It can hurt. It can make you feel as though you've had sand thrown in your eyes. It looks pretty awful, too. It can also injure your eyes and, if caused by bacteria or a virus, can spread like the plague. So what are you supposed to do? Start by seeking the help of your doctor. If you have a bacterial infection, you may be given antibiotic eye drops that will speed up healing and shorten contagion time. Meanwhile, you can take steps to ease the itch and control the crusting.

Get an eyeful of relief

• **Hot or cold compresses** can help. If you have considerable discharge from your eyes, run a flannel under warm water and use it as a compress to prevent the sticky secretions from drying on the lashes. Use a cold compress (soak a flannel in iced water) to shrink swelling and reduce itchiness, especially if your conjunctivitis is caused by allergies. Do either one – or both – for 5 minutes three or four times a day. Use a clean flannel each time.

• Wipe away the secretions and crusty material with a cotton wool ball soaked in 1 part **baby shampoo** to 10 parts warm water. The warm water loosens the crust, and the shampoo cleans the area where your eyelid and eyelashes meet.

• Use an eyewash made of lightly **salted water.** Bring a pint of water to a boil, add a teaspoon of salt and let it simmer for at least 15 minutes. Let the solution cool down. Use a sterile eye-dropper or eye-bath to apply the wash. After each treatment, sterilize the eye-dropper or eye-bath again in boiling water.

• A **goldenseal** eyewash will help fight infection. Goldenseal contains a compound called berberine that has antibacterial properties. To make the wash, steep 1 teaspoon of dried goldenseal in boiling water for 10 minutes, strain and let it cool. Apply with a sterile eye-dropper three times a day.

Prepare your eyes for bed

• If your doctor has prescribed antibiotic or steroid **eye drops** or ointments, use them each night before you go to bed to ensure that your eyelids don't get glued shut while you sleep.

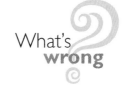

What's wrong

When eyes are red, irritated and glued shut with a gummy secretion, you've probably got conjunctivitis. It's an inflammation of the conjunctiva, the transparent membrane that lines the inner eyelids and sheathes the globe of the eye. Commonly known as pink-eye, conjunctivitis is usually caused by a bacterial or viral infection or an allergic reaction to pollen, cosmetics, contact lens cleaning solution or other substances. Depending on the type, conjunctivitis can cause your eyes to burn, itch, run profusely and become intensely sensitive to light. A sticky discharge glues your eyelashes and eyelids together while you sleep.

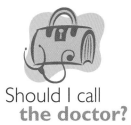

Should I call the doctor?

Call your doctor if your symptoms are severe. While mild cases of pinkeye, especially those caused by viruses, should go away on their own within a week, some forms of the condition can lead to potentially serious eye damage. You will want to get your doctor's advice as soon as possible if your vision is blurred, if spots or blisters develop near the eye, if conjunctivitis doesn't go away on its own in a week or if you don't see any improvement after three to four days of steady treatment. If you have bacterial conjunctivitis, quick treatment will prevent complications.

Make sure the tip of the eyedrop bottle or tube does not touch your eyes. Otherwise, you might contaminate the medicine and potentially re-infect your eyes the next time you use it.

Soothers for sore eyes

• Soothe your eyes with a **camomile** compress. Place a camomile tea bag in warm (not hot) water for 2 or 3 minutes, squeeze out the excess liquid, then place the teabag over your sore eye or eyes for ten minutes. Repeat three or four times a day with a fresh teabag. Keep your eyes closed so the wash doesn't come into direct contact with your eye.

• Practitioners of Ayurveda, the traditional medicine of India, treat conjunctivitis with a pulp of fresh **coriander** leaves. Whizz a handful of coriander leaves with 100ml water in a blender. Strain off the juice and apply the pulp to your closed eyelids. Leave it on for a few minutes, then wipe away the mixture before you open your eyes.

• Another Ayurvedic treatment for conjunctivitis is to steep 1 teaspoon of **coriander** seeds in 1 cup of boiling water for at least 15 minutes. Strain, cool and use the water to bathe your closed eyes. Wipe away any excess before you open your eyes.

Contain the contagion

• To avoid re-infection, **don't wear eye make-up** or **contact lenses** until the infection is completely gone. Discard any eye make-up you were using when the infection developed.

• **Try not to touch your eyes.** If you happen to touch them accidentally, wash your hands with soap and water, then dry with a paper towel or hot-air dryer instead of a hand towel.

Three types of pink-eye

The three main types of conjunctivitis are viral, bacterial and allergic. There is some overlap of symptoms, but a doctor can distinguish one from the other:

VIRAL
• Infection usually begins with one eye, but may spread to the other
• Watery discharge
• Irritation/redness

BACTERIAL
• Usually affects only one eye, but may spread to the other
• Irritation, redness and/or a gritty feeling
• Copious discharge

ALLERGIC
• Usually affects both eyes
• Itching and watering
• Swollen eyelids

- If you have to dab your eyes, use a **separate tissue** for each eye. Immediately throw both tissues in a plastic bag and wash your hands. When it's time to throw out the plastic bag, do it yourself and wash your hands thoroughly afterwards.

- Carry a small bottle of **antibacterial hand gel** with you and use it often.

- If you wear **contact lenses**, do not wear them at all while you've actually got conjunctivitis, then sterilize them properly before wearing them again when it's cleared up. Always wash your hands before you put in or take out your lenses. And never, ever clean a contact lens with saliva.

- Put your towel, flannel and pillowcase **into the washing machine** every day to help to prevent you from re-introducing the bacteria or virus to the same eye or spreading it to the other eye. (And other people can pick up conjunctivitis by using the same flannel or towels that you've used.)

- **Let someone else make the beds**. Conjunctivitis can be spread from your hands to the sheets.

- If you have young children with conjunctivitis who are too young to follow the rules about not touching their eyes and washing their hands, they should **stay at home from school or nursery**. Most daycare nurseries and pre-schools will not admit a child with symptoms of conjunctivitis.

If you have allergic conjunctivitis…

If your eye itches and produces a stringy discharge, your conjunctivitis may be the result of an allergy. Try taking an **oral antihistamine** to relieve the itching and swelling.

- Avoid **whatever's causing it** if possible – whether pollen, animals or cosmetics. It may be a new pet, new type of eye make-up or a different shampoo.

- To help combat inflammation caused by allergies, try a combination of **vitamin C** and **quercetin.** Take 1000mg a day vitamin C in divided doses, together with 1500mg quercetin. Quercetin is one of a class of nutrients called bioflavonoids – derived from a range of fruits and vegetables – that have anti-inflammatory properties.

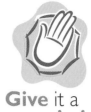

Give it a miss!

Some herbal healers recommend eyebright (euphrasia) to treat conjunctivitis, based on its traditional use among Native American Indians for relieving eye problems. However, recent studies have shown that eyebright can actually cause watering, itching and redness if it comes in contact with the eye. Its therapeutic value has never been proved.

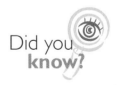

Did you know?

Tears themselves contain antibacterial substances, which is why most eye infections eventually clear up unassisted.

Constipation

Your first instinct when you're in this predicament might be to reach for a laxative. But the chances are you don't need one. The best way to become regular again is simply to eat more fibre – 20g to 35g a day. Fibre absorbs water and makes stools softer and bulkier, which speeds the products of digestion through your system. To cope with all that fibre the body needs more fluids too. And don't forget about exercise, which can also help to keep things moving. Do all three things and everything will begin to work smoothly once more.

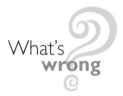

What's wrong

You hear nature's call, and you want to answer, desperately. But your body won't respond – or when it does, your stools are hard, dry and difficult or painful to pass. The most common reason bowels go on strike is because the body is lacking in dietary fibre or water. Another common cause is ignoring the 'call to stool' – or being too busy to go, especially if you're rushing out of the house in the morning – better to get up 10 minutes earlier. Constipation may also be due to lack of exercise, using laxatives too often, and health conditions such as hypothyroidism, diabetes, depression or irritable bowel syndrome. Certain prescription or over-the-counter medications may be to blame as well.

Fix it with fibre

- Start your day with a high-fibre bran cereal. Some brands contain as much as 15g of insoluble fibre per serving. This is the fibre that adds bulk, spurring the body to move it through the digestive tract more quickly. A word of advice: if you are not used to eating this much fibre, start with a smaller serving – say, half-and-half bran and cornflakes, served with skimmed milk or low-fat yoghurt – then work your way up. Otherwise you may experience wind, bloating and stomach cramps.
- Fill up on cooked **dried beans**, **prunes**, **pears**, **figs**, **oats** and **nuts**. All are good sources of soluble fibre, the kind that turns to gel in the intestines and helps to soften the stool.
- Mix 1 to 2 teaspoons crushed **psyllium** seeds (also known as ispaghula) into a cup of hot water. Let it infuse for 2 hours, add lemon and honey to taste, then drink. Psyllium adds bulk and is the main ingredient in many over-the-counter bulk forming laxatives. You'll find the seeds in most pharmacies and health-food shops. You can also try this with flax seeds (linseed).
- **Flax seeds** are high in fibre and also contain omega-3 fats, known to be beneficial to the heart and circulatory system. Have a tablespoon of the ground seeds, which are sold in health-food shops, two or three times a day. Some people like the taste of flax seed (it faintly resembles walnuts). If you don't, you can stir it into your breakfast cereal, add it to stewed apple or blend it into a fruit smoothie. Or grind the seeds in a spice mill or coffee grinder, keep the ground seeds in the fridge and sprinkle half a teaspoon into your orange juice.

• As you increase your intake of fibre, also be sure to drink **lots of water** – at least eight 250ml glasses a day. Fibre is extremely absorbent, and if you don't drink enough, your stools may become small, hard and painful to pass.

Have a hot cup to loosen up

• Have a morning cup of coffee. If you're a coffee drinker, you may have already discovered that the **caffeine** in coffee has a bowel-loosening effect. It induces a bowel movement by stimulating the colon. Just don't drink too much of it – caffeine is also diuretic and will eliminate fluid from your body.

• If you don't like coffee, try any other **hot drink** first thing in the morning. Herbal or decaffeinated tea or a cup of hot water with a little lemon juice or honey may stimulate the colon as well. (Lemon juice is a natural laxative.)

• **Dandelion tea**, which has a mild laxative effect, may also help bowel movements to become regular again. Steep a teaspoon of dried root in a cup of boiling water and drink 1 cup three times a day. You'll find dried dandelion root in health-food shops.

Wrinkled fruit gets things moving

• The humble **prune** is one of the oldest home remedies for constipation. It's high in fibre (roughly 1g per prune). Also, prunes contain a compound called dihydroxyphenyl isatin, which stimulates the intestinal contractions that make you want to go.

• If you don't like prunes then try chewing **raisins**. They, too, are high in fibre and contain tartaric acid, which has a laxative effect. In one study in which people ate a small box of raisins a day, doctors found that it took half the time for digested food to make it through the digestive tract.

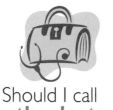

Should I call the doctor?

Although bothersome, constipation is usually not grave. However, it can sometimes signal a serious condition such as colorectal cancer or bowel obstruction. Tell your doctor if it lasts two weeks or more, or if you see blood in your stool, or if constipation is accompanied by fever, severe abdominal pain, or weight loss, or if constipation alternates with diarrhoea. If you've recently started a new medication that seems to be causing constipation, you need to talk to your doctor. Antihistamines, diuretics, blood-pressure drugs, some tranquillizers, codeine or morphine-based painkillers, calcium supplements, certain antidepressants and antacids that contain calcium or aluminium can all cause constipation.

Constipation – reality or illusion?

The advertising world would have us believe that daily elimination is the pinnacle of perfect health. Untrue, say doctors. Many of us have what doctors call 'perceived constipation' – that is, we think we are constipated, but our bodies don't. People have varying body rhythms, and it is just as healthy (for some people) to go once every three days as it is (for others) to go three times a day.

Fibre providers

If you're wondering how to increase the fibre in your diet for an improved digestive system, here are some foods that contain soluble and insoluble fibre.

Food	Portion size	Grams of fibre	Food	Portion size	Grams of fibre
Bran cereal (All Bran)	1 bowl	15	Muesli	1 bowl (90g)	8
Bran Flakes	1 bowl	8	Shredded Wheat	2	4.5
Wholemeal bread	2 slices	5	Hummus	60g	2
Raspberries	15	6	Peanuts	25g	2
Lentils, boiled	150g	3	Prunes, dried	8	4
Blackberries	15	5	Apricots, dried	8	10
Baked beans	200g can	13	Dates	9	2
Figs, dried	2	5	Apple	1	2
Wholemeal spaghetti, boiled	150g	6	Pear (with skin)	1	4
Red kidney beans, canned	100g	7	Banana	1	1.5
			Porridge	1 bowl	2
			Brussels sprouts	10	3

Get up and go

● Get regular **exercise**. There's good reason for a morning walk being known as a daily constitutional: when you move your body, you also help to move food through your bowel more quickly. Aim for a daily walk at the very least.

Put the pressure on

● Practitioners of **acupressure** say that the technique can help to stimulate your digestion and, therefore, your bowels. Apply pressure with your thumb and forefinger to the fleshy web between the thumb and forefinger of the other hand. Do this for two minutes every day while the problem persists. (*Alert* This technique should not be used in pregnancy.)

Last resorts

● The herb *cascara sagrada* is so effective that it is even added to several over-the-counter laxatives. It's known as a 'stimulant laxative' because it stimulates the intestinal tract. The herb comes in a variety of forms and, because it is so powerful, and because it also interacts with numerous medicines, it should be used only under medical supervision. In any case, don't take it for more than eight to ten days; it can make your body lose too much water, potassium and salt – and with regular use, you can become dependent on it. (*Alert* Do not use if you have any other abdominal condition. Drink plenty of water while taking it. Cascara must not be used by pregnant women or children.)

● If other remedies fail, try the mother of all natural laxatives, **senna.** It should work in about 8 hours, so most people take it before bedtime. Take 20 to 40 drops of the tincture at night, but don't plan on making it a long-term cure. With repeated use, senna can cause stomach cramps and diarrhoea. As with *cascara sagrada*, long-term use can cause dependency.

● For a gentler alternative, use a glycerol suppository, available over-the-counter from pharmacies. Again, don't rely on this method or your constipation could end up worse than it was in the first place.

Final pointers

● **Never ignore nature's call.** If you do, you're asking for a case of constipation.

● **Never** try to **force a bowel movement.** You may give yourself haemorrhoids (piles) or anal fissures. These not only hurt, they aggravate constipation because they narrow the anal opening. Also, straining on the toilet can strain your heart: it reduces your heart rate and pushes up blood pressure and can sometimes even cause a sudden heart attack.

Coughs

Coughing not only annoys you but also irritates anyone nearby – whether a loved one, someone in the row in front at the cinema, or the entire auditorium during a quiet solo at a classical concert. But if you have a productive cough, you don't want to suppress it; it's the body's way of clearing out mucus. You actually want to encourage it so you can get rid of the phlegm quickly and get the coughing over with. If you have a dry cough, on the other hand, the trick is to coat the throat and tame the tickle.

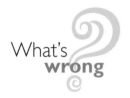

Suck something soothing

- Suck any cough drops or boiled sweets. The hard sweet increases saliva production and causes you to swallow more, suppressing coughs.
- For 'productive' coughs, try **white horehound**. A bittersweet herb, it acts as an expectorant, triggering the coughing reflex and helping to bring up phlegm. Potters produce a horehound and aniseed cough mixture, available in pharmacies.
- For 'dry' coughs, try and get hold of **slippery elm lozenges** (sold online and in some health-food shops). Made from the bark of the slippery elm tree, these were once medicine-chest staples. Slippery elm is loaded with a gel-like substance that coats the throat and keeps coughing to a minimum.

Dose a cough with homemade syrups

- Blend 2 tablespoons **lemon juice** with 1 tablespoon **honey** and add a pinch of **cayenne pepper**. The honey coats your throat, soothing irritated tissues, while the lemon reduces inflammation and delivers a dose of infection-fighting vitamin C. The cayenne boosts circulation in the area, hastening the healing process. Or, instead of cayenne, add a little freshly **grated onion**. Onions contain irritating compounds that trigger the cough reflex and bring up phlegm.
- Another **onion remedy** is to peel and chop 6 medium onions and put them with 4 tablespoons of **honey** into a bowl set over a pan of boiling water (or a double boiler). Cover and simmer for 2 hours. Strain the mixture and take 1 tablespoon every 2 or 3 hours.

- At bedtime, mix a little **blackcurrant cordial** (choose a 'high-juice' version) with a tot of port – the alcohol is purely therapeutic to help you sleep.
- For a throat-soothing syrup, mix 5 or 6 **cloves** with a cup of **honey** and leave in the refrigerator overnight. In the morning, remove the cloves and take a teaspoon as needed. Cloves dull the pain and honey soothes inflammation.
- Earlier generations swore by **rock candy** (sweets similar to seaside rock). One recipe combined '1 box rock candy, 1lb [450g] raisins, the juice of 3 lemons, ½ cup of sugar and enough whisky to form a syrup'. However, it takes a few weeks for the rock candy to dissolve.
- More readily available helpful products include **lobelia** cough syrup (from Napiers herbalists, by mail order or from www.napiers.net); **Galloway's** cough syrup, which contains ipecacuanha, squill vinegar, peppermint oil and chloroform, and **glycerin and blackcurrant** linctus (both from chemists).
- **Raspberry vinegar** can be taken by the spoonful, alone or with juice if you wish to disguise the taste. The vinegar is also useful as a gargle if the cough is accompanied by a sore throat.
- An old-fashioned 'cure' is **rosehip syrup** – it sweetly coats the throat and is loaded with vitamin C.
- **Camomile** is a comforting herb: it aids sleep when taken as a tea and helps a cough with catarrh when used as an inhalation. Or leave a few drops of camomile tincture in a bowl on a radiator in the bedroom overnight.

Brew a cough-calming tea

- **Thyme** is an expectorant and also contains substances that relax the respiratory tract. To make thyme tea, place 2 tablespoons of fresh thyme (or 1 tablespoon dried) in a cup of hot

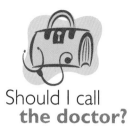

Should I call the doctor?

Most coughs clear up on their own within a week to 10 days. But if yours lasts more than 4 weeks, or you cough up green or bloody phlegm, see your doctor. Coughing can be a symptom of a more serious illness, such as chronic obstructive airways disease or asthma. It can even indicate heart failure, especially if it's accompanied by wheezing, shortness of breath or swelling of the ankles. If you have sharp chest pains, chills, or a fever higher than 38°C (101°F) for more than three days as well as a cough, you may have pneumonia. See a doctor sooner if the cough affects a baby or a weak elderly person.

Steam away croup

A child with croup has a barking cough that often worsens at night. Caused by a viral or bacterial infection, croup is not usually dangerous but it can be extremely frightening to parents. To treat it, take your child into the bathroom and run a hot, steamy shower or fill a bath with hot water so that the air is humid. Keep the child in the steam until the croup subsides. If it doesn't improve – or if the child is struggling to breathe – call a doctor, dial 999 or take your child to your nearest A&E department.

Could heartburn be the problem?

If your cough troubles you mainly after meals, at night or while lying down, your problem might not be in your chest but in your digestive system. Heartburn results when stomach acids back up into your lower oesophagus, irritating the delicate tissue – which can lead to coughing. If you can control any symptoms of heartburn (see page 205), you may find that you take care of the cough as well.

water. Allow it to infuse for 5 minutes, then strain out the herb, add honey if you wish and drink.

● Aromatic **hyssop** has been used in liqueurs and medicines since Biblical times. An infusion of hyssop's dried flowers can be taken three times a day for coughs, asthma and bronchitis.

● Sip a cup of **marshmallow tea**. When combined with water, marshmallow leaf yields a gooey mucilage that coats the throat and also thins mucus in the lungs, making it easier to cough up. To make the tea, steep 2–3g of the dried leaf in a cup of hot water for 10 minutes and strain before drinking. Drink a total of 3 cups a day.

● Add 45 drops of **liquorice** tincture to a cup of hot water and sip. Take three times a day. Liquorice loosens phlegm and relaxes bronchial spasms. (*Alert* Don't take liquorice for more than a few weeks, as it can raise blood pressure.)

● Practitioners of Ayurveda, the traditional medicine of India, recommend a **spice tea** that you can drink several times a day. To make the tea, add ½ teaspoon of powdered **ginger** and a pinch each of **clove** and **cinnamon** powder to a cupful of boiling water, stir and drink.

Rub on relief

● Buy a **chest rub** that contains **camphor** or **menthol** and apply it to your throat and chest. It can help you to breathe more easily by relieving congestion. Vicks VapoRub is very comforting at bedtime. Or prepare an infusion of **eucalyptus** leaves and essential oil and inhale the steam through your mouth and nose as often as you like. The essential oil can be rubbed into the throat and chest twice a day.

● If you don't have anything to use as a chest rub, try making a **mustard poultice** to loosen up chest congestion. Mix 1 part mustard powder and 2 parts flour in a bowl. Add just enough water to make a paste. Spread the paste on a tea towel and fold the towel in half. Protect your skin with a layer of petroleum jelly, then press the poultice in place. (Never put a mustard mixture directly onto your skin as it can burn.) Check your skin often and remove the poultice if your skin becomes too red or irritated. Some people recommend using egg white instead of water to make a plaster that's less likely to burn.

Learn a new coughing technique

- If your throat is strained and irritated from nonstop coughing, try this technique to head off a coughing fit. The next time you feel a cough coming on, **force yourself to take a series of small, gentle coughs**, finally ending with a large one. The tiny coughs help move mucus toward the upper part of your air passage so you can expel more of it with that last, big cough.

Put some rhythm in your remedy

- If you're at home and you have a partner who can help, use a chest percussion technique to help clear chest congestion. Lie on your stomach on a firm bed or mat. Ask your partner to **slap cupped hands rhythmically** over your back, progressing from the lower back up towards your neck. Repeat several times until your congestion starts to loosen up.

Lights out, vapour on

- To help prevent nocturnal coughing, use a **humidifier** in your bedroom to moisten the air, particularly in winter.

Choosing a cough syrup

When you go to the chemist to buy a cough mixture, which one do you choose? Your pharmacist is qualified to give the best advice, so ask. If you are bringing up phlegm, buy an expectorant cough syrup – such as Robitussin Chesty Cough – that contains guaifenesin and take it during the day. It will loosen the mucus and make it easier to expel. Take a cough suppressant only if you have a dry cough. Look on the label for codeine (such as in pholcodine) or dextromethorphan (such as Benylin Dry Cough). As an alternative to these cough medicines, try Nelson's Sootha (Bryonia) Cough Syrup, a homeopathic cough preparation.

Cuts and grazes

If you can stop the bleeding and keep the wound clean to prevent infection, you've done your part; nature will take over from there. What you will need are cotton wool and water for cleaning, surgical spirit or an antiseptic spray or liquid, bandages, sticky plasters and antiseptic cream. Other wound remedies that work when you've nothing else to hand are within easy reach – from honey to garlic to your own saliva.

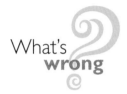

What's wrong

You have just sliced yourself with a sharp object – a kitchen knife, your razor, a broken drinking glass, even a piece of paper. Or you've had a sudden encounter with a tarmac pavement and lost a bit of skin on your elbow or knee. There may be visible bleeding – and perhaps an invisible invasion of bacteria into the wound, bringing a risk of infection.

Clean, disinfect and cover

● To stanch bleeding, apply **pressure** to the wound with a clean cloth or piece of gauze. At a pinch, use your hand.

● Once bleeding has stopped, gently clean the area around the wound with soap and water. Then apply a bandage.

● You can also cleanse a cut with a tincture of **calendula**, a bacteria-killing herb known for its wound-healing powers. Look for calendula succus, which is a low-alcohol formula. If you can't find this, use the standard tincture and dilute it with a little water. To heal grazes even faster, try applying calendula cream, sold in health-food shops and pharmacies.

● Twice a day, you can clean your cut with **myrrh**, which stimulates the production of white blood cells. These are the infection-fighting cells that gather at the wound site. Mix a teaspoon of myrrh tincture (available at health-food shops) with 100ml water. Pour a little over the cut or graze and leave the wound exposed to the air until it dries.

● Try **tea tree oil**. It contains a strong antiseptic compound and is popular all over the world for treating wounds. Stir 1½ teaspoons of the oil into a cup of warm water and use this to rinse cuts and grazes twice a day.

Cures from your kitchen

● If you have no access to antiseptic cream, then dab on a little **honey** and cover the wound with a clean cloth or bandage. Honey has antibacterial properties, and studies have shown that it can speed up wound healing. If you don't have any sticky plasters or bandages immediately to hand, don't worry – honey dries to form a natural covering.

- **Garlic** is another of nature's antibiotics. Try taping a crushed clove over the cut. If it irritates your skin, take it off right away.

Grazed knee? Keep the scab soft

- Children seem to manage to graze their knees almost every day. One helpful solution is **Vaseline or any other petroleum jelly.** It protects grazed skin and keeps scabs soft so that they're less tempting to pick. Vaseline or any other **petroleum jelly,** will also do the trick.

A lesson from your canine companion

- If you can't wash a wound – you're on a walk in the middle of nowhere, for example – then **lick it.** A report in *The Lancet* described the beneficial effects of licking a wound – but it must be your own spit. Anyone else's would be highly likely to cause infection.

Glue it together

- The warning label on **Super Glue** tells you that it 'bonds skin instantly'. But if you've got a very small slice in your finger (like a paper cut), maybe an instant skin glue is just what you want. Super Glue is effectively the same as Histoacryl, a tissue glue, used in medicine to seal wounds. This is available without prescription, as is a similar product called LiquiBand. However, you need to press the edges of the cut together properly so this may not work for very deep or ragged wounds, or for wounds over a joint that gets moved a lot. If used improperly, the glue may simply create a 'wedge' in the wound that prevents the skin edges from joining, potentially leaving a bigger scar. Make sure you don't touch the glue while it's drying, or you'll end up sticking bits of you together that you don't want stuck.

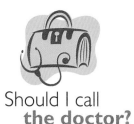

Should I call the doctor?

Call the doctor if your wound won't close or stop bleeding, or if you have any signs of infection (pus, unusual discharge, fever, red streaks that spread outwards from the wound). If you have a deep puncture wound – especially if it is contaminated with farm manure – your doctor may advise you to have a tetanus booster.

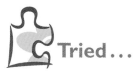

Tried...

Some people claim that shaking black pepper on a cut will stop the bleeding in a trice.

...& true

It may or may not stop the bleeding any faster, but black pepper does have painkilling, antiseptic and antibiotic properties.

Dandruff

D o your shoulders look as if you've been in a snowstorm? Are you blinded by a blizzard every time you comb your hair? Dandruff isn't a serious health problem, but it can certainly be embarrassing. To control those flakes, use the right shampoo. You can also whip up a homemade scalp rinse that will tackle the yeast behind many cases of dandruff and help to stop the dreaded itching.

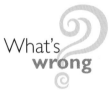

What's wrong

People continually shed outer layers of dead skin. When those skin cells flake off the scalp at turbo speed, you have a case of dandruff. The condition has many possible causes. Stress is one. Others include overactive oil glands and seborrhoeic dermatitis – an itchy, scaly rash that can affect the face and chest as well as the scalp. There's evidence to suggest that dandruff is often caused by an overgrowth of a common yeast, called *Pityrosporum orbiculare*. The yeast feeds on skin oils – which may explain why people who have oily scalps are more susceptible to dandruff.

Wash dandruff away

● Look for shampoos that contain **selenium sulphide, zinc pyrithione** or **tar.** The first two ingredients slow down the rate at which the cells on your scalp multiply. They are used in shampoos such as Head and Shoulders. Tar based formulas, such as Polytar and T Gel retard cell growth. These shampoos are all more effective than products that are formulated with sulphur or salicylic acid, which simply loosen flakes so they can be washed away.

● If your dandruff doesn't respond to a shampoo like Head and Shoulders, try one that contains **ketoconazole**, such as Nizoral. Ketoconazole is an antifungal medication that will kill the yeast that may be causing your dandruff.

● If your dandruff shampoo stops working after a few months, your scalp has probably got used to the active ingredient and started to ignore it. Just switch to a shampoo made with a **different active ingredient.** You may need to switch back in another few months.

● Leave dandruff shampoo on your scalp for **at least 10 minutes** before you rinse to let it do its work. For a serious case of dandruff, it is worth taking a bit more time. Lather up, put a shower cap on your head and leave the shampoo on for an hour.

Rely on rinses

● Make a dandruff rinse using the herb **goldenseal**. It contains berberine, which has strong antibacterial and antifungal properties. Pour a cup of boiling water over 2 teaspoons of chopped root. Steep, strain and let it cool. Use this as a rinse after you've shampooed, or any time during the day. If you can't find goldenseal root, add a few drops of goldenseal tincture to a little shampoo.

- Brew up a fragrant **rosemary** rinse. Like goldenseal, rosemary fights bacteria and fungi. And rosemary is a lot easier to find. To make the rinse, pour 1 cup of boiling water over 1 teaspoon of chopped rosemary. Let it sit for a few minutes, then strain. Use the infusion as a rinse once a day. If you find that the rinse irritates your skin, try a different remedy.

- Another herbal anti-dandruff rinse is made with **bay leaves**. Add a handful of crushed bay leaves to a litre of very hot (just boiled) water. Cover and let steep for 20 minutes. Strain, allow to cool and apply. You can leave it in your hair for an hour or so before rinsing.

- **Cider vinegar**, which kills a variety of fungi and bacteria, is frequently recommended as a home remedy for dandruff. Mix 1 part water with 1 part apple cider vinegar. Apply as a rinse after you shampoo.

Try tea tree

- **Tea tree oil** has strong antifungal properties. Dilute 7 drops of tea tree oil in 1 tablespoon of carrier oil (such as olive or grapeseed oil) and apply to your scalp. Leave it overnight. Or add a few drops to your normal shampoo. Several shampoos are now available with tea tree oil already in them.

A cultured cure

- It's not pretty, but it may work: Spread **live yoghurt** on your scalp and leave it there for half an hour, then rinse. Yoghurt contains 'friendly' bacteria that keep yeast in check. That's why it's also a traditional remedy for yeast infections.

Take some helpful fatty acids

- Take 1 or 2 teaspoons of **flax seed oil** (linseed) a day. It contains essential fatty acids, which seem to help itchy skin conditions such as psoriasis and eczema – and perhaps dandruff. Be patient; you may need to take the oil for up to three months before you notice a difference. One additional benefit is that flax seed oil helps to guard against heart disease.

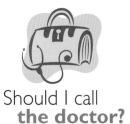

Should I call the doctor?

Normally, a mild case of dandruff will respond to self-treatment, so give home remedies or over-the-counter dandruff shampoos about two weeks to work. Consult your doctor if there's no improvement or if you have severe itching along with a red, irritated scalp. You also need a doctor's advice if you notice thick scaling, yellowish crusting or red patches along your neckline. These symptoms suggest seborrhoeic dermatitis, a condition that requires medical advice and treatment.

Depression

What did Ludwig van Beethoven, Winston Churchill and Vincent van Gogh have in common? They all, at one time or another, suffered from depression. In fact, depression is so widespread that some psychologists call it the common cold of emotional disorders. If you're depressed, you're not alone. Neither do you have to let depression control your life. For severe, chronic depression, there are effective prescription medications as well as various forms of therapy. For mild to moderate depression that comes and goes, there are plenty of strategies for combating depression that you can try out on your own.

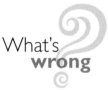

What's wrong

Maybe you've experienced a traumatic event. Or maybe, for no reason you can put your finger on, you just feel sad and empty. Depression is usually linked to a combination of medical, genetic and environmental factors. There are four types: major depression, in which the emotional low is severe and lasts for more than two weeks; mild depression, or dysthymia, which has milder or fewer symptoms; bipolar disorder, which causes extreme mood swings (manic depression); and post-natal depression, which sometimes affects a mother after giving birth.

Work it out

● Get out and move your body. Numerous studies have confirmed that **frequent exercise** can be a powerful mood enhancer. For mild or moderate depression it may even work as well as antidepressants. All you need is at least 20 minutes' worth of aerobic exercise three times a week. Walk, lift weights, jump a skipping rope, cycle – any form will do. Work up a sweat to get the best effect.

Look to food to change your mood

● If you're on a high-protein diet to lose weight, **lack of carbohydrates** could be contributing to your miserable mood. Foods like fruits, vegetables, beans and whole grains help your brain to make the mood-regulating brain chemical serotonin.
● Aim to **eat fish** three times a week or more. Researchers in Finland found that people who ate fish less than once a week had a 31 per cent higher incidence of mild to moderate depression than people who ate fish more often. Fresh tuna, salmon, sardines and mackerel are top choices; they're rich in omega-3 fatty acids, essential to normal brain function. There's early evidence that they also influence serotonin production.
● If you drink **coffee** or **cola**, cut back or even **give it up**. Caffeine suppresses serotonin production and has been linked to depression.
● **Avoid alcohol.** While wine, beer or spirits may initially lift your mood, alcohol is actually a depressant.

Put it in writing

• **Record your feelings** on paper – especially painful feelings. Research shows that people who write about their most painful emotions for 20 minutes a day dramatically improved their psychological well-being after just four days. Sit with a blank piece of paper in front of you and write nonstop about the most distressing event happening in your life at the moment. Don't think; just write.

Lift your spirit

• **Go to church** or any other place of worship. In a study of 4,000 older people, researchers found that those who frequently attended religious services were half as likely to be depressed as those who didn't.

Try taking 'sammy'

• Take **SAM-e**, pronounced 'sammy'. In many European countries, the effectiveness of SAM-e against depression is so widely accepted that the supplement is often prescribed by doctors. SAM-e is a naturally occurring substance found in every living cell, and low levels have been linked with depression. Dozens of studies have shown that taking SAM-e produces significant improvement after just three weeks. In animal studies, SAM-e was found to boost the levels of three neurotransmitters – serotonin, dopamine and noradrenaline – involved in mood changes. Look for enteric-coated capsules, which are easier to digest. The recommended dose for mild depression is 200mg twice a day. If you don't notice any improvement after two or three weeks this dose can be gradually increased up to a maximum of 400mg three times a day. (*Alert* Do not take SAM-e if you have manic depression – it can precipitate episodes of mania.)

• Three times a day, with meals, take 300mg of **St John's wort**. In folk medicine, it was originally believed to ward off witches. Now that witches are more or less a thing of the past, more than 20 scientific studies have shown that St John's wort can help to ease mild depression, possibly by allowing certain brain chemicals to build up between nerve cells, as some antidepressants do. Opt for a brand standardized to 0.3 per cent hypericin and give it at least four weeks to begin working before you

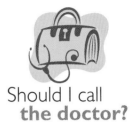

Should I call the doctor?

A divorce, a death, a move, or a career change can give you temporary feelings of sadness, as you experience a loss or confront new challenges. Almost everyone experiences a mild depression at some point in life. But if your sadness lasts more than two weeks, or is accompanied by sleep and appetite changes (eating and sleeping too much or not at all), loss of interest in sex and a reduced ability to concentrate, the chances are that you need treatment. Your doctor will be able to advise you whether you need psychotherapy, medication, or both.

make any judgment about its effectiveness. Because this herb can cause sensitivity to sunlight, try to stay out of the sun as much as possible while you're taking it. *Alert* Always tell your doctor if you're taking St John's wort and before taking any other medicine – it interacts with many other drugs.

• **5-HTP**, one form of the amino acid tryptophan, is thought to work in the same way as Prozac, by increasing serotonin levels. Start with 50mg of 5-HTP once a day and, if necessary, build up to a maximum of 100mg three times a day. It is best not to drive or do hazardous work until you determine how 5-HTP affects you as it can cause drowsiness. Consult your doctor first if taking any other medication as it interacts with many drugs and don't take this supplement for more than three months unless you have your doctor's approval. *Alert* Do not take 5-HTP if you're pregnant or planning a pregnancy

• Take 1000mg, three times a day, of **acetyl-L-carnitine** an amino acid that is chemically similar to acetylcholine – a neurotransmitter that acts in the muscles as well as the central nervous system. Acetyl-L-carnitine helps to increase energy production in brain cells, protect nerve cell membranes and improve both mood and memory.

Feel better about yourself and your life

Is your inner monologue depressing you? Here's how to turn your thinking around:

1 Take a factual approach. Challenge irrational beliefs that chip away at your confidence. If you think people are laughing at you, look for evidence. Could they be laughing at something else?

2 Don't be perfect. It isn't possible – but you knew that. So why worry if someone doesn't like you or if you're not in control and able to deal with every situation?

3 When something bad happens, don't automatically think the worst ('I failed the test because I'm stupid'). There are usually many reasons things go wrong. Look at them objectively and focus on what you can change ('I'll do better next time if I revise harder').

4 If self-examination does reveal a personal weakness, don't dwell on it. Try to keep the implications from spiralling ('I'm useless. I can't do anything well'). And remember: that recognizing that perhaps you're weak in one area doesn't make you a weak person. Instead, that knowledge can help you to identify where to invest more effort and guide you to your strengths.

5 Loosen your grip on the controls. Inevitably, things won't always go your way, nor can they be expected to. Accept that the world is not and cannot ever be under your control and strive to be calm in the face of adversity. That way, two problems – the upsetting situation and your reaction to it – are whittled down to just one.

- The mineral **magnesium** is very important for restoring and maintaining healthy nerve function. Magnesium is a key component in the production and function of serotonin. Supplements may help to alleviate anxiety and depression. Take 150mg of magnesium, preferably as magnesium citrate (the form most easily absorbed), twice a day. If you take magnesium supplements, be sure to take calcium supplements as well. Imbalances in the amounts of these two minerals in the body can reduce their beneficial effects.
- Take **1 vitamin B-complex** supplement each morning with breakfast. Low levels of B vitamins have been linked with depression and fatigue. Look for a brand with 50mcg of vitamin B_{12} and biotin, 400mcg of folic acid and 50mg of the other B vitamins (but note that the maximum recommended dose for B_6 *in the longterm* is 10mg a day).

The power of prevention

- **Get enough sleep**. Studies have shown that people who get less than 8 hours of sleep, night after night, tend to have lower serotonin levels than those who get full nights of rest. To help ensure a good night's sleep, try to go to bed at the same time every evening and rise at the same time every morning – even at weekends.
- **Turn the telly off**. Research suggests that the longer you watch television, the more your mood suffers. Watching hours of sitcom repeats, movie marathons or game shows may seem a good way to relieve stress and revel in entertainment. But studies have shown that, on the contrary, people who watch a lot of television tend to have intensified feelings of isolation.

Diarrhoea

When a case of the runs has you running to the loo, your aims are twofold: stave off dehydration and avoid anything that will make the diarrhoea worse. If you can stay close to home, simply let the problem 'run' its course (and don't forget to drink plenty of fluids). If you can't, try astringent teas, eat more soluble fibre (which soaks up excess fluids in the intestine) or try an ancient Chinese remedy.

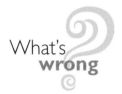

What's wrong

Normally, as food goes through your digestive tract, the large intestine soaks up extra water. Sometimes, though, it doesn't, and you get rid of the fluid in your stool – a bothersome problem we call diarrhoea. Common causes include viral infections, such as flu, exposure to parasites or foreign versions of the bacterium *E. coli* while travelling, bacterial food poisoning and intolerance to an ingredient in dairy foods. Diarrhoea that lasts for days or weeks, however, may suggest irritable bowel syndrome. And diarrhoea that's not quickly resolved can cause dehydration, which is especially dangerous in infants and the elderly.

Tame diarrhoea with tannins

• Drink **black tea** with **sugar**. Tea will rehydrate the body and contains astringent tannins that help to reduce intestinal inflammation and block the absorption of toxins by your intestines. The sugar improves sodium and water absorption.

• Tannin-rich **blackberries** have long been used in folk remedies for diarrhoea. To make **blackberry tea** place 1.5g of dried blackberry leaves in a cup of boiling water; leave to infuse for 10 minutes and strain. Take 3 cups a day between meals. Or bring 2 tablespoons of fresh blackberries to the boil in 250ml water, simmer gently for 10 minutes, then strain. Drink 1 cup several times a day. You can also buy blackberry tea bags in health-food shops; check that they contain blackberry leaves. **Raspberry leaf tea** is also said to be effective. It is rich in minerals and some vitamins. It's widely used in pregnancy but possibly best avoided in the early stages (up to about 12 weeks).

Root out the problem

• Capsules of **goldenseal**, made from the bright-yellow root of a perennial herb, appear to kill many of the bacteria, such as *E. coli*, that cause diarrhoea. The key compound in the herb is berberine, which is so effective that goldenseal is sometimes called a 'herbal antibiotic'. Take two or three 125mg capsules a day until the diarrhoea subsides.

Infuse your body with fluids

• When your diarrhoea is profuse, you need to replace your body's supply of water and electrolytes, which include sodium, potassium and chloride. They keep your heart beating properly and play many other crucial roles as well. Mix up the perfect **electrolyte drink** by stirring ½ teaspoon of salt and 4 teaspoons of sugar into 1 litre of water. Add a little orange juice, lemon juice or salt substitute for potassium. During the day, drink a full litre. Don't use more than this amount of sugar or salt as more of either could dehydrate your body.

• Some proprietary sports or energy drinks can also replace lost electrolytes.

• It is especially important for a mother to continue feeding a breastfed infant who has diarrhoea. For bottlefed babies or older children, use an oral rehydration solution such as **Dioralyte** or **Rehidrat**, which are designed specifically to replace children's electrolytes.

• If your diarrhoea is mild and you're not dehydrated, start sipping **bottled soft drinks** (if the drinks are fizzy, stir briskly to get rid of the bubbles – you don't want the carbonation to give you wind). These will keep your fluid levels normal. Take sips for a few hours, then start drinking as much as you can comfortably until you're getting 500ml of fluid each hour. Avoid diet versions – your body needs the sugar. Try also to drink more nutritious liquids such as **clear chicken stock**.

Rebuild your diet

• Start by eating only foods that contain no solid content, such as **chicken stock** or a little **jelly**. Stock is an especially good choice, as it supplies your body with water, electrolytes from the salt and protein. Stick with these 'clear' foods for a day or two. But **avoid fruit juices**. They can contain large amounts of a sugar called fructose, which many people have trouble digesting even when they're feeling well.

• Spoil yourself with the **BRAT diet**. BRAT stands for bananas, rice, apple (purée) and toast. All are bland and soothing, and the bananas and apple contain pectin, a type of soluble fibre that soaks up excess fluid in your intestine and slows down the passage of stool. (Avoid apple juice, however, which can make diarrhoea worse.)

• **Carrots** are another soothing source of pectin. Cook some carrots until they're soft, then drop them in a blender with a little water and purée into a baby-food consistency. Eat a table-spoon or two each hour.

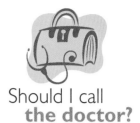

Should I call the doctor?

If diarrhoea lasts longer than two days, recurs frequently, or is accompanied by lightheadedness, a fever, intense cramping or blood or pus in the stool, see a doctor. The following instances also require medical attention:

• the person is very young, very old, otherwise ill or has a compromised immune system;

• the diarrhoea alternates with constipation;

• the person is taking drugs that could cause diarrhoea, such as some antacids or laxatives, anti-malarials and antibiotics;

• the person is taking drugs whose action is vital and may be impaired by diarrhoea, such as the Pill, anti-malarials, drugs for diabetes and epilepsy, and anticoagulants;

• if symptoms do not clear up in a couple of days and you have just returned from abroad.

• if an elderly person or young child has been taking antibiotics and develops a particularly foul-smelling form of diarrhoea, this might be due to overgrowth of the bacterium *Clostridium difficile*, which requires immediate treatment.

Deal with Delhi belly

Traveller's diarrhoea, known by many other names – Delhi belly, Montezuma's revenge or Tiki trots – is the bane of international travellers. It is usually caused by exposure to foreign strains of bacteria in the food or water. Before you leave for remote places, learn what steps you can take to avoid it.

• Take Pepto-Bismol before, during and after the trip. A number of studies have shown that this over-the-counter remedy can help to prevent traveller's diarrhoea. Even if it has started, Pepto-Bismol can help reduce the severity of the symptoms. Following the directions on the package, chew 2 pills four times a day or (if you are taking the liquid) 1 tablespoon four times a day. Don't worry if your stool or tongue turn black, it's a normal side-effect of Pepto-Bismol.

• Before you leave, start taking acidophilus capsules twice a day to boost the number of beneficial bacteria in your intestine. Continue taking them while you're abroad. Follow the dosage instructions on the bottle. But make sure you're getting live bacteria.

• Only drink water or other drinks that come in sealed bottles or cans, or water that has been boiled for 3 to 5 minutes. Use bottled water to brush your teeth and cook, and never have ice cubes in your drinks (you don't know what water was used to make them).

• Acidic drinks like orange juice and colas are also good for diarrhoea prevention because they help keep the bacterium E. coli in check.

• Eat only freshly cooked and piping hot foods and make sure you avoid any foods that have been cooked and then re-heated, or kept warm.

• Eat only fruits that you can peel yourself and avoid salads as the leaves will possibly have been rinsed in local water.

• Have a glass of wine with meals. In laboratory experiments, wine has been shown to kill the bacteria that cause traveller's diarrhoea. There's no research to say whether drinking wine actually helps, but if you enjoy wine (in moderation) anyway, why not? You're on holiday!

● **Avoid** foods that are rich in **roughage**, which can be hard to digest. That means no beans, cabbage or Brussels sprouts.

● It may be worth avoiding **milk-based produce** for a few days as a bout of diarrhoea can damage the intestinal lining, causing temporary lactose intolerance.

● An exception is **live yoghurt,** which contains **beneficial bacteria** such as *Lactobacillus acidophilus* and *Bifidobacterium*. Eating yoghurt with live cultures helps to restore healthy levels of these bacteria to your intestine and may speed up recovery from diarrhoea. If your diarrhoea is related to taking antibiotics, which kill good and bad bacteria indiscriminately, it's especially important to replenish your stock of good bacteria. If you don't like yoghurt, you could buy **acidophilus capsules** and follow the label instructions or dose yourself with probiotics such as Yakult or Actimel.

Solve it with psyllium

• One good treatment for diarrhoea is also a remedy for the opposite problem – constipation. Ground-up **psyllium seeds** (ispaghula) soak up excess fluid in the intestine, making the stool bulkier. They are the key ingredient in Fybogel and Isogel and other natural-fibre products. Take 1 to 3 tablespoons mixed in water each day.

An ancient Chinese treatment

• Here's an old Chinese remedy for diarrhoea. We have no idea if it works, but it can't hurt. Peel and crush 2 cloves of **garlic**, add 2 teaspoons **brown sugar**, boil in ¾ cup water and drink two to three times a day. Garlic is a potent antibacterial and may kill the bacteria that cause many cases of diarrhoea.

The power of prevention

• If you find that you frequently get diarrhoea after consuming milk and other dairy produce, cut those foods from your diet. They contain **lactose**, a sugar to which some people are **intolerant**. Try dairy substitutes such as soya milk. You may find that you can eat certain low-lactose dairy foods, such as butter, mature cheddar or products labelled 'lactose-free'.

• **Steer clear** of any products containing **xylitol, sorbitol** and **mannitol**. These sweeteners are often found in sugar-free gum and confectionery, and also in strawberries, cherries, prunes and peaches. Our bodies cannot easily digest the sweeteners.

• **Wash your hands** with soap and warm water before you prepare foods and after you handle raw meats. And be sure to wash thoroughly all plates and cooking implements that have come in contact with raw meat.

• To prevent food poisoning, **defrost foods in your microwave** or the **refrigerator**, not on the worktop.

• Large doses of **vitamin C** may give you diarrhoea.

• If you regularly take antacids that contain **magnesium**, such as magnesium trisilicate or Maalox, consider **switching to another brand**. This ingredient can cause diarrhoea.

Dry hair

If you believe what you see on television, you may be convinced that only brand-name shampoos and conditioners can give you the buoyant and swirling strands that make life such fun. What those advertisements won't tell you is that something as simple as mayonnaise can add just as much lustre to over-dry locks, giving you the bounce and flounce that those models flaunt.

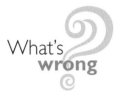

What's wrong

Your hair can become dry, rough, brittle and frizzy for many reasons. It's a non-living material, similar in composition to your fingernails, but each strand has an outer layer of cells that protects the inner hair shaft. If this coating becomes damaged, hair loses moisture and lustre and the ends become frayed. Excessive use of hair dyes, chlorine exposure, excessive sunlight and heat from hair dryers, hair straighteners and curling tongs can all damage it. And some people have dry hair just because they don't have an abundance of oil-producing glands on their scalps.

Start in the shower

- Only wash your hair **every other day**. Your hair will stay clean enough and you'll leave in more of its natural oils.
- Use **baby shampoo**, which is less drying than some other shampoos.
- Wash and rinse your hair with **warm water** rather than hot. Hot water strips protective oils from your hair. The best temperature for your hair is just slightly warmer than your body temperature.
- Thoroughly **rinse** your hair after you shampoo it. Shampoo can leave a residue, which dries out the strands.

Salad solutions

- **Avocado** moisturizes hair shafts and loads them with protein, making them stronger. Thoroughly mix a ripe, peeled avocado with a teaspoon of wheatgerm oil and a teaspoon of jojoba oil. Apply it to freshly washed hair and work it all the way to the ends. Cover your scalp with a shower cap or a plastic bag, wait 15 to 30 minutes, then rinse thoroughly.
- **Mayonnaise** is an excellent alternative to avocado; the egg it contains is a good source of protein for your hair. Rub the mayo into your hair and leave in for anything up to an hour, then wash it out.

Stay in condition

- If you use a store-bought conditioner, pick one with a 'thermal protector' ingredient such as **dimethicone** or **phenyl trimethicone**. These protect your hair from heat, which is especially important if you blow-dry.

Make your own conditioner by mixing 60g **olive oil** and 60g **aloe vera gel** with 6 drops each of **rosemary** and **sandalwood** essential oils. Olive oil is a natural emollient, aloe vera hydrates, while rosemary adds body and softness to hair. (The sandalwood, which is optional, just adds fragrance.) Leave the mixture on for an hour or two, then rinse it out.

When you use a conditioner, first apply it liberally to the **ends**, where hair is the driest. Then work your way towards your scalp.

In a frizz emergency, simply use a little bit of **hand lotion** and smooth it through dry hair.

Deft drying

Let your hair **air-dry** whenever possible. If you must use a hair dryer, use it sparingly. The same goes for curling tongs, straighteners or hot rollers. When you apply heat, it's like drying out a leaf in sunlight – you're inviting brittleness.

When you do use the hair dryer, make sure you use a **warm**, not hot, setting.

Brush up on your brushing technique

Use a brush that has **natural bristles** rather than synthetic ones. Synthetic materials generate static electricity, which will make your hair more brittle.

First **brush the ends** to remove tangles. That way, you won't pull and break your hair when you take full strokes with the brush.

After you've brushed the ends, make long, full strokes all the way from the roots of your hair to the ends to **spread hair's natural oils**.

Strengthen your strands

B vitamins may make your hair stronger. Take a 50mg B-complex supplement twice a day with food.

The mineral **selenium** is also helpful for maintaining healthy hair. Take 200mcg a day – or eat Brazil nuts: 30g of dried nuts contains 840mcg selenium. (*Alert* Excessive intake of selenium can be toxic and one of the symptoms is … hair loss!)

A beneficial oil that may help to keep hair lustrous from inside your body is **evening primrose**. Try taking 1000mg of

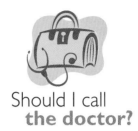

Should I call the doctor?

If your hair's appearance suddenly changes on its own – and you start feeling fatigued, chilled, irritable and you are constipated – talk to your doctor. These could be signs of hypothyroidism. It's also worth consulting your doctor if you have dry hair and also a crusty or itchy scalp, which could be a sign of psoriasis.

evening primrose three times a day with meals. The oil is high in gamma-linolenic acid, an essential fatty acid.

The power of prevention

- When you swim in a chlorinated pool, wear a **swimming cap** to keep the chlorine off your hair. As soon as possible after getting out of the pool, wash your hair.
- Use a **humidifier** in your bedroom. In cold weather, your central heating probably keeps the air very dry, which in turn dries out your hair.
- Get your hair **trimmed** at least every six weeks to eliminate dry, split ends.

Dry mouth

If a lack of saliva makes it hard for you to lick envelopes or even to talk comfortably, you'll definitely want to moisten your mouth. First, talk to your doctor about what might be causing your mouth to be so parched. Consider an over-the-counter saliva substitute such as Saliveze, Glandosane, Salivix pastilles or BioXtra gel. Simply by drinking plenty of water you will keep your mouth moist, as will the other tricks in this chapter.

Check your medicine cabinet

- Dozens of medications can cause you to have a dry mouth. **Check the label** of any that you're taking and if a dry mouth is listed as a side effect, ask your doctor if you can switch to another drug. Frequent culprits include many anti-histamines and decongestants as well as enalapril (Innovace), fluoxetine (Prozac), amlodipine (Istin) and paroxetine (Seroxat).

Just add water

- Carry a **water bottle** with you and sip water frequently. Swirl each sip around in your mouth before you swallow.
- To stimulate saliva flow, squeeze in some **lime** or **lemon juice** or add half a teaspoon of **apple cider vinegar**.

Make your mouth water

- Chew **sugar-free gum** or suck on **sugar-free boiled sweets** to stimulate the flow of saliva. Sugar-free gums that contains xylitol can also help to reduce cavity-causing bacteria.
- Keep a **chilli-pepper** shaker on the dinner table. The same 'hot stuff' that makes your eyes water and your nose run can make your saliva pour forth. Add just a touch to spice up your meals.

Avoid these drought-inducers

- **Limit** your intake of **coffee** and other **caffeinated drinks**, as well as **alcohol**. Drinking these to excess will cause you to urinate more frequently, making your body lose more fluids.
- **Forgo fizzy drinks**, even those without caffeine. If your mouth is dry, you don't have enough saliva to break down the acid they contain.

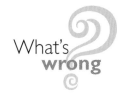

What's wrong

The mucous membranes in the mouth have become abnormally dry due to a lack of saliva. A dry mouth can be caused by medications or by the radiation, chemotherapy and surgery used to treat oral cancer. And sometimes it's the result of an autoimmune condition called Sjögren's syndrome, in which the immune system attacks moisture-producing glands in the body. Having a dry mouth is also related to ageing: About 40 per cent of people over the age of 65 have it. Because saliva protects us from oral infections and tooth decay, having a dry mouth can lead to bad breath, mouth sores, cavities and fungal and bacterial infections in the mouth.

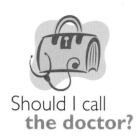

Should I call **the doctor?**

If you notice that your mouth is unusually dry for more than a few days, talk to your doctor or dentist. A consultation is especially important if the condition prevents you from eating or speaking normally or your mouth is red and irritated. When you discuss the problem with your doctor, be sure to mention any medications you are taking, as they may be contributing to the problem.

- **Say no to salty foods** or **highly acidic drinks** like orange juice and lemonade. These can cause pain if your mouth is too dry. Choose apple or pear juice or milky drinks instead.
- Keep **sugary snacks** to a minimum.
- **Stop smoking.** Tobacco smoke dries up saliva.

Add a little night moisture

- To avoid your mouth drying out at night, use a **humidifier** or **vapourizer** in your bedroom.

Swishing well

- If you use a proprietary mouthwash, choose one like Corsodyl that **doesn't contain alcohol**, which dries your mouth and can irritate already-sensitive gum tissues.
- For a homemade mouthwash, mix a large pinch of **salt** and large pinch of **bicarbonate of soda** in a cup of warm water. Rinse your mouth and spit. This solution will counteract acids in your mouth and rinse away infectious agents.

Teeth treatments

- Choose a toothpaste that **doesn't contain sodium lauryl sulphate (SLS),** which can irritate mouth tissues. Most brands contain it, but health-food shops sell brands without SLS.
- Make sure you **brush** and **floss** thoroughly. Saliva is important for clearing away food debris in your mouth, and when your mouth is dry this food can cling.

Keep your mouth shut

- When you inhale through your nose, you moisturize the air going into your body. But when your sinuses are blocked, you naturally do a lot of mouth breathing, and that means you're taking in a lot of dry air. Take steps to treat a **sinus condition** (see page 338) or **allergies** (see page 34) and you will also help to prevent a dry mouth.

Dry skin

The outer layer of your skin works like a self-oiling machine, but sometimes oil production can't keep up with demand. Trouble occurs when you shower a lot, use skin-drying soap or live in a house where the air is Saharan. What is the best refreshment for parched skin? Most moisturizers (which don't actually *add* moisture to the skin but work by locking in moisture that's already there) will do the trick. Or try one of the home remedies below.

Exfoliate for softer skin

- Give your skin a **milk bath.** The lactic acid in milk exfoliates dead skin cells and may also increase the skin's ability to hold in moisture. Soak a flannel in cold milk. Lay the flannel on any area of skin that is particularly dry or irritated. Leave it there for 5 minutes and when you rinse off the milk, do so gently, so some of the lactic acid stays on your skin.
- To soften rough patches of skin, fill a bath with warm water and add 2 cups of **Epsom salts**, then climb in and soak for a few minutes. While your skin is still wet, you can also rub handfuls of Epsom salts on the rough areas to exfoliate the skin. You'll be amazed at just how good your skin feels when you get out. If you have any **dried seaweed**, you can also add a few strips to your bath to boost the softening effect.
- Apply **aloe vera gel** to help your dry skin heal more quickly. It contains acids that eat away dead skin cells. To obtain the fresh gel, cut off a leaf at the base and split it open with a knife. Scrape out the gel with a spoon.
- Use a moisturizer that contains **alpha-hydroxy acids** (AHAs) or a lotion that contains **urea**, such as Eucerin. These remove loose, flaky skin cells, leaving the skin softer.

Add more moisture

- Purée a ripe **avocado** and pat the flesh onto your face as a moisturizing mask. The oil acts as an emollient. It also contains beneficial vitamin E.
- Turn to any of these inexpensive products to trap in your skin's own moisture: **lanolin** (obtained from wool), **mineral**

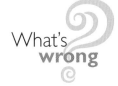

What's **wrong**

When all is well with your skin, its glands are constantly producing an oil called sebum that keeps skin moist and supple. During winter, however, dry air (both outdoors and in) can cause your skin to become flaky, itchy, cracked and rough. Hands and face suffer worst because they are the most exposed. And hands produce the least amount of protective sebum.

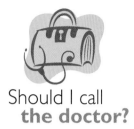

Should I call the doctor?

If your skin is so dry that you're still intensely uncomfortable after two weeks of self-help techniques, consult your doctor. Also seek medical care if you develop a severe, itchy rash or if your skin shows signs of infection, such as redness, crustiness or oozing. In rare instances, dry skin can be a sign of an underlying medical condition such as hypothyroidism or diabetes.

oil, petroleum jelly, peanut oil or even cooking margarine. Just use them sparingly to avoid feeling greasy.

Switch soaps
- If you use a **deodorant** soap, **stop.** These soaps dry the skin. And they contain perfumes, which are irritants.
- Use a **cream soap** such as Dove, Oilatum or Neutrogena. These have extra oil or fat added late in the soap-making process. They leave a beneficial oily film on the skin.
- Try gentle cleansers like **Cetaphil** and **Alpha-Keri**. The milder soaps in general have a pH (a measure of acidity) which is closer to that of your skin and remove dirt without stripping away too much natural oil.
- **Liquid soaps** also tend to be gentler on your skin. Choose one labelled 'moisturizing' and keep bottles next to your kitchen sink and beside the basins in the bathroom and loo for washing your hands.

Short showers; brief baths
- Never stay in the bath or shower for more than 15 minutes. When you have a long soak, you're washing away your skin's protective oils. And use **warm water**, not hot. Hot water tends to strip the oil from your skin.
- **Add an emollient,** such as bath E45, to the bath water.
- Use **soap extremely sparingly** – in other words, only on the armpits, groin area and feet, and wash the rest of your body with simple water.
- Take a **bath or shower in the evening,** so your skin can replace protective oils overnight while you're asleep.

Dampen your domestic environment
- In the winter, try to make sure the **humidity** in your house remains comfortable. Stand a bowl of water by the fire; hang water reservoirs on radiators; leave the bathroom door open when you bath or shower; put a humidifier beside your bed and keep your bedroom door closed at night when the machine is switched on.
- If you have a **fireplace** or **wood-burning stove,** use it sparingly. The heat generated from these sources is extremely drying.

Homemade moisturizer

To make your own skin moisturizer, melt 1 teaspoon of white beeswax and 2 table-spoons of lanolin in a double boiler. Stir in 3 tablespoons of olive oil, 1 tablespoon of fresh aloe vera gel, and 2 tablespoons of rose water (sold in pharmacies). Let cool.

Eat, drink and be moister

• Be sure to drink at least eight 250ml glasses of **water** each day. **Herbal teas** and **juices** also count, but not caffeinated beverages like tea or coffee and colas containing caffeine, or any drinks that include alcohol. All of those have a diuretic effect, which means you'll lose body fluids because you'll have to urinate more frequently.

• At least twice a week, eat some oily fish such as **mackerel, sardines, herring** or **salmon.** These are rich in **omega-3 fatty acids**, which help to keep your skin-cell membranes healthy. Other good sources of these fatty acids are **walnuts, avocados** and **flax seed** (linseed) **oil.** Mix up to 2 tablespoons of flax seed oil each day into your salad dressing or your morning porridge. (If you add it to hot cereal, do so only after the cereal is cooked. Flax seed oil breaks down into less useful compounds if you cook with it.)

Get your fill of vitamins and minerals

• Certain vitamins, in particular the B vitamins and vitamin C, along with various minerals help to maintain healthy skin. Every day take a B-complex vitamin supplement containing **thiamin, riboflavin and pantothenic acid;** or **brewers' yeast.**

• Look for a multivitamin/mineral **supplement** that offers a range of skin-enhancing nutrients in one pill. One brand is DermaVite. It contains vitamins A, B_6, C and E, riboflavin, folate, zinc, selenium and other minerals and nutrients.

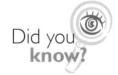

Did you know?

Having a lot of houseplants can help to prevent dry skin. Plants add moisture to the air in two ways: through photosynthesis (their leaves produce water) and also via evaporation from their well-watered soil.

REMEDIES FROM THE SEA

If you're looking for a respite from stress, few things can match a lazy day on the beach. Blue skies, warm sand and lapping water have a way of melting away tension. But did you know that the world's oceans are balm for the body as well as the mind? Marine plants and animals are the source of various drugs, and many more marine-based pharmaceuticals are under development, including cancer drugs from starfish eggs, the world's most powerful sunscreen from a species of jellyfish and an osteoporosis drug derived from coral.

Fish oil for your health

You've probably heard that a diet rich in oily fish like sardines, mackerel and tuna can help to protect you against the blood clots that cause heart attacks. That has been demonstrated again and again in clinical trials initiated after researchers noticed a curiously low incidence of coronary artery disease in natives of Greenland, for whom fish is a dietary staple.

Now it appears that the same omega-3 fatty acids in fish that protect against blood clotting also seem to be effective against a host of other health problems, including depression and inflammatory conditions such as psoriasis, rheumatoid arthritis and Crohn's disease, as well as lupus and eczema. They may even ease menstrual cramps. If you don't like the taste of fish, take fish oil capsules instead. For more information about fish oil capsules, see page 416.

Seaweed superfoods

Seaweed, too, is more than a great wrap for sushi and health farm clients. Nori, kelp, laver, dulse and other seaweeds – more than 2,500 varieties – are good sources of protein and dietary fibre. They also contain up to 20 times the vitamin and mineral content of vegetables that grow on land.

Unlike terrestrial plants, seaweed contains vitamin B_{12}. That is significant because as more people reduce their consumption of meat and dairy foods – the usual sources of B_{12} in the diet – so more people are becoming deficient in the vitamin. This lack can cause fatigue, depression, numbness and tingling.

Seaweed is also a rich source of alginic acid, which helps to rid the body of toxic heavy metals such as lead. In addition, it contains compounds that may help to prevent cancer.

Nori, for example, is rich in the anti-oxidant beta-carotene which, like all anti-oxidants, can neutralize harmful molecules known as free radicals before they cause the DNA damage that may eventually lead to malignant tumours. Seaweeds are as popular in Asian cuisine as potatoes are in Britain; that may help to explain why cancer rates in Asia are just a fraction of what they are in the UK.

Help for an underactive thyroid

As with cancer, obesity is much rarer in Japan than in most Western countries. One theory suggests that the abundance of iodine-rich seaweed in traditional Japanese cuisine helps to boost meta-bolism. Metabolic processes are governed in part by thyroid hormones. And an underactive thyroid gland can be caused by an iodine deficiency. If that's the case, eat more iodine and you will boost your thyroid hormone production and, along with it, your meta-bolism. Signs of an underactive thyroid gland include fatigue, lethargy and dry skin. You should see your doctor if you think your thyroid isn't performing as it should.

Most people in developed countries get plenty of iodine from iodized salt. But if your doctor advises you to consume more iodine – to help an underactive thyroid, for instance – then find out about adding seaweed to your diet.

Sea salt for healthy skin

For thousands of years, people have been bathing in the super-salty waters of the Dead Sea to cure their ailments. While the waters of the Dead Sea may not work miracles, there is no doubt that bathing in salt water is a great way to moisturize dry, damaged skin.

Even severe cases of psoriasis can some-times be cleared up by bathing repeatedly in water to which sea salt has been added. Whether it's the minerals in the sea salt or the salt itself isn't clear, though there is no doubt that salt is a very effective natural exfoliant.

Seaweeds to savour

Once an important part of the British diet, seaweed is in fashion once again and can now be found on the menus of many top restaurants. Seaweed is sold fresh or dried: dried varieties need reconstituting by soaking in water before use.

Dulse The red leaves are popular in Ireland where it is often mixed into potatoes mashed with butter and then fried to make 'champ'.

Kelp Its long brown ribbons and hand-shaped fronds are chopped up and added to soups or dried and sprinkled over food.

Laver Harvested on the coast west of Swansea, puréed 'laverbread' is rolled in oatmeal and crisply fried for breakfast.

Nori This Japanese seaweed is sold in paper-like sheets and used to wrap rice or sushi. Or you can cut it into strips and use it as a decorative flavouring in soup.

Wakame Another Japanese variety, wakame (or alaria) is now cultivated in Brittany. It is used mainly to flavour soups, but you can also add strips to stews, stir-fries or salads.

Seaweed is full of salt. If you need to limit your intake of sodium – due to high blood pressure, for example – then soak the leaves before adding them to recipes.

When simple dry skin is the problem, a salt scrub is often the answer. Make a paste with about a cup of sea salt and enough glycerine (sold in pharmacies) to get the salt to stick together. After a shower, while your skin is still wet, rub this mixture over your body using your hands or a loofah sponge. Once you rinse away the salt and dry off, you'll be amazed at how soft your skin feels.

Ear problems

There's nothing like an earache to bring back the less pleasant memories of childhood. Put simply, earaches are no fun. You can approach the problem from the outside in, using carefully chosen eardrops or even a little garlic juice, or from the inside out, with soups and gargles that help to drain mucus and expand the Eustachian tubes. Warm and cold treatments can also help you to weather the pain.

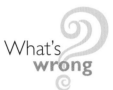

What's wrong

An earache means something has probably gone awry in the middle ear, which is the tiny space located behind the eardrum. A thin canal called the Eustachian tube runs from the middle ear to the back of the throat. It allows fluid to drain away, and it's also where the pressure inside your ear adjusts to meet outside air pressure. The common cold virus can cause fluid to accumulate in the Eustachian tube, triggering significant pain. Bacteria thrive in the fluid, leading to middle-ear infections. These are all too common in children, but can strike adults as well. If you get an earache from flying, the cause is probably excessive air pressure rather than infection.

Drop in

● Warm a teaspoon of **baby oil**, **mineral oil** or **olive oil** over a saucer of hot water for a minute, test the temperature on your wrist, then drip a few drops of the warm oil into your ear to help ease discomfort. (*Alert* Never drop fluids into the ear if you think the eardrum may be ruptured. This is usually indicated by a discharge from the ear.)

Drain it, dry it

● Try a **spicy chicken soup** or fiery bowl of **chilli**. The spiciness gets your mucus flowing and can help your ears to drain, relieving painful pressure.

● Gulp down plenty of **water** every day. The muscles that work when you swallow help your Eustachian tubes to open up, allowing your ears to drain.

● Gargle with warm **salt water.** It helps to increase blood circulation to the Eustachian tubes and decreases any swelling that may be blocking them.

● Try **echinacea** and **goldenseal**. Echinacea helps your body to fight off infection and goldenseal helps to dry out the fluid in the ear. Add a full dropper of each tincture to a little water and drink every 2 to 3 hours.

● Use an **extra pillow** to prop your head up slightly more than normal while you sleep. This will help your ears to drain, easing pressure.

Warm and chill

● Lie on your side and place a comfortably warm **hot-water bottle** or **heating pad** over your ear. Or use a towel dampened with hot water. The soothing warmth increases circulation to the ear and also helps to relieve pressure.

- Use a **hair dryer** as another source of warmth. Set the dryer on the lowest warm temperature, hold it at least 15cm (6in) from your ear, and direct the airstream down into your ear.
- To draw inflammation away from the affected ear, wear **ice-cold socks** on your feet and apply a **warm compress** to your ear. Saturate cotton socks in iced water, wring them out and place them against the soles of your feet. Then pull wool socks over the cold socks to hold them in place. Simultaneously, place a hot damp compress over the painful ear.

Ease the ache with garlic

- Eat one or two raw cloves of **garlic** every day. The pungent bulb helps to fight viruses and bacteria. Some brave souls just chew on the cloves. Or crush fresh garlic, mix it with olive oil and spread it on your favourite bread.
- If raw garlic upsets your stomach, take a **garlic capsule** with each meal instead.
- Make **antibacterial eardrops**. Squeeze a clove of garlic and mix a few drops of the antibacterial juice into a teaspoon of olive oil. Drop into your ear to fight the infection.

Do away with earwax

When your ears produce too much wax (or cerumen), or you inadvertently push it into the canal by trying to clean it out, it can form a plug deep in the ear. This can cause earaches, ringing in the ears, hearing loss and balance problems. Easy-does-it earwax removal is usually a two-part project – first the insertion of something to soften up the wax, then an ear wash to flood the gunk and carry it out.

- Gently **massage** the area directly behind your earlobe to help loosen the wax. Then **tug the earlobe** while opening and closing your mouth.

Soften and rinse

- At bedtime, fill an eyedropper with warm **olive oil** and pour into the affected ear. Let the softening fluid work its way down into your ear. Put a **cotton wool plug** in the ear after insertion (to avoid staining the pillow).

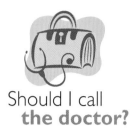

Should I call the doctor?

See your doctor if your ear is extremely painful, if it hurts for more than a few days, or is accompanied by a fever. You should also tell the doctor about any fluid discharge from your ear, feelings of dizziness or pain when you chew. Sudden, intense pain, followed by some relief, could indicate a ruptured eardrum. Other common signs of ruptured eardrum are discharge (sometimes with blood), muffled hearing, a ringing in the ears, and a feeling of dizziness or vertigo. *If you have these symptoms, see your doctor before trying any of the remedies in this chapter.* Also, consult your doctor if your ear is blocked because of impacted wax, and attempts to loosen it at home have not produced any relief. The doctor may suggest ear drops or syringing.

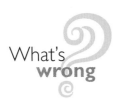

• Repeat the warm olive oil treatment daily for three or four days. If the wax is soft, **it will come out on its own** or with normal washing or cleaning (gently) with a cotton bud.

Air your ear

• After you finish washing the wax out of your ears, use a **hair dryer** to air-dry them. Set the hair dryer on its coolest setting and hold it about 30cm (12in) away.

To clean – or not?

• Whenever you wash, wipe a damp flannel around the loops and whorls of your outer ear. Unless you are removing wax following softening with oil (as described above), **never stick a cotton bud** or any other type of probe into your ear. You'll ram the wax in deeper, and because there are no oil glands deep in the ear canal to keep the wax soft, it will harden like a rock. You could also puncture your eardrum or scratch your ear canal.

• Some experts believe that **saturated fats** prompt your body to produce greater amounts of earwax and also make the wax stickier. **Cut down** on fatty meats, butter and hard cheeses and minimize your consumption of hydrogenated fats found in processed foods. Replace these dietary fats with healthier ones, such as those found in oily fish, nuts and seeds.

• If you wear a **hearing aid**, wipe it with a tissue every night at bedtime when you remove it. This gets rid of wax residue before it has time to accumulate.

• For people who have a lot of ear hair – particularly some older men – it helps to trim the hair with a battery-operated **ear-hair trimmer.** This will help to prevent earwax from getting enmeshed in hair around the opening of the ear canal.

Strategies for swimmer's ear

• First **see your pharmacist.** Explain your symptoms and ask for a suitable over-the-counter remedy. If your ear is still at the itchy stage, some drops may clear it up before infection sets in.

• Alternatively, mix equal parts of **surgical spirit and white vinegar** and use a clean eyedropper to put a few drops in your itchy ear. Tilt your head so the mixture flows into the ear canal, then tug your earlobe to make sure it flows all the way in. Keep your head tilted, or lie down, for a few minutes, then sit up and tip your head towards your shoulder to drain it. The acidity of the vinegar creates a hostile environment for bacteria and fungi, while the alcohol in the surgical spirit evaporates quickly, helping to dry out the ear canal fast.

The power of prevention

A few simple steps can keep you from having to worry about aching ears or swimmer's ear.

- When you have a cold, **blow your nose gently.** If you blow too forcefully, you can push bacteria back into your middle ear from your sinuses and trigger an infection.
- Frequent ear infections can be a sign of **food allergy.** Most often, the troublesome foods are dairy products, wheat, corn, peanuts or oranges. Try removing these foods from your diet for several weeks to see if you feel any better. Then add them back one at a time. If your ears start aching, ban that particular food from your diet for good.
- Chew **sugar-free gum** that contains the sweetener xylitol, which comes from silver birch trees (and is also found in strawberries and plums). In one study, children who chewed two pieces of the gum five times a day for two months had 40 per cent fewer ear infections. The xylitol may cut down the growth of bacteria that causes middle-ear infections.
- **Wear earplugs for swimming** and when washing your hair or showering to keep the water out. Choose wax or silicone plugs that can be softened and moulded to fit the ear canal, or buy earplugs specially designed for swimmers, which are available in children's sizes, too.
- After swimming or showering, **blow-dry your ears**. Set the dryer on low and direct warm air into your ear for about 30 seconds. Hold the nozzle at least 30cm (12in) away.
- Don't try to get all the wax out of your ears. In normal amounts, **earwax** coats the ear canal, which protects your inner ear from moisture.
- Avoid exposure to **loud noises** – if you are doing a noisy job, wear ear defenders available from DIY stores.

Eczema

Experts are unanimous – the best way to deal with itchy patches of eczema is to keep the skin well moisturized. That means keeping out of the water as much as possible: no dishwashing, frequent hand washing, or long showers. Protect your skin with a thick, heavy-duty cream – not a watery lotion. Avoid eczema aggravators, such as harsh soaps and any other triggers. And, hard as it may be, don't scratch.

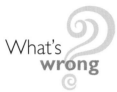

What's wrong

There are several types of eczema. Atopic eczema, the most common, usually occurs in people with a family history of allergies or asthma. Symptoms – red, itchy skin – generally begin before the age of five, then reappear periodically during childhood and sometimes into adulthood. During acute flare-ups, the skin may be marked with small, fluid-filled blisters. Over time, excessive scratching causes patches of skin to look thick and scaly. Skin damaged by eczema and scratching is prone to bacterial infections. Another type of eczema, called contact dermatitis, stems from contact with an irritating substance such as detergent, soap and cosmetics.

Rash relief

- To soothe itching, soak a flannel in **ice-cold milk** and lay it over the itchy area. Repeat several times a day.
- Add **colloidal oatmeal**, such as Aveeno, to the bath. This finely ground oatmeal floats suspended in the water and is soothing to itchy skin. It is available from pharmacies.
- Keep baths and showers to under 10 minutes. Use **lukewarm water** and **don't bath every day** if you don't have to. Eczema can get worse when skin is dry and excessive bathing washes away the protective oils that keep your skin moist.
- After bathing, use a **heavy cream-based moisturizer** to guard the skin against irritants. Ask your pharmacist for an aqueous cream or emulsifying ointment. Even petroleum jelly or solid cooking margarine works well. Avoid water-based lotions, scented lotions and even baby lotions, which have a high water content.

Try these foods and supplements

- Eat more foods rich in omega-3 fatty acids, which help to reduce inflammation and allergic reactions. You'll find these in **walnuts, avocados, salmon, mackerel** and **tuna**.
- Another good source of omega-3s is **flax seed oil**. Take up to 1 tablespoon each day; its beneficial properties are lost in high cooking temperatures, so add it to salad dressing, mix it with yoghurt or blend it into other foods.
- To ease itchy skin, try **evening primrose oil**, which supplies gamma-linolenic acid (GLA), an essential fatty acid that people with eczema sometimes lack. Take 1,000mg three times a day with food for three to four months.

• Take 250mg **vitamin E** each day to help counteract itchy, dry skin. Good dietary sources of vitamin E include wheat-germ, vegetable oils, nuts and seeds. (*Alert* Do not take vitamin E supplements if you take blood-thinning drugs unless you have your doctor's approval.)

• Make sure you get enough vitamin A. The recommended daily amount for vitamin A is 600mcg for women and 700mcg for men. However, as it can be toxic in high doses, it is far better – especially for children, who make up the majority of eczema sufferers – to obtain vitamin A from foods rather than supplements. Good sources include liver, fish-liver oil, carrots, green leafy vegetables, egg yolks, enriched margarine, milk products and yellow fruits.

Go to gotu

• The herb **gotu kola**, used externally, can help to ease itchy skin conditions. Look for a commercial cream or tincture. If you use the extract, dilute it first (five parts water to one part extract). Alternatively, you can make a cup of the tea, soak a cloth in it, and use the cloth as a compress. To make the tea, steep 1 to 2 teaspoons of the dried herb in a cup of very hot water for 10 minutes, then strain.

• As an alternative to gotu kola, look for a cream containing **camomile**, **liquorice** or **witch hazel**. All of them reduce skin inflammation.

Ways to stop scratching

• If the itchy area is somewhere far too accessible, such as the wrist or the back of the hand, **cover it with a small plaster** as a deterrent to scratching.

• Some people scratch in their sleep. If you (or your child) wake up with scratched skin, **put on thin cotton gloves** (or even a pair of lightweight socks) at night.

• **Keep fingernails short** to minimize skin damage from scratching.

The power of prevention

• Many experts believe that **food allergies** play a significant role in eczema, particularly in children under the age of two. In children, the problems often come from eggs, orange juice,

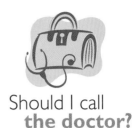

Should I call the doctor?

If your eczema is widespread or keeps recurring despite your self-care treatments, contact your doctor. You need to see a doctor as soon as possible if an itchy patch of skin begins to show signs of infection. These include crusting sores, pus, red streaks on the skin, excessive pain, swelling or fever.

New medicine

Tacrolimus (Protopic), a new topical treatment for eczema, has recently been licensed in the UK. Its active ingredient is an immunosuppressant – it damps down the activity of the body's immune system, reducing inflammation. Tacrolimus is not a cure for eczema, but another treatment. Your specialist consultant may prescribe it if your eczema is still severe after exploring other avenues of treatment – emollients, steroids (either topical or short-term oral), antibiotics or UV light.

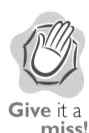

Give it a miss!

Over-the-counter corticosteroid creams, like hydrocortisone, can help to tame eczema. But if you use them too often – say, every day for more than three weeks – they can thin and damage the skin.

milk and nuts. In adults, the troublesome foods are usually dairy foods, wheat, eggs, yeast and citrus fruits or juices. Try eliminating these foods from the diet for about a month, then bring them back one at a time for three days to see if the skin reacts. In children, this food-elimination diet may produce a visible change in a short time. Dramatic change is much rarer in adults but still you might note some improvement. It's best to talk to your doctor before experimenting with elimination diets – for yourself or for a child.

• Try to minimize exposure to **house dust mites** and **pet dander** (see *Allergies* page 34). This means keeping the house – especially children's bedrooms – as dust free as possible. Good strategies include using allergy-protective mattress and pillow covers, avoiding soft furnishings and carpets whenever you can, keeping pets out of bedrooms and laundering bed linen in a hot wash (60°C or higher).

• In winter, run a **humidifier** in the bedroom.

• If you have a **dishwasher**, use it as much as possible to avoid contact with detergents and water. When you do wash up, wear **lined rubber gloves** or wear rubber gloves over a pair of thin cotton gloves. **Avoid direct contact with latex**, as it can cause allergic reactions – and make eczema worse.

• Keep your use of laundry chemicals to a minimum. Use a **fragrance-free** and **dye-free** detergent. **Avoid bleach, fabric softeners** and **tumble dryer sheets**.

• Give your clothes an **extra rinse** in the washing machine to remove all traces of detergent.

• Have you touched anything that might have caused a reaction? **Contact dermatitis** can be caused by nickel used in earrings and other jewellery, as well as latex, cosmetics, perfumes and cleaning agents.

Eye irritation

Redness, scratchiness and sensitivity to light occur when your eyes are too dry. A speck of dust no bigger than the full stop at the end of this sentence can feel like a jagged-edged boulder if it lodges beneath your eyelid. And if your eyes dry out in the wind or cry out against chlorine, it's hard to focus on anything else. Fortunately, you can often sort out the problem in the blink of an eye.

Dust begone

- If there's a particle in your eye, gently pull the upper lashes to lift the lid away from your eyeball. Roll your eye around. If you don't produce enough tears to wash out the particle, use **sterile eyewash** or **artificial tears**.
- Some people take that technique one step further and flip an **upper eyelid inside out**. Sometimes that's all it takes to flick out the particle.
- If that manoeuvre doesn't work, or you don't want to attempt it, try a simple **eyewash.** Wash and rinse your hands at the sink, cup some warm water in your palms and then put your closed eye into your cupped hands. Open your eye underwater to flush away the particle.

Lose contact with your contacts

- If you wear contact lenses and get something in your eye, **remove the lens** and clean it, using normal cleaning techniques. Examine it closely to make sure the particle has not stuck to it. If you do have to remove a speck, clean the lens once more before putting it back into your eye.

Soothe itchy eyes

- Soak a flannel in **cool water** and lay it over your closed eyes for as long as needed. This is particularly effective if your eyes are red and itchy from allergies. The cold constricts blood vessels, while the moist cloth keeps your eyes damp.
- Soak **tea bags** in cool water and place one over each closed eye for 15 minutes. Any kind of tea bag will do: it's the cool dampness that soothes the eye – not what's inside the bag.

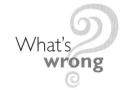

What's wrong

The world can be a dusty, gritty place, and when a speck lands in your eye, it can be very uncomfortable. Usually, tears come to the rescue, cleaning the surface of the eyes, nourishing their cells and countering the desiccating effects of dry air. Without tears, your eyes become irritated and red. As we age, we produce fewer tears, which is one reason older people tend to have more eye irritation. Allergies can cause red, itchy eyes, as can exposure to dry air and cigarette smoke.

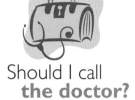

Should I call **the doctor?**

Give it a **miss!**

Moisten your eyes

- Buy a **humidifier** and run it the room where you spend most time – the sitting room during the day and the bedroom at night, for example.
- For eyes that are dry and irritated, use **artificial tears**. They come in different thicknesses: more viscous ones last longer but can blur your vision temporarily; runnier ones need putting in more often. Ask your pharmacist for advice on the best type for you, and look for a product that doesn't contain preservatives, such as Tears Naturale or Viscotears. Read the label for directions.

The power of prevention

- **Get more sleep**. Lack of sleep can cause eyes to become dry and red because the blood vessels are swollen.
- Eat a **banana** every day to help relieve dry eyes. Bananas are rich in potassium, which helps to control the balance of sodium and the release of fluid in your cells.
- Add a tablespoon of **flax seed oil** to juice or cereal. It's a good source of omega-3 fatty acids, which are essential for keeping your eyes well lubricated. Teardrops contain not only water but fat and mucus. To have a healthy tear film, you need to eat plenty of omega-3 fatty acids, also found in walnuts and certain oily fish, such as tuna or salmon.
- If your eyes are frequently dry, review the **drugs** you take. Common culprits include antihistamines, antidepressants, blood pressure medications and tranquillizers.
- Wear **eye-protectors** when you're doing chores that raise airborne debris – sweeping the patio or vigorous dusting, say.
- Wear watertight **swimming goggles** whenever you're swimming in a chlorinated pool.
- In the sun, wear **sunglasses** to protect your eyes from ultraviolet radiation. Sunglasses can also keep eyes from drying out on windy days.
- Eye make-up is a common cause of irritation – choose hypoallergenic brands. And if you use a **cream** or **ointment** on your upper eyelids, make sure it won't irritate your eyes.
- Stay away from **tobacco smoke**. If you do smoke, you'll probably find that your eyes feel a lot better if you give it up.

Eye strain

Your eyes may be the windows to your soul, but when overworked, they become doorways to pain, headaches and blurred vision. Unfortunately, eye strain is all too common when people spend countless hours staring into the glare of computer monitors and televisions. There are several things you can do to lessen the problem. Give the eyes as much rest as possible. And make some adjustments to your computer and your work habits to make life easier on the eyes.

Rest them, blink them, close them

- Whenever you're working on a task that requires close concentration, **take a break** every 20 minutes or so. Look at a faraway object – a picture on the opposite wall or a view out of the window – for at least 30 seconds. By allowing your eyes to shift focus, you give them a rest.
- Try to **blink often** – every few seconds or so – when you're paying close attention to your television or computer screen. Blinking moistens your eyeballs and relaxes your eye muscles.
- If you have a long task that involves prolonged staring, **close your eyes** periodically. Even if you just shut your eyelids for a few seconds, you'll get some immediate relief.

Warm and cool relief

- Another way to **relax your eye muscles**: Briskly rub your hands together until they grow warm, and gently place the heels of your palms over your closed eyes. Hold them there for a few seconds.
- If you soak a flannel or hand towel in **cool water**, wring it out, and lay it over your eyes for 5 minutes to relieve strain.
- Cool your eyes with sliced **cucumber.** Lie on your back and place a slice over each closed eye. Leave on for 2 or 3 minutes, or replace the first pair with another, cooler set of slices.

Tear up

- For eyestrain that is related to dry eyes, use **artificial tears**, available at pharmacies. Two brands are Viscotears and Tears Naturale.

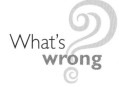

What's **wrong**

If you hold a dumbbell in your outstretched hand, your muscles soon get tired. The same happens to eyes when you overtax them. If the eye muscles that focus your vision don't have a chance to relax, you'll soon feel the strain. You may even have trouble focusing. And if you're squinting against bright sunlight, eye pain can come on very quickly.

Glasses for your neck?

If you wear bifocals, you can get neck strain from working at a computer. That's because with bifocals, the 'reading' lens is at the bottom of the glasses, so you have to tilt your head back in order to see the computer screen. Ask your optician to prescribe another pair of glasses that will give you clear vision at a distance of 50cm (20in), so you can read what is on the monitor without awkward head tilting.

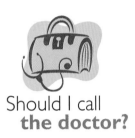

Should I call the doctor?

If your eyes frequently feel strained and home remedies don't work, if your vision becomes increasingly poor or you're very sensitive to light, consult an ophthalmologist. Also, if dizziness or double vision occur suddenly and don't go away when you rest your eyes, be sure to consult your doctor promptly.

Adjust your monitor

- **Turn the contrast** on your computer monitor to high. You will find that letters and images become crisper.
- Adjust your **chair height** so you're looking slightly downwards at the screen. Tilt the screen to meet your gaze.
- Ensure your eyes are at least 50cm (20in) from the screen.
- Adjust your computer screen or close the curtains or blinds near your work area so that you **don't have window-glare** on the screen.
- **Clean the dust** off the screen regularly to improve clarity.
- If you're mildly short sighted, try reading or viewing the computer screen **without your distance glasses.** Your eyes might be more comfortable that way.
- Choose a **bigger font** so that your eyes don't have to work as hard to focus, or use the **zoom** option to enlarge what you're viewing.

Wear shades

- In any bright sun – even in winter – **wear sunglasses.** They will reduce eyestrain that comes from screwing up your eyes. The best sunglasses have yellow, amber, orange or brown lenses. Light in the blue part of the spectrum is what makes us squint, and these lenses block it.

Light up your life

- When you're reading, be sure the light is adequate so you don't strain your eyes. The best results are with a **flexible gooseneck lamp** directed so that the light falls on the page. Generally, a lower-watt bulb in a gooseneck lamp is more effective than a higher-watt bulb in a table lamp. A 40 to 60-watt spotlight bulb should give plenty of illumination.

- Don't settle for one reading lamp in an otherwise dark room. Make sure that **other lights are also switched on**. If there's too much contrast between the light where you're reading and the rest of the room, your pupils will constantly have to narrow and widen to adjust for the difference.
- **Avoid** reading or working under **fluorescent lights.** They may flicker, contributing to eyestrain. The incandescent light from ordinary light bulbs is your best bet – or try natural daylight-imitating bulbs, especially for close work.

Check out cheap specs

- After the age of 40 or so, many people have trouble focusing on close objects – such as threading a needle or reading the list of ingredients or cooking instructions on packaged foods – a condition called presbyopia. If your distance vision is still fine and both eyes are focusing equally, try buying an inexpensive pair of **reading glasses** from your local pharmacy, a supermarket, or another outlet that stocks them. It is important to continue to go to your optician for regular eye tests even if these glasses sort out your eyesight problems, because other eye problems could easily go unnoticed.

Fatigue

Feeling dog-tired, as so many people do, is disheartening, demoralizing and frustrating. You want to race like a thoroughbred, but you feel stuck in the mud. Half the time you're struggling just to stay awake. Life is passing by and you can't keep up with it. Willpower doesn't work, so what does? Sometimes your best bet is a total energy makeover – changes in the way you eat, drink and exercise. Certain supplements can also help. Or maybe your solution is simple: sleep, beautiful sleep. And it wouldn't hurt to see your doctor who may test your blood for hypothyroidism, anaemia, vitamin B_{12} deficiency and other conditions that can cause fatigue.

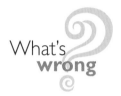

What's wrong

People complain of feeling drained and exhausted so often that doctors call fatigue the number one health complaint. Often fatigue is accompanied by lack of motivation and low sex drive. A long list of medical conditions and lifestyle issues can contribute to fatigue, including lack of sleep, inadequate nutrition, flu, obesity, allergies, infections, anaemia, alcohol abuse, hypothyroidism, heart disease, cancer, diabetes and AIDS.

Quick fixes

● For a quick pick-me-up, put 2 drops of **peppermint oil** on a tissue or handkerchief, hold it to your nose and breathe deeply. If you have more time, try adding 2 drops of the oil to bathwater along with 4 drops of **rosemary oil** for an invigorating soak.

● Lie on your back and use pillows to prop your feet at a level higher than your head or, better still, lie on an adjustable exercise bench or other surface that slants. In India, yogis fight fatigue through such practices by encouraging **bloodflow to the brain**, which is thought to boost alertness.

High-octane eating

● **Eat a good breakfast** along with several small meals and healthy snacks throughout the day. That is better than eating two or three large meals. Try to limit the size of your meals to 300 calories. This will keep your blood sugar levels steady and help to prevent your energy levels plunging.

● **Go easy on** foods high in **refined carbohydrates** – that is, lots of white sugar or white flour. These foods make your blood sugar rise rapidly, then crash quickly. French bread, spaghetti and cake are not your best choices. You'll end up feeling weak and tired.

● Eat more high-fibre foods that are rich in **complex carbo-hydrates**, such as wholegrain cereals, wholemeal bread and vegetables. These help to stabilize blood sugar.

- **Cut down on** your intake of **fatty foods.** To improve the function of your adrenal glands – which influence the way you metabolize nutrients – you should have no more than 10 per cent saturated fat in your diet.
- Cut a washed, **unpeeled potato** into slices and leave the pieces to soak in water overnight. In the morning, drink the juice for a natural tonic brimming with potassium. Your body needs this mineral for transmitting nerve impulses and making muscles move, along with other vital functions; in fact, some natural healers maintain that deficiencies are common in people with fatigue.

Supplement your energy stores

- Ginseng is an ancient cure for that rundown feeling. Look for a supplement containing extracts standardized on ginsenoside content (in the case of Panax ginsengs) or eleutheroside content (in the case of Siberian ginseng). Take 100-250mg Panax ginseng extract (or 300-400mg Siberian ginseng) once or twice a day. This herbal remedy stimulates your nervous system and will help to protect your body from the ravages of stress. (*Alert* Do not take ginseng if you have high blood pressure.)
- Try taking 150mg of **magnesium** (preferably as magnesium citrate) twice a day. This mineral is involved in hundreds of chemical reactions in the body. It plays a role in changing protein, fat and carbohydrates into energy sources. A mild deficiency may be the cause of fatigue in some people.
- **Ginkgo** improves bloodflow to the brain, which can make you feel more alert and less fatigued. Take 15 drops of ginkgo tincture in the mornings.
- Consider supplements of the amino acid **carnitine.** This amino acid helps to fuel the activity of mitochondria, cell components that produce energy. It's found in some foods, but most people don't get enough in their diets. Follow the dosage directions on the label.
- **Coenzyme Q_{10},** a substance produced by the body, also helps your mitochondria make energy. Take 50mg twice a day, at breakfast and supper. It's best absorbed when taken with food. It may take eight weeks before you notice any effect. Coenzyme Q_{10} is also found in certain foods, including nuts and oils.

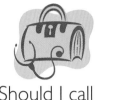

Should I call **the doctor?**

If you feel 'tired all the time' even after taking steps to treat fatigue, make an appointment to see your doctor. Fatigue can be a symptom of thyroid problems, depression, diabetes, anaemia and many other conditions. If you have fatigue along with the sudden onset of abdominal pain, shortness of breath or severe headache, seek immediate medical attention.

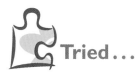

Tried...

Eating spinach once a day is a time honoured remedy for relieving fatigue and we all know what it did for Popeye...

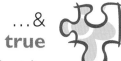

...& true

You can't go wrong. Spinach contains potassium as well as many B vitamins, all of which are important to energy metabolism.

What to drink

- Sip **water** all day long, at least eight glasses. Don't wait until you're thirsty, because your 'thirst alarm' isn't always accurate. Even a little dehydration can make you feel tired.
- **Keep caffeinated drinks to a minimum.** The caffeine in coffee and some colas can give you a short-term burst of energy, but following that rush, there's usually a 'crash'.
- **Limit alcohol consumption.** Alcohol depresses your central nervous system. It also reduces your blood sugar level.

Get your engine moving

- Most days of the week, try to do at least 30 minutes of **aerobic exercise**. Not only does exercise help you to shed pounds (carrying extra weight is tiring), it also gives you an energy boost. People who exercise regularly find they also tend to sleep better.
- Consider taking up **yoga** or **tai chi.** These ancient forms of exercise allow you to get physical activity, but they also include relaxation components that can be reinvigorating.
- Fit in 10 minutes of **low-level exercise** when you feel sluggish. Usually people with fatigue have a decreased supply of adenosine diphosphate (ADP), an intracellular 'messenger' involved in energy metabolism. Translated, it means there's not enough 'spark' in the engine. Almost any kind of activity will help – singing, taking deep breaths, walking or stretching.

Nod off to switch on

- Always **get up at the same time**, even at weekends. Your body will eventually get the hang of a regular sleep routine.
- **Go to bed earlier** than normal if you need extra sleep. As long as you're getting up at the same time every morning, it's fine to have a flexible going-to-bed schedule.
- **Keep naps short.** If you snooze for more than half an hour during the day, your body will want more and you'll feel groggy when you wake up.

Complete the picture

- Take a daily **multivitamin** to ensure you're getting the minimum amount of nutrients your body needs. Deficiencies can deplete your energy stores.

Fever

If your forehead is fiery with fever, you could reach for paracetamol or ibuprofen to lower your temperature. But if your fever is 38.5°C (101°F) or below, don't be afraid to let it run its course; you have a raised temperature for a reason – a fever enhances the body's defence mechanisms. If you are uncomfortable and want to take action, try these cooling tips. (*Never give anyone under the age of 16 aspirin for a raised temperature; doing so can trigger a potentially fatal disease called Reye's syndrome.*)

Be cool

- Take a **bath in lukewarm water.** This temperature will feel pretty cool when you have a fever and the bath should help to bring your body temperature down. Don't try to bring a fever down rapidly by plunging yourself into cold water; that will send blood rushing to your internal organs, which is how the body defends itself from cold. Your interior actually warms up instead of cooling down.
- Give yourself a **sponge bath.** Tepid sponging of high-heat areas like the armpits and groin with cool water can help to reduce a temperature as the water evaporates.
- When you're not bathing, place **cold, damp flannels** on your forehead and the back of your neck.

Sweat it out

- Brew a cup of **yarrow tea.** This herb opens your pores and triggers sweating, helping to move a fever on. Steep a tablespoon of the herb in a cup of boiling water for 10 minutes. Let it cool and strain. Drink a cup or two until you start to sweat.
- Another herb, **elderflower**, also helps you to sweat. And it happens to be good for other problems associated with flu and colds, like overproduction of mucus. To make elderflower tea, mix 2 teaspoons of the herb in a cup of boiling water and let it steep for 15 minutes. Strain out the elderflower. Drink three times a day as long as the fever continues.
- Drink a cup of hot **ginger tea**, which also induces sweating. To make the tea, steep ½ teaspoon of minced root ginger in a cup of boiling water. Strain, then drink.

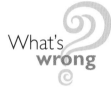

What's **wrong**

A fever is often a sign that your body is fighting off infection. As your white blood cells battle with microscopic invaders, they release chemicals that raise your body temperature, making the environment less friendly to viruses and bacteria. In adults, a temperature higher than 38°C (100°F) is generally regarded as a fever. In older children and adults, a fever below 38.5°C (101°F) doesn't necessarily need to be treated unless sweating, shivering or both is causing severe discomfort. But in babies and very young infants, any fever should be treated.

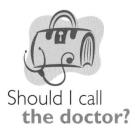

Should I call the doctor?

Contact your doctor if you have a temperature of 39.5°C (103°F) or higher or if a temperature of 38.5°C (101°F) lasts longer than three days. Also, call your doctor **immediately** if the fever is accompanied by a stiff neck, severe headache or rash that does not fade when pressed beneath the side of a glass. Other symptoms that need medical attention are extreme drowsiness, shortness of breath, burning on passing urine, red streaks near a wound or sensitivity to light. And consult your doctor about any fever in infants younger than six months.

Old **wives'** tale

Forget the old saying about 'starving a fever' to make it go away. (Actually, the original saying was 'feed a cold, *stave* a fever', *stave* meaning to prevent.) Fasting will weaken you just as you should be preserving your strength. Even if you don't feel like eating, at least have some chicken soup and toast or other soothing foods.

Fight fire with fire

- Sprinkle **cayenne pepper** on your food when you have a fever. One of its main components is capsaicin, the fiery ingredient found in hot peppers. Cayenne makes you sweat and also promotes rapid blood circulation.

Soak your socks

- Try the **wet sock treatment**, a popular folk remedy for fever. First warm your feet in hot water. Then soak a thin pair of cotton socks in cold water, wring them out and put them on just before going to bed. Pull a pair of dry wool socks over the wet ones. This approach helps to ease a fever by drawing blood to the feet, which dramatically increases blood circulation. Don't try this cure if your bedroom is uncomfortably chilly.
- Another way to draw blood to the feet is with a **mustard footbath**. In a basin large enough for your feet – a washing-up bowl is ideal – add 2 teaspoons of mustard powder per litre of hot water, then soak.

Roll up in a wet sheet

- An old folk remedy for treating a fever is to **soak a sheet in cold water** and wrap yourself in it. Modern doctors advise against lowering your body temperature too quickly, so if you try this remedy use tepid rather than cold water. Cover the wet sheet with a large beach towel or blanket, then lie down for about 15 minutes. Unwrap yourself when the wet sheet starts to get warm.

Fill up on fluids

- When you have a fever, it's easy to become dehydrated. Drink 8 to 12 glasses of **water** a day or enough to make your urine pale. A sports drink like Lucozade Sport can also be helpful. It not only replaces fluids lost to dehydration but lost minerals as well.
- Orange juice and other fruit juices rich in **vitamin C** are good choices, because vitamin C helps your immune system to fight off infection.
- Cold **grapes** provide hydration – and a soothing treat.

Food poisoning

Summer picnics, barbecues and al fresco eating should be, and usually are, fun. It's the aftermath that isn't always such a laugh. Nausea, vomiting, diarrhoea and stomach pain are all symptoms of food poisoning, a form of gastroenteritis caused by eating or drinking something contaminated with micro-organisms or by the toxic substances produced by them. If you are suffering, here are some ways to feel better. And, just as important, some tips to make sure it never happens again.

Rehydrate your body

- One of the potential dangers of diarrhoea and vomiting is dehydration. Particularly at risk are young children and people who are frail, elderly or have a weakened immune system. **Drink lots of water** or water-based fluids. If you're vomiting, take **plenty of sips** rather than gulping down a glassful.
- **Replace salts and sugars** lost through diarrhoea, especially if you can't keep any food down. Try sipping this balanced drink: squeeze the juice of 2 oranges; add ½ teaspoon of salt and 2 teaspoons of honey. Top up with water until you have 500ml. Try to drink a glass every half hour, in little sips if necessary, until your symptoms improve.
- You can also buy **oral rehydration sachets**, such as Dioralyte or Rehidrat, over the counter from a pharmacy.
- **Experiment** to see whether you keep down warm drinks better than cold ones.
- Drink **herbal teas** such as camomile, thyme, ginger, peppermint and fennel. These soothing herbs are mildly antiseptic and will help to relieve stomach cramps.

External comforters

- Have a warm bath laced with essential oils. Sprinkle 3 drops each of geranium and ginger oils and 2 of peppermint oil into the bathwater. Soak for about 20 minutes, keeping the bath topped up with warm water.
- **Massage your tummy** with soothing oils – or ask a loved one to do it for you. Add 3 drops of tea tree oil and 2 drops each of peppermint, geranium and sandalwood oils to

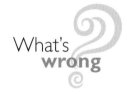

What's **wrong**

You've eaten something that has given you food poisoning. The trouble is, it could be anything from ten days ago to as little as an hour earlier, which can make it difficult to pinpoint the source. It may have been a piece of slightly pink chicken from the barbecue, or a lukewarm burger from a van at the football ground or an egg mayonnaise sandwich from the local deli. You feel sick and shivery, your muscles are aching and all you want to do is to curl up in bed and sleep until the nightmare goes away. Micro-organisms have entered your body in one of two ways – either the food containing them hasn't been cooked thoroughly, or the person preparing your food is carrying the bug and has not washed his or her hands properly before handling the food.

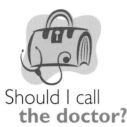

Should I call the doctor?

5 teaspoons of a carrier oil, such as almond oil BP (sold at pharmacies). Put the oils into a glass and stand it in a pan of hot water so as to warm the oil to body temperature. Use the oil to massage your abdomen in smooth, firm, clockwise circles for as long as it feels comfortable.

Find the pressure points

● There is an **acupressure point** on your outer calf that can help to relieve diarrhoea. Find it eight finger-widths below the lower edge of the kneecap, one finger-width outwards from the front of the shinbone. Press the point with your thumb for 2 minutes on each leg.

● For **nausea and vomiting**, the point is located on your arm. Press the point between the tendons two thumb-widths above the crease of your inner wrist. This is the area that acupressure bands, sold for motion sickness, are designed to stimulate.

Ginger – the miracle worker

Ginger counters nausea and vomiting. If you can manage it, try chewing a piece of fresh root ginger (hot!) or crystallized ginger; or drink ginger tea – available in sachets from supermarkets and health-food shops; or take ginger tablets.

Bind it up

● Make a binding drink. Mix a tablespoon of **arrowroot** with a little water to form a smooth paste, then add 500ml boiling water and stir it as it thickens. Flavour with honey or lemon juice. Drinking this at regular intervals throughout the day will help to solidify bowel contents.

Back to normal

● **Start with rice**. Once you begin to feel better, you need a non-irritating food that will help to bind your bowels. Simple boiled white rice is just what the doctor ordered. The water in which the rice has been boiled is an easily digested post-tummy-upset food for very young children.

● Once you can hold down a little rice, introduce other bland foods such as clear **chicken stock** (easily made by simmering cooked chicken bones for 30 minutes, straining and adding salt to taste), low fat yoghurt, toast without butter and apple purée.

Heinz babyfoods make a good pure apple purée if you feel too weak to make your own.

- As you recover, eat some **live yoghurt** each day to help restore the balance of micro-organisms in your intestines.
- Add a daily **vitamin and mineral supplement** to restore your body's nutrient balance.

The power of prevention

In order to prevent food poisoning at home, cleanliness is vital. This involves personal hygiene and careful choosing, storing and using of food.

- Always **wash hands** thoroughly with soap and warm water after using the toilet and before preparing food or eating. Be especially careful handling raw chicken and wash hands afterwards, and before touching anything – especially other foods such as salads that are not going to be cooked.
- Keep **kitchen work surfaces**, the fridge, freezer and chopping boards clean, and **scrub tin openers**.
- Keep one chopping board that you use only for **raw meats**.
- **Keep pets away** from food and off work surfaces.
- Disinfect sponges, dishcloths and washing-up brushes in a **diluted bleach solution** at least twice a week, and get out **clean tea towels** every day.
- **Defrost** food **completely** in the refrigerator, not on the worktop, before cooking, and **do not refreeze**. Or thaw frozen meat in the microwave and cook as soon as it's thawed.
- **Cook raw meats thoroughly** and reheat leftovers until piping hot.
- Store **raw foods** covered up at the bottom of the fridge, and keep cooked and uncooked meats on separate shelves.
- Store all perishable foods at 5°C (41°F) or colder.
- Rinse fruit and vegetables carefully before eating.
- Throw away food that is **past its 'use-by' date**, that smells odd or has fungus on it. Be especially careful with chicken and shellfish. Don't buy or use dented or swollen cans or jars whose lids appear swollen.

(See also *Diarrhoea*, page 144 and *Nausea*, page 296)

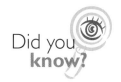

Did you **know?**

Eggs with hairline cracks may be harbouring salmonella bacteria. Don't use them – put them straight in the bin.

Foot odour

Do people hold their noses when you kick off your shoes? Has the family dog fallen in love with your trainers? There are plenty of solutions that go much further than bicarbonate of soda to stop the sweat, eat the odour and keep your feet from smelling like … smelly feet. In particular, many people swear by changing their socks at least twice a day and using antiperspirant on their (washed) feet.

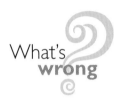

What's wrong

Your feet are the natural habitat of millions of bacteria, which thrive on your sweat and shed skin cells. By-products produced by these bacteria are what give feet that stinky smell. When you seal your feet in a pair of shoes and they pour out sweat, you give the bacteria more food to feast on. Foot odour can also be caused by poorly controlled fungal infections, such as athlete's foot. People with diabetes or heart disease, as well as elderly people in general, are often more prone to foot infections and foot odour due to inefficient blood circulation.

Give feet the armpit treatment

● It shouldn't come as a surprise that the same **antiperspirant** as you use on your armpits can also keep your feet less sweaty (and therefore less smelly). Simply spray or roll it on before putting on your shoes and socks.

● Wash your feet every day in warm water using a **deodorant soap** or **antibacterial soap**.

Turn up the heat

● After a bath or shower, blow dry your feet with a **hair-dryer** set to its lowest temperature. This is especially good advice if you are prone to athlete's foot or nail fungus as it helps to prevent infection and reduces moisture.

Soak them and scent them

● Try a **black tea footbath.** Simmer two teabags in 500ml water for 15 minutes. Remove the bags and dilute the tea with 2 litres of water, then soak your feet for 30 minutes. Repeat every day. The tannic acid in strong black tea kills bacteria and closes pores to help your feet sweat less.

● Make an odour-fighting foot soak by adding a cup of **vinegar** to a basin of warm water. For more odour-fighting force, add a few drops of **thyme oil.** The oil contains a strong antiseptic that kills odour-causing bacteria. Soak your feet for 15 to 20 minutes a day for a week. (*Alert* Do not use this remedy if you have any open sores or broken skin.)

● If you don't have access to thyme oil, you can easily buy a product that contains it: **Listerine** mouthwash. Try adding a splash to your footbath. (Again, don't use on broken skin.)

Fragrant foot rub

- **Lavender oil** not only smells good, it can also help to kill bacteria. Rub a few drops onto your feet and massage it in before you go to bed at night. Cover your feet with socks. Before trying this remedy, you should check to make sure that the oil will not irritate your skin by putting one drop on a small area.

Epsom salts soak

- Mix 2 cups of **Epsom salts** with 4 litres of warm water in a bucket or basin. Soak your feet for 15 minutes twice a day. The astringent Epsom salts will help to reduce sweating and may kill bacteria.

Try an acne treatment

- Apply a **benzoyl peroxide** gel (sold over the counter in pharmacies as an acne treatment) to the bottom of your feet in order to fight bacteria. It can be effective, working in the same way as it does on the bacteria that cause acne.

Powder power

- Dust your feet with **talcum powder** or **foot powder** before you put on your shoes and socks. It will absorb odour-causing sweat.
- Two other good foot powders to try are **bicarbonate of soda**, which neutralizes odour, and **cornflour**, which absorbs moisture.

Dress well for a better smell

- **Change your socks** at least once and preferably two or three times a day, replacing them with a clean pair each time.
- Alternate between at least **two pairs of shoes**. After you've worn one pair, set them aside and let them air out for at least 24 hours.
- Wear shoes with **open-mesh** sides or open sandals that allow your feet to 'breathe'. Your feet will also breathe better if you wear **cotton socks** rather than synthetic blends.
- The best cure, of course, is to stop wearing shoes – so dump those smelly old slippers and pad around the house (at least) **barefoot whenever possible**.

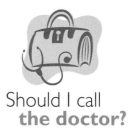

Should I call the doctor?

See your GP if you have athlete's foot that does not clear up with home treatment, excessive sweating even without trainers, or any signs of fungal infection of the nails. You may have an infection that requires a prescription antibiotic or antifungal medication.

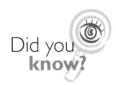

You have more than 250,000 sweat glands on your feet, which pump out as much as half a pint of sweat each day.

Treat trainers too

● Check the care instructions on your sports shoes. If they're washable, chuck them into the **washing machine** at least once a month.

Sweet-smelling shoes

● Store your shoes in a place that's **bright** and well **ventilated** – not in a dark wardrobe or cupboard where bacteria thrive.

● Each time you put your shoes away, insert a sachet filled with **cedar chips** into them. You can buy cedar chips packed in breathable cotton bags designed to fit into shoes (try a shoe repair centre). They absorb moisture, neutralize embarrassing odours and keep shoes dry and comfortable.

● You can also buy shoe inserts that consist of mesh pouches filled with **zeolite** (available online). Zeolite is a natural volcanic mineral that attracts odours and moisture and traps them. Expose the reusable pouch to the sun for six hours to discharge the collected odours.

● Another option is to put a couple of handfuls of **dried lavender** into a hanky and tie it up with a rubber band. Place one lavender bag in each shoe over night.

● Apparently **cat litter** (clean) works a treat too. Scoop some into an old pair of socks and pop these into your shoes whenever you take them off. After all, that's what litter is designed to do – neutralize odours and absorb moisture…

● Buy odour-absorbing **insoles** that contain activated charcoal and cut them to fit. Replace them every three to six months.

● If your shoes have removable insoles, **take them out to dry** every time you remove your shoes. And put them in the washing machine from time to time.

Foot pain

Sometimes foot pain has an obvious cause, such as a fungal infection (athlete's foot), corn, callus or ingrowing toenail. But if the discomfort you feel stems simply from fatigue or ill-fitting shoes, your best friend may be water – warm or cold, with or without herbal extras – or an invigorating foot massage. If no one is willing to give you a foot massage then read on – here are some easy ways to give your feet a treat.

Pamper your feet with water and oils

- For a refreshing and stimulating treat for the feet, fill one basin with **cold water** and another with water as **hot** as you can comfortably stand. Sit in a comfortable chair, and place your feet in the cold water. After 5 minutes, switch to the hot water. Repeat. This 'hydromassage' alternately dilates and constricts blood vessels in your feet, boosting circulation.
- To pamper your feet with essential oils – a ritual dating back to biblical times – fill a bowl with hot water and add 2 drops of **peppermint oil**, along with 4 drops each of **eucalyptus** and **rosemary oil**. Soak your feet for 10 minutes.
- If you don't have any essential oils at home, brew up a very strong cup of **peppermint tea** and add it to the water.
- Soak your feet in a warm-water footbath spiked with 15g **arnica tincture**. The improved bloodflow almost instantly results in less pain.

Massage magic

- In health-food shops, you can buy a **roller** that is specially designed to massage the soles of the feet. Or you can simply roll your bare foot over a **tennis ball**, **golf ball** or **rolling pin** for several minutes.
- To make a **stimulating massage oil** to soothe your foot pain, combine 3 drops of clove oil, which is thought to be a mild circulation booster, and 3 tablespoons of sesame oil. Mix the ingredients well and massage the oils into your aching feet. Another foot-rub recipe calls for 3 drops of lavender oil, 1 drop of camomile oil and 1 drop of geranium oil mixed into 2 teaspoons of olive oil.

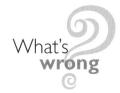

What's **wrong**

You spend up to 80 per cent of your waking hours on your feet and each day, on average, an adult takes 8,000 to 10,000 steps. So it's hardly surprising that, from time to time, your feet end up hurting. Virtually anything can cause foot pain, including shoes that don't fit properly, diseases such as arthritis and diabetes, and poor circulation.

Should I call **the doctor?**

Aid to the fallen

• Shoe inserts, or **orthotics**, help to relieve foot pain caused by flat feet or fallen arches. These are custom-made to fit into your shoes – a podiatrist can measure your feet for fit.

Give feet a workout

• Scatter a few **pencils** on the floor, and pick them up with your toes. This little exercise helps to relieve foot ache.
• Wrap a thick **rubber band** around all the toes on one foot. Spread your toes and hold the stretch for five seconds. Repeat ten times to relieve shoe-bound feet.

Heal your heel

• Heel pain, especially in the morning, may signal plantar fasciitis, an inflammation of the tough band of tissue that connects your heel bone to the base of your toes. To obtain relief, **stretch the Achilles tendon**. Stand about a metre from a wall. Place your hands on the wall, and move your right leg forwards, knee bent. Keep your left leg straight, with your heel on the floor. You should feel a gentle stretch in your heel and foot arch. Hold for 10 seconds, switch sides and repeat.
• Apply an **ice pack** to the sore heel for about 20 minutes three times a day.
• Buy a **heel cup** from a pharmacy. It fits inside the shoe, cushioning the heel and protecting it from a pounding.

The power of prevention

• Whenever you have to stand in one place for a long time – when you're running a stall at a school fete, for instance – **stand on a rubber mat**.
• **Wear running shoes** whenever possible, even if you don't run. They provide the best cushioning and arch support. If you don't want to wear running shoes, at least choose shoes with thick soles.
• **Shop for new shoes in the afternoon**, when your feet have expanded to their maximum size. If you wear insoles, be sure to take them shopping with you, so as to make sure your new shoes will fit with the insoles in position.

Fungal infections

Any fungal infection spreads easily. Most women will suffer the itching and discomfort of a vaginal yeast infection at least once in their lives and no one is immune from tineal infections such as ringworm and athlete's foot. In most cases, fungal infections are easily treated with over-the-counter antifungal creams or an oral antifungal drug (available over the counter or on prescription). Whatever medication you're using, other measures can also help in treating and preventing a recurrence.

Dealing with thrush

Probably the most common fungal infection, thrush, or candidiasis, is caused by the yeast organism *Candida albicans*. It usually occurs in the vagina but can also appear in the mouth and in damp skin folds. Couples may also pass a yeast infection back and forth during sex. If you have a vaginal yeast infection, be sure your partner isn't also infected, which most often happens in uncircumcised men.

- For vaginal infections, douche twice a day, for two days in a row, with a mixture of 2 tablespoons white **vinegar** in a litre of water. This slightly acidic solution creates an unfriendly environment for yeast. But you should do this only for two days, and only when you have a yeast infection. If you use a vinegar douche when it is not necessary, you rinse out the beneficial bacteria that keep infections at bay.
- Infections in both men and women can be easily treated with over-the-counter creams, such as Canestan. Applying natural yoghurt can also relieve the pain.
- Sprinkle a cup of **sea salt** into a warm bath, stir the water around until the salt dissolves and have a nice soak. You can do this every day, as long as it helps to relieve itching and pain. The saltwater soak also speeds up healing. Rinsing with a saltwater solution can be useful for treating oral thrush too.

Try infection-fighting garlic

- Eat a few cloves of **garlic** each day. The pungent cloves have been used since ancient times to combat everything from colds to intestinal infections. Its antifungal action makes it useful

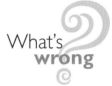

What's wrong

We all carry small amounts of yeast. Called *Candida albicans*, it inhabits various moist parts of our bodies, usually without causing problems. But occasionally something triggers yeast cells to multiply. One trigger is antibiotics, which can kill off beneficial bacteria that keep yeast populations in check. Most women will have a vaginal yeast infection at some point in their lives and the infection can be spread to a sexual partner. In women, symptoms include itching, redness and a thick white discharge, often said to resemble cottage cheese. In men, who have become infected, the foreskin and penis head is usually red and inflamed. It is best to avoid sex until the infection has cleared.

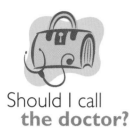

Should I call the doctor?

against yeast infections. It's most effective if crushed and eaten raw. If you don't fancy the idea of munching a whole clove, crush it and add to a salad dressing or stir into pasta sauce.

- Some people recommend inserting a gauze-wrapped garlic clove into the vagina. But most women will prefer using an **antifungal cream** – especially as garlic can sting.

Battle yeast with bacteria

- Every day, eat a cup of plain, unsweetened **yoghurt** containing live *Lactobacillus acidophilus* bacteria. This has been shown to reduce yeast overgrowth in the vagina and the intestines. However, if you have a bacterial as opposed to a yeast infection, yoghurt might make matters worse.

Other fungus fighters

- Prepare a solution of **cinnamon**, which research suggests has strong antifungal properties. (In fact, some German researchers concluded that impregnating toilet paper with cinnamon would completely suppress the fungus responsible for yeast infections.) Add 8 broken sticks of cinnamon to 4 cups of boiling water and simmer for about 5 minutes. Take off the heat and leave to steep for about 45 minutes. Some herbalists advise using the lukewarm solution as a douche; others say that drinking cinnamon tea helps to control yeast infections.
- To help your immune system fight the infection, take three 200mg doses of **echinacea** three times a day, or a dropper of tincture in half a cup of water four times a day. Take echinacea daily for up to two weeks, then stop taking it for two weeks.

Keeping thrush at bay

- Contrary to popular belief, a diet high in carbohydrates or **sugar does not increase your risk** of a yeast infection. There's no benefit to be gained from eating a yeast-free diet, either. The yeast that is used in breadmaking is not the same type as that responsible for yeast infections.
- **Go without underwear at night.** As yeast flourishes in warm, moist environments, the ventilation will help you to avoid infection. **During the day**, go knickerless, too, whenever you can. Otherwise, choose cotton knickers, which allow better air circulation than synthetic fabrics.

- For the same reason, **avoid tight trousers**.
- **Don't stay in a wet bathing suit** after swimming. Shower promptly and change into dry clothes.
- Use a **hair dryer** on its cool setting to dry the external vaginal area completely after a bath or a swim.
- **Don't use soap** or hot water to clean the vaginal area. This removes healthy natural skin barriers that help to control yeast.
- **Keep away from scented tampons**, feminine deodorants and douches. Chemicals in fragrances can upset the delicate environment in the vagina and allow yeast to take over.
- Also **avoid perfumed talc**. Some women find that powder irritates the skin and this additional irritation makes them more prone to yeast infection.
- Go to the toilet **after you make love**. Mucous membranes of the vagina are normally slightly acidic, but semen is alkaline, making it friendlier to yeast. Passing urine will help to make the area less inviting to infectious growth.

Repelling ringworm

Ringworm – once thought to be an actual worm lurking beneath the skin – is a common fungal infection of the skin.
- At the first sign of infection, look for over-the-counter **antifungal remedies** that contain ingredients such as miconazole or clotrimazole. Brands include Canesten AF and Daktarin. Most need to be applied twice a day. If you follow the package directions, ringworm should start to clear within a week. Apply twice a day for at least eight weeks to be sure of getting rid of the infection completely.
- Be sure you keep the affected patch **clean and dry**.
- If the infection starts to ooze or blister over, apply cool or warm **moist compresses**. Or soak in water with dissolved **Epsom salts** to help dry up the oozing rash. Take care not to break the blisters, and see a doctor as soon as possible.

In a nutshell

- If ringworm strikes in autumn, you might be able to cure it with the outer casing of a **walnut**. Walnut trees bear fruits that look like large pale green plums. The walnut, in its shell, is surrounded by a distinctive-smelling thick green rind. Crush the rind into a pulp and apply it to ringworm up to four

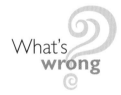

What's wrong?

Ringworm is a fungal infection of the skin that tends to creep insidiously along the groin, scalp, feet and face. It often begins as a round, itchy red patch that grows outwards. As it expands, the middle area heals, but all round it is a red scaly ring where infection continues to spread. If it's on your scalp, there will be some flaky skin and patches of hair loss. The condition is contagious, ringworm thrives in warm, moist environments and is often spread when people touch an infected surface such as a shower floor.

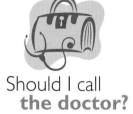

Should I call the doctor?

times a day until the condition clears up. (*Alert* The pulp is poisonous to eat, so make sure it only goes on your skin.)

The curry cure

• Cure ringworm with **turmeric**. The main ingredient in curry powder, turmeric contains curcumin, which has helped many people who have inflammatory conditions, such as arthritis. It's not clear why turmeric should work so well on a fungal skin problem, but Asian medicine has long used this spice to fight ringworm. Stir enough water into a teaspoon or two of powdered turmeric to make a paste. Spread it on the affected area and cover it with a piece of gauze. After 20 minutes to an hour, remove it. You can repeat this three or four times a day, but stop the treatment if turmeric irritates your skin.

The power of prevention

• **Don't share shoes or used towels** with other people – they can spread an infection.

• If family members have ringworm, make sure that **no one shares clothes** or **hairbrushes**.

• Wash in **hot water** any clothes, towels, flannels and bed-clothes that may have come in touch with the infected area.

• Be sure to dry your feet completely soon after swimming or bathing, using a **hair dryer** whenever possible. The area between the toes is the most common place for fungus to start growing.

• Instead of going barefoot at a public swimming pool, wear **flip-flops** or **sandals** to avoid picking up fungus.

• Use an **antifungal powder** in your shoes or your groin area to absorb excess moisture.

• Pets can carry ringworm that can be transferred to humans. If you see a **hairless spot on your dog or cat**, take the animal to the vet as soon as possible for ringworm treatment.

(See also *Athlete's foot*, page 52 and *Itching*, page 255.)

Gout

The agony of gout can start very quickly. One minute, you're skipping along with a smile on your face and a song in your heart. The next, you're in excruciating pain. Your first instinct might be to reach for aspirin – bad move. Aspirin slows down the excretion of uric acid, which only makes things worse. A much better bet is ibuprofen. Like aspirin, this is an anti-inflammatory painkiller, but it does not aggravate the condition. Then you can turn to these home remedies to further reduce pain. Make sure you are strict with yourself about drinking plenty of water, as this will dissolve uric acid crystals.

Lift off and ice down

- During an acute attack, try to **stay off your feet** as much as possible and keep the affected joint elevated. This probably won't be a problem. When gout is at its worst, most people can't even bear the weight of a sheet on the painful joint.
- If you can stand it, apply an **ice pack** for 20 minutes or so. The cold will dull the pain and bring down the swelling. Wrap the ice in a cloth to protect your skin. Use the ice pack three times a day for two or three days.

Try the cherry remedy

- **Cherries** are an old folk remedy for gout. They contain compounds that help to neutralize uric acid in the blood. Cherries are also a source of anti-inflammatory compounds. So if you feel an attack of gout coming on, try eating a handful or two or cherries right away. If they aren't in season, buy canned. Studies suggest that you need about 20 cherries to get the same pain relieving effects as one aspirin. Fresh or dried cherries work equally well.
- If you don't like cherries, **strawberries** and **raspberries** have a similar effect to cherries, but you need to eat a lot more.

Supplements to the rescue

- Daily doses of **fish oil** or **flax seed oil** can ease the inflammation in the joints. These oils are rich sources of a potent anti-inflammatory agent known as eicosapentaenoic acid (EPA). The recommended dose of flax seed oil is 1–3g a day

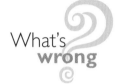

What's **wrong**

When too much uric acid (produced in the liver and excreted in the urine) builds up in your system, needle-sharp crystals of the compound can form in the fluid that cushions your joints. You may feel like you have shards of glass jammed into your joints. This painful inflammatory condition, known as gout, usually occurs in men over age 40 (it takes years for uric acid crystals to build up). Though it most often affects the big toe, gout can strike the wrist, knee, elbow or another joint. Besides pain, gout can cause severe swelling.

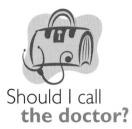

Should I call the doctor?

(1g oil is about a tablespoon). Buy flax seed oil rather than capsules – more than a dozen capsules are needed to equal 1 tablespoon of oil. The recommended dose for fish oil is 6000mg a day in capsule or oil form. (*Alert* At this dose, it must be fish oil, *not* fish liver or cod liver oil. This amount of fish liver oil would contain the right level of anti-inflammatory agents but far too much vitamin A and D.)

● Another way to ease inflammation is with pills containing **bromelain**, an enzyme found in pineapple. To achieve a therapeutic effect, a product must contain 2000MCUs (milk clotting units) per gram. Check the label information before you buy. The usual dosage for acute gout attacks is 500mg three times a day between meals.

● Fresh celery, or tablets containing **celery seed extract**, seem to help eliminate uric acid. The usual dose is 2 to 4 tablets a day.

● Long advocated by herbalists to treat joint inflammation, **nettle leaf** also helps to lower uric acid levels. Experts usually recommend 300 to 600mg of a freeze-dried extract a day. Don't use nettle for any longer than three months at a time. (*Alert* Avoid nettle in tincture form. Tinctures contain alcohol, which aggravates gout.) Another way to use nettle is topically. Soak a clean cloth in a tea brewed from the leaves of nettle and apply it to the tender joint. If you pick this common weed yourself, wear gloves, long trousers and long sleeves to protect yourself against nettle's stinging leaves.

Live on water, not beer

● Drink lots of **water** – at least eight 250ml glasses a day. Fluids will help to flush excess uric acid from your system. As a bonus, the water may help to discourage kidney stones, which disproportionately affect people with gout.

Foods to avoid

High-protein foods, as well as foods that contain chemical compounds known as purines, can raise levels of uric acid in the body. If you have gout, the list of foods to avoid includes meat-based gravy; offal – such as liver, kidneys and sweetbreads; shellfish, such as mussels; anchovies, sardines and herring; game; fried foods; refined carbohydrates (such as white flour); oatmeal; yeast-containing foods like beer and baked goods; and certain vegetables including asparagus, peas, beans, spinach and cauliflower.

- **Avoid alcohol.** It seems to increase uric acid production and inhibit its excretion. Beer is particularly bad – it contains more purines (see panel below left) than other alcoholic beverages.

Check your medicines

- If you take diuretics – for high blood pressure, for instance – ask your doctor about **alternatives.** Diuretics eliminate excess fluids from the body; as a side effect they reduce the amount of uric acid that passes in the urine. Less passes, more remains in your body – and the worse your gout.
- Gout can also be **triggered by niacin** or **nicotinic acid,** which is sometimes prescribed for high cholesterol. If your doctor has prescribed niacin for you, ask about alternatives.

Fast not, hurt not

- Losing weight can help to keep gout at bay, but going on a crash diet or fasting is a big mistake. Drastic dieting causes cells to release more uric acid. If you're overweight, **lose weight slowly** and sensibly – a kilo (2lb) a week at most.

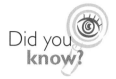

Did you **know?**

Because only the wealthy could once afford foods like herring, prawns and fatty meats, known to trigger gout attacks, gout used to be known as a rich man's disease.

Greasy hair

Does it look as if someone's oiled your hair? Is it lank and unappealing? Don't blame your hygiene habits, because your problem is probably hereditary. Fight back with the right shampoo – make sure you wash and rinse your hair twice – and try a special grease-stopping rinse you can make yourself.

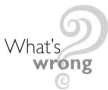

What's wrong

Your hair is lank, limp and stuck to your head. It may even look dirty, although you washed it yesterday (or just hours ago). But don't blame your hair. Blame the oil-producing sebaceous glands that lie just beneath the surface of your skin. They secrete sebum, a mixture of fatty acids that protects your scalp. Some people's sebaceous glands pump out so much sebum that each hair becomes coated with the stuff. Genetics, stress, hormones – especially the male hormone, androgen – or a poor diet can contribute to the problem, as can certain contraceptive pills.

Read your shampoo bottle

● Choose a shampoo that's high in sodium lauryl sulphate and low in any type of conditioner, such as lanolin. What you want are **clarifying shampoos** that tend to strip oil from the scalp and the hair shaft.

● Even if you don't have dandruff, you might get good results with a dandruff shampoo containing **coal tar**. The formulas used for these shampoos tend to dry out even the oiliest hair.

Do the daily double

● It may seem obvious that you need to shampoo every day – maybe even twice a day in hot, humid weather. But on top of that, you should **shampoo twice** every time you wash your hair. Lather up, leave the shampoo on your hair for several minutes (that gives it time to remove the oil), rinse thoroughly, then repeat. Even on the second round, leave the shampoo in your hair for a few minutes before you rinse.

● **Don't use conditioner.** All this does is put back the oil you've so carefully washed away.

Change the rinse cycle

● Rinsing your hair with water is fine, but you'll get even better results if you use a strong **rosemary tea**. Wonderfully aromatic, this herb contains essential oils that help control overproduction of oil on the scalp. To make the rinse, pour a cup of boiling water over 2 tablespoons of dried rosemary. Steep for 20 minutes, strain, cool and pour into an empty plastic bottle. Keep this in the bathroom and splash your hair with the tea after the final clean water rinse. There's no need to rinse off the tea afterwards, as long as you like the fragrance.

Emergency talc 'shampoo'

You're running late – there's no time to shower. But your hair looks like an oil slick. For an emergency 'dry' shampoo, turn to your bottle of talcum powder. Part your hair and sprinkle on a small amount, one section at a time. Lightly massage the powder first into the scalp, then through your hair. The powder will absorb some of the oil. Voilà – an instant 'shampoo'. Remember, only use a small amount. If you use too much, you'll end up with dull tresses that look somewhat whitish.

• Make a **lemon juice** rinse. Blend juice from 2 lemons into 2 cups of distilled water and pour into an empty shampoo bottle. After washing and rinsing your hair, blot it dry and apply the mixture to your scalp. Leave it on for 5 minutes, allowing the acidic lemon juice to work on the oil. Then rinse with cool water.

• **Vinegar**, which is also acidic, can de-grease your hair too. Mix a cup of vinegar with a cup of water, then pour it over your hair as a final rinse. Don't worry about smelling like a salad – the smell will quickly fade.

Extreme measures: mouthwash

• If your hair is extremely oily, you can mix a solution that will help slow your scalp's production of sebum. In a small cup, mix equal parts **witch hazel** with any commercial **mouth-wash**. Both ingredients are astringents, which means they help to tighten skin pores as they dry. Dip a cotton wool ball in the solution and then dab it onto your scalp (not your hair) after you've finished shampooing and rinsing.

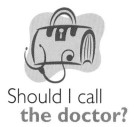

Should I call the doctor?

As physical challenges go, greasy hair isn't a serious problem, but it can be embarrassing. If you hate the look of your hair, and the advice in this chapter doesn't help, you may want to talk to your doctor about the possibility of being referred to a dermatologist.

Gum problems

If your gums are sore and you want instant pain relief, you can go to any chemist and buy a tube of gel containing the topical anaesthetic benzocaine. Or try a gargle or a soothing gum massage as described below. But your real battle is against plaque. Control plaque with regular visits to the dentist or hygienist and diligent brushing (use a soft-bristled brush and pay special attention to your gum line) and flossing, and you should be able to forget all about gum problems.

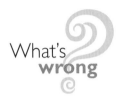

What's wrong

Are your gums puffy? Do they bleed when you brush? You probably have gingivitis, a form of gum inflammation caused by plaque, the sticky film of food particles and bacteria that accumulates on your teeth. Plaque irritates gums. If it isn't removed by brushing and flossing, it can turn into hard mineral deposits that are even more irritating (and which can be removed only by a dentist). Left untreated, gingivitis eventually leads to full-blown gum disease, in which the gums pull away from the teeth. The resulting germ-filled pockets can lead to painful abscesses and chronic bad breath, and can even cause your teeth to loosen and fall out.

Numb those gums

- To soothe gum pain and reduce swelling, rinse your mouth for 30 seconds with **salt water** (1 teaspoon mixed into a glass of warm water).
- Alternatively, rinse your mouth with **hydrogen peroxide** diluted in an equal amount of warm water. Like salt, hydrogen peroxide dulls the pain and helps to kill bacteria.
- Put a wet **teabag** on the painful area. Tea contains tannic acid, a powerful astringent that shrinks swollen tissues and helps to staunch bleeding. Think of it as a styptic pencil for your gums.
- Apply an **ice pack** (wrapped in a cloth) to your cheek near the painful area. Ice helps to reduce swelling and the cold also acts as a local anaesthetic. **Clove oil** and **baby teething gel** are also helpful in an acute episode.
- Dab your gums with a paste of **bicarbonate of soda** and water. Bicarb kills germs and helps to neutralize the acids they secrete, although too much of it can damage tender gum tissue.

Rub for relief

- What do you do when your muscles are sore? **Massage** them. And your gums benefit from massage too. Just grip them between your thumb and index finger and give a series of gentle squeezes. That helps to boost circulation to painful, irritated tissue, helping gums to heal faster.
- To enhance the soothing effect of a gum massage, try doing what practitioners of Ayurvedic medicine recommend – massage your gums with **coconut oil**.

• Another way to massage your gums is with a soft wooden **dental stimulator**, which you can buy at any chemist. Insert it between two teeth, point the tip so that it's at a 45-degree angle to the gum line, circle gently for a few seconds, then move on to the next two teeth.

• Buy an oral irrigation device such as Interplak and use **water pressure** to clean and massage your teeth and gums where your toothbrush cannot reach. **Electric toothbrushes** are a good buy, too. The small, spinning head can get at those hard-to-reach bits right at the back of your mouth.

• A time-tested wound healer, **calendula** may help sore gums by reducing inflammation. Simply rub the tincture directly onto the gums.

Rinse and gargle

• Try a product called **Gengigel** made by Oraldent. It's sold in some pharmacies and online. This is a biological mouth and gum-care gel based on a natural substance found in the connective tissues of the body (cartilage, synovial fluid, and skin) that is said to help stimulate the production of new, healthy tissue when applied to the gums.

• Rinsing your mouth with **camomile tea** is said to be highly effective against gingivitis. Simply pour a cup of hot water over 3 teaspoons of the herb, steep for 10 minutes, then strain and cool. Mix up a large quantity and keep it in the fridge.

• Over-the-counter mouthwashes can also help to heal your gums. Choose a brand that contains **cetylpyridinium chloride** or **domiphen bromide**. These ingredients have been shown to have a significant effect on reducing plaque. Anbesol liquid contains cetylpyridinium chloride and Scope contains both ingredients. Note that these are alcohol-based rinses and therefore prolonged use is inadvisable as it may increase the risk of oral cancer.

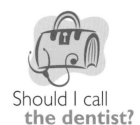

Should I call the dentist?

If you are having your teeth professionally cleaned and examined twice a year, minor gum irritation does not require a visit to the dentist. Consider your irritated gums as an alert that you need to pay more attention to brushing and flossing. Do make a dental appointment if you notice a change in the appearance of your gums or if they start bleeding. For intense pain, book an immediate appointment, especially if you have a raised temperature and swollen glands in your neck. You could have an abscess that needs prompt treatment.

Haemorrhoids

They're a common problem yet some people are still too embarrassed to seek help for the painful burning, itching and bleeding caused by haemorrhoids. Pharmacies sell many products that help – creams, pads, ointments and suppositories. As a rule of thumb, doctors say you should avoid over-the-counter products that have ingredients ending in 'caine'. These contain an anaesthetic that provides immediate relief but, if used regularly, causes increased irritation. In addition to OTCs, however, there are plenty of household remedies you can try.

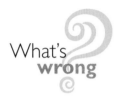

What's wrong

Haemorrhoids are swollen veins in or around the anus that cause pain, itching and, occasionally, bleeding. Internal haemorrhoids, the most common type, develop inside the anus. You might have some bleeding, but no pain. External haemorrhoids are the painful ones and they too can cause some bleeding. Either kind may turn into a prolapsed haemorrhoid, a soft lump that protrudes from the anus. Prolonged sitting, pregnancy and ageing can all contribute to haemorrhoids. If you often have constipation and strain when you're having a bowel movement, you can create haemorrhoids or make them worse.

The comfort of warmth

• Fill a bath with **warm water**, then ease yourself into it. You should be sitting with your knees raised, allowing maximum exposure of the anal area to the warm water. You'll find that this eases the pain. What you can't feel is how the warm water encourages increased bloodflow to the area, and that, in turn, helps to shrink swollen veins.

• Try adding a handful of **Epsom salts** before you plunge into the bath to help constrict the haemorrhoids. Stir the water well to dissolve the salts.

• Rather than fill up a whole bath every time you want relief, you can buy a **'sitz bath'**. These baths, designed solely for sitting in, are available from medical supply stores. Or if you have a bidet – and you are not too large – you can simply immerse your rear in the bowl. Filling a basin is a lot faster than filling a whole bath and, as it's more convenient, you'll probably use it more often.

• For external haemorrhoids, apply a warm, wet **teabag.** You can do this while sitting on the toilet. The warmth soothes and you get added benefit from one of tea's main components, tannic acid. It helps to reduce pain and swelling and also promotes blood clotting, which helps to stop the bleeding.

Sit on ice

• Fill a sturdy plastic bag with **ice**, wrap the bag in a thin cloth – an old pillowcase is ideal – and sit on it. Or use a bag of frozen peas (also wrapped in a cloth), which will mould itself more comfortably to your contours. The cold shrinks the swollen vessels, providing enormous relief. Sit in the chilly saddle for up to 20 minutes. There's no limit on how often you can do this, but give yourself at least a 10-minute break between applications. **Alternating hot and cold** – using a sitz bath between ice applications – is also helpful.

Do dab, don't scratch

● Soak a cotton wool ball with undistilled **witch hazel** and apply to the haemorrhoids. It's rich in tannins, which cause the blood vessels to contract.

● A dab of **Vaseline**, also contained in many over-the-counter haemorrhoid treatments, can help to soothe the area.

● Liquid **vitamin E** and **wheatgerm oil** are both reputed to be effective. Put them on a cotton wool ball and apply it a few times a day.

● If you can find it in a health-food store, try a salve that contains **comfrey** or **calendula,** which will both soothe and promote healing.

● Strange as it sounds, a poultice made from **grated potato** is astringent and soothing.

Lounge around

● A couple of times a day, find a comfortable sofa, stretch out, and **put your feet up.** What's good for your frayed nerves is also good for your haemorrhoids. In this supine posture, you take the weight off your overstressed anal area. At the same time, you improve circulation to the area that needs it. Ideally, allow at least 30 minutes for this 'task'. If you sit or stand for long periods, make sure you change position regularly.

Go with the grain

● Get more roughage into your diet. Research shows that **a high-fibre diet** can significantly reduce haemorrhoid symptoms, including pain and bleeding. Foods that are rich in fibre include wholegrain breads and cereals, fresh fruits and vegetables, brown rice and nuts.

● When you're getting more fibre, you need to stay well hydrated to prevent constipation. Be sure to **drink enough fluids** so that your urine is pale, not dark, yellow.

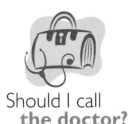

Should I call the doctor?

Haemorrhoids don't require immediate medical attention. If you see bright red blood in the stool – a telltale sign – you can first try some home treatment. But inflammatory bowel disease or a bowel infection can cause haemorrhoid-like symptoms. So if you see very dark blood or the stool looks black, contact your doctor right away, as this is often a sign of intestinal bleeding. Also see your doctor immediately if you have significant rectal bleeding, persistent faecal incontinence or the pain suddenly intensifies.

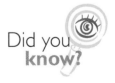

Did you know?

Hippocrates, the famous Greek physician who lived more than 2,400 years ago, knew that haemorrhoids were dilated anal veins. But he recommended burning them away with a red-hot iron.

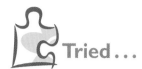

Tried...

Vicks VapoRub is a little-known home remedy for haemorrhoids.

**...&
true**

There's no harm in trying this, but it should only ever be applied externally – to the outside of the anus – as camphor, one of its ingredients, can be toxic. Its proponents say it doesn't sting (but others disagree) – so you'll have to try it to find out.

Limit sitting and lifting

● Anyone who does a lot of sitting needs to do some standing as well. If you're tied to your desk most of the time, take a **five-minute walk** every hour or so. Every time you get up, you ease the rectal pressure that leads to haemorrhoids.

● Heavy lifting puts pressure on the anal area. If there's a sofa or dresser that needs lifting, claim that you have a bad back and ask for volunteers.

● If you usually lift weights when you work out at the gym, make sure you **skip the squat thrusts**. Every time you crouch down, then lift up again, you put direct pressure on your rectum. Also avoid any exercise that involves sitting for long periods, such as cycling on an exercise bike.

Throne room policy

● The key to avoiding haemorrhoids is not straining, so excuse yourself and **go to the loo whenever you have to go**. The trouble with waiting is that it leads to constipation. And that, of course, means you have to strain more when you do go. And that invites haemorrhoids.

● After a bowel movement, wipe with **plain**, **white**, **unscented toilet paper** that's been dampened under running water. Scented, coloured loo paper may have some aesthetic attractions but any additional chemical can be an irritant.

● Follow the paper wipe with **facial tissues coated** with an **unscented moisturizing cream**.

Hangover

'I will never, ever drink again!' So says anyone who has ever woken up with a hammering headache and a stomach rolling around like an old trainer in a washing machine. The first piece of advice is, if you feel like being sick, do so. Vomiting is the body's way of ridding itself of toxins. If you can't survive without a painkiller, then choose aspirin or ibuprofen. Avoid paracetamol, which can harm your liver if you've been drinking. To reduce a horrible hangover, try the tips below. As for brave resolution … well, if you do drink again, take steps to limit the alcohol's impact on your system.

First steps for fast relief

- As soon as you wake up, drink 2 large glasses of **water** to undo the dehydration.
- Have a large glass of **grapefruit**, **orange** or **tomato juice**. Fruit juice contains the simple sugar fructose, which speeds up the metabolism of alcohol.
- If you drink **coffee**, have a cup or two as soon as possible. Caffeine is a vasoconstrictor, meaning it narrows the swollen blood vessels in your head. Just don't go overboard. Like alcohol, caffeine is a diuretic, and if you drink too much you'll become even more dehydrated.
- **Kudzu** is a traditional Chinese remedy for alcohol poisoning, usually taken as a 'morning after' tea. You can buy kudzu tincture at some health-food shops, though it's hard to find. You can also buy it online but would need to do so in anticipation … Follow the dosage directions on the package.

Recovery snacks

- Once you overcome the queasiness, make yourself a nice bowl of hot **chicken soup** or stock. Either will help to replace the salt and potassium the body loses when you've been drinking.
- A **banana milkshake** is an especially good way to replace potassium and other nutrients lost during a night of heavy drinking. Mix ½ cup of milk with a banana and 2 teaspoons of honey in a blender and drink up. Banana is a good source of potassium, which is lost in urine. And honey is rich in fructose.

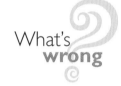

What's **wrong**

You had too much to drink last night and you've woken up with a wicked hangover. Your head is pounding. You're drenched in sweat. You feel like being sick. Maybe you feel shaky or anxious too. What's going on? The alcohol in your system has left you dehydrated and depleted of minerals. It's also caused the blood vessels in your head to dilate; that accounts for the headache. Finally, alcohol makes your blood abnormally acidic (a condition called acidosis), which causes nausea and sweating.

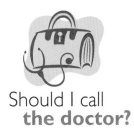

Should I call the doctor?

Even without treatment, a hangover should last for no more than 24 hours. If you're still feeling bad after that, call a doctor. Of course, if you can't remember what happened while you were drinking, or if you get hangovers on a regular basis, you may have a drinking problem. Call your doctor to discuss treatment options.

Old **wives' tale**

The 16th century English dramatist John Heywood suggested that the best way to recover from a hangover was to have the 'hair of the dog that bit you' – meaning, another alcoholic drink. The expression is a spin-off from the misguided notion that you could recover from a dog bite by plucking a hair from the dog and holding it to the wound. Unfortunately, the advice doesn't work any better for hangovers than it does for dog bites. Drinking your way out of a hangover will only postpone and prolong your misery.

• If you feel well enough, eat a light meal – fresh fruit, toast and honey. **Fruit** and **honey** are good sources of fructose. Save the bacon and eggs for another day.

Homeopathic help

• The homeopathic remedy **nux vomica** is considered an antidote to alcohol hangovers. Dissolve 3 to 5 pellets of the 30C potency on the tongue every four hours.

Get moving

• Although your instinct might be to stay in bed, you're better off if you can take a brisk walk or go for a run. That will boost your production of **endorphins**, the body's natural painkillers. Heavy drinking can lower endorphin levels.

The power of prevention

• If you're off to a social occasion where alcohol will be served, **eat something** – ideally something a bit greasy – before you go. Fatty substances help to coat the intestines, slowing down the absorption of alcohol. Slow absorption means less chance of inebriation – and a smaller chance of developing a hangover the following day.

• If you drink spirits, choose **vodka** or gin over whiskey, rum or brandy, and white wine over red. Clear spirits such as vodka don't contain congeners – naturally occurring compounds that contribute to morning-after nausea and headache. White wine contains fewer congeners than red wine.

• **Drink slowly.** Your body burns alcohol at a regular rate of roughly 30ml (1oz) an hour. Give it more time to burn that alcohol and less will reach your brain.

• Alternate alcoholic drinks with **sparkling water**, **fruit juice** or other **alcohol-free** drinks.

• Avoid champagne or any other alcoholic drink with **bubbles** in it (gin and tonic or rum and coke, say). Fizz puts alcohol into your bloodstream more quickly.

Headaches

In our stressful world of traffic jams, tight deadlines and high-speed everything, it's no wonder we find ourselves taking an occasional painkiller. For a bad headache, take two 500mg paracetamol tablets or two 200mg ibuprofen tablets. Aspirin is also an effective painkiller but is not suitable for anyone under 16 years, or who has an allergy to aspirin. However, painkillers are only part of the solution. There's much more you can do to escape the thump of a throbbing head.

Give it some acupressure

• With a firm, circular motion, **massage** the web of skin between the base of your thumb and your forefinger. Continue massaging for several minutes, then switch hands and repeat until the pain clears up. Acupressure experts call this fleshy area trigger point LIG4 and maintain that it is linked to areas of the brain where headaches originate.

Heat up and cool down

• Believe it or not, soaking your feet in **hot water** will help your head to feel better. By drawing blood to your feet, the hot-water footbath will ease pressure on the blood vessels in your head. For a really bad headache, add a bit of mustard powder to the water.

• For a tension headache, place a **hot compress** on your forehead or the back on your neck. The heat will help to relax knotted-up muscles in this area.

• It might sound contradictory, but you can follow up the heat treatment (or substitute it) by applying a **cold compress** to your forehead. Wrap a couple of ice cubes in a flannel or use a bag of frozen peas wrapped in a tea towel. Cold constricts blood vessels and, when they shrink, they stop pressing on sensitive nerves. Because headache pain sometimes originates in the nerves in the back of your neck, try moving the compress to the muscles at the base of your skull.

• Here's an alternative to a cold compress: soak your hands in **iced water** for as long as you can stand it. While your hands are submerged in the water, repeatedly open and close your

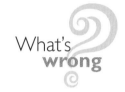

What's **wrong**

Specialists have identified a few major types of headache. Tension headaches seem to be caused by muscle contractions in the head and neck, and they're characterized by dull, steady pressure. Migraines originate with constriction and expansion of blood vessels in the head. They cause throbbing pain often accompanied by nausea and sensitivity to light or sound. Agonizing cluster headaches are sometimes triggered by drinking or smoking. They come episodically in groups, or 'clusters', followed by periods of remission.

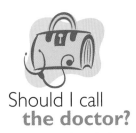

Should I call the doctor?

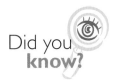

Did you know?

fists. This treatment works on the same principle as an ice pack on your head – the cold narrows your dilated blood vessels.

Try the caffeine cure
• Have a cup of **strong coffee.** Caffeine reduces blood-vessel swelling, and thus can help to relieve a headache. This is why caffeine is an ingredient in some extra-strength painkillers like Anadin Extra. If you are already a heavy coffee drinker, don't try this tip. Caffeine withdrawal can cause headaches, creating a vicious cycle.

Do something constrictive
• Tie a **headband**, **scarf** or **tie** around your forehead, then tighten it just to the point where you can feel pressure all around your head. Reducing the flow of blood to your scalp can help to relieve the pain caused by swollen blood vessels. You might try soaking the headband in **vinegar**, a traditional headache remedy.

Ease the pain with lavender and peppermint
• Certain essential oils – especially **lavender** – can help to ease tension and relieve the pain of a headache. Gently massage a little lavender oil onto your forehead and temples, then lie back and enjoy the relaxing scent. For maximum relief, slip away to a room that's cool, dark and quiet. The longer you can lie there quietly breathing in the aroma, the better.
• In addition to lavender oil – or instead of it – use **peppermint oil.** The menthol it contains can help dissolve away a headache. Its fragrance at first stimulates, then relaxes, the nerves that cause headache pain.
• If you have a vapouriser, add 7 drops **lavender oil** and 3 drops **peppermint oil**, then breathe in the relief. Alternatively, try sprinkling a few drops of peppermint oil onto a tissue. Inhale deeply several times.
• Wring out two wet **peppermint tea bags** and place them on your closed eyelids or forehead for five minutes.

Sip something soothing
• **Ginger** has anti-inflammatory properties and has long been used as an effective remedy for headaches. To make an

effective solution, grind up ½ teaspoon of ginger, stir it into a glass of water and drink. Or, alternatively, pour a cup of hot water over a teaspoon of freshly ground ginger, allow the tea to cool a little and drink. Ginger is especially effective against migraines, though how it works is not properly understood. Doctors do know that ginger has an effect on prostaglandins, hormone-like substances that contribute to inflammation. Ginger also helps to control the nausea that so often accompanies migraines.

Migraines

Migraines are characterized by throbbing, excruciating pain, often accompanied by nausea, vomiting, sensitivity to light or visual disturbances. Doctors aren't sure what causes migraines, but they suspect an association with abnormal constriction and dilation of the arteries that supply blood to the brain. The problem tends to run in families. There are many possible triggers, including sensitivities to foods or food additives, stress, hormonal fluctuations during the menstrual cycle, oral contraceptives, caffeine withdrawal, changes in the weather or season, bright lights and certain smells. Migraines are more common in women than in men.

It is easier to prevent a migraine than it is to treat one. Try these techniques:

• Avoid foods that contain a lot of the amino acid tyramine. Such 'trigger' foods include cured and processed meats, like pepperoni and salami, frankfurters and other sausages, aged cheeses such as Cheddar, nuts and peanuts. Chocolate and red wine, notorious migraine triggers, are also rich in tyramine.

• The herb feverfew has the power to reduce the intensity and frequency of migraines. Take 250mg extract (standardized to contain at least 0.4% parthenolide) every morning. It may be several months before the herb reaches its maximum preventative power. The fresh leaves are also effective, but they can cause mouth ulcers so are best eaten sandwiched in some bread.

• Flax seed oil is rich in essential fatty acids, which help your body produce fewer inflammation-causing prostaglandins, hormone-like chemicals that can constrict blood vessels. Take 1 to 2 tablespoons a day. Buy the cold-pressed oil and keep it in the refrigerator to protect it from light and heat. Take it by mixing it into a smoothie or adding it to salad dressing.

• Although experts aren't sure how, the B vitamin riboflavin can help to prevent migraines. The Food Standards Agency recommends a maximum dose of 40mg a day, although the effective dose used in trials of migraine prophylaxis is much higher – 400mg – with no apparent side effects.

• A magnesium supplement may also help. In some studies, people reported that their symptoms were much improved by taking 200mg of magnesium a day. But if you do take magnesium, be sure to take 500mg calcium as well – imbalances of the two minerals can reduce their beneficial effects. The two supplements should not be taken at the same time – allow at least three hours between.

• At the first sign of a migraine, take 1-2g of fresh powdered ginger or a 1cm chunk of fresh ginger root. Danish researchers discovered that ginger can help to prevent migraines by blocking prostaglandins.

• Try drinking a cup of **rosemary tea**; some people say it helps to prevent a headache from getting worse. Pour a cup of boiling water over a teaspoon of the dried herb, steep for 10 minutes, strain and drink.

• One grandmother's remedy was strong **black tea** with a few bruised whole **cloves** added. Tea contains caffeine and cloves have anti-inflammatory properties, so this brew might indeed help a headache.

• Drink a large glass of **water** and see if it helps. Dehydration often causes a headache.

The power of prevention

• If you grind your teeth or clench your jaw – either when you're awake or asleep – take steps to prevent the problem. You might need to wear a **mouthguard** at night. (See *Jaw problems*, page 260, for advice.)

• **Eat at regular intervals**. There's evidence that a drop in blood sugar – the result of going too long without eating – can set the stage for headaches.

• At least three days a week, spend 30 minutes walking, cycling, swimming or performing some other kind of **aerobic exercise**. These exercises are great stress-relievers.

Head lice

The notice on the school door warns parents that: 'some children in your child's class have head lice. Please be extra vigilant'. Once lice are in the hair, even a clipper cut won't get rid of them. You have to remove the lice eggs that attach themselves to the hair shafts about 5mm from the scalp. You can choose a chemical treatment (although there is increasing resistance – among lice and parents – to these) or more laborious, but quite effective, home remedies. Treat the affected scalp, and check the family while you're at it.

Be a nit-picker

• **Wet combing** is the most effective way to deal with head-lice and is better for your child's scalp than using chemicals. It is also the only treatment with anything like proven efficacy. For easier combing, coat the wet hair with conditioner.

• Time-consuming as it is, combing for headlice needs to be undertaken meticulously, for at least 30 minutes, at least every four days for at least two weeks, **until no live lice have been found for at least three consecutive combs.** Metal lice combs are sold in pharmacies and some supermarkets. If your child's head is infested, you may have to put on a video to persuade him or her to sit still through this process. Nits are yellowish-white, oval-shaped and adhere to the hair shaft at an angle. They look a bit like dandruff, but they don't drift out of the hair the way dandruff does. Mature lice can grow to about the size of sesame seeds. Freshly hatched lice are clear; those approaching midlife (about a week old) are reddish-brown. If you see lice, ideally the comb will remove them – wipe it on a sheet of white kitchen paper after each stroke.

• If your child's hair is **very curly or prone to tangles**, it's best to coat the hair with conditioner, then brush out tangles before combing through it with a lice comb . Rinse the comb in a basin of hot water after each pass so you can see any lice caught, and to stop the insects getting back into the hair.

The natural approach

• If you're wary of synthetic pesticides, you may be able to smother lice overnight. First, 'shampoo' the hair and scalp with

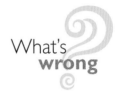

What's **wrong**

An itchy head is driving your child, or you, mad. The trouble is, itching is not usually an early symptom; lice may have been around for three months before they cause itching. Just 1-2mm long, these wingless insects live close to the scalp, laying their eggs (nits) and feeding on blood. When head lice appear in young children, word usually gets around quickly. The main route of spread is close head-to-head contact among children and between family members. Lice rarely spread by other means (combs, hats, ribbons), as they generally don't leave the body (except for another warm, living host). In fact, they die quickly without warmth and a host to feed on.

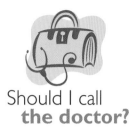

Should I call the doctor?

The remedies in this chapter will usually take care of a run-of-the-mill case of head lice. But you'll need a doctor's help if self-treatment fails, or if the skin on the scalp becomes cracked or inflamed.

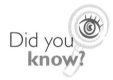

Did you know?

Before effective head lice shampoos came on the market, some said that the best way to kill lice was to rinse the hair with paint thinner or paraffin. These methods were probably effective when nothing else was available, but you should *never* attempt such risky treatment. There is the danger of maiming through fire and also the potential lung damage to any child inhaling these volatile chemicals.

mayonnaise, then put on a shower cap. The next morning, lice should be dead. Unfortunately, you can't smother louse eggs (nits) – you'll still have to remove them with a nit comb.

- **Petroleum jelly** can stifle roaming lice. Apply a thick layer of petroleum jelly, such as Vaseline, to the scalp, then cover with a shower cap. Leave on overnight. In the morning, use **baby oil** to remove the petroleum jelly – and the lice with it. Repeat for several nights in a row. (One warning: it may take quite a lot of shampooing to remove all the petroleum jelly from the hair.)

- Essential oils can kill lice and help to soothe the itching. There are many different 'recipes'. One effective combination is 20 drops **tea tree oil**, 10 drops **rosemary oil** and 15 drops each of **lemon** (or **thyme**) and **lavender oil** mixed into 4 tablespoons of **vegetable oil**. Rub the mixture into dry hair, cover with a plastic shower cap then wrap that with a towel. After an hour, unwrap, shampoo well and rinse.

- After any of the treatments above, **rinse** with a solution of equal amounts of **white vinegar** and **water**. This will help to kill off eggs and to remove oil residues from the hair.

A chemical cosh

- You may decide to go for a chemical 'cure', but don't waste your money on shampoos. They are not regarded by doctors as effective. **Lotions and liquids** work better but need to be left on for 12 hours – even the one that states only 2 hours on its label! (*Alert* Many lotions are flammable – a nasty accident can occur if a child being treated goes near *any* source of open flame, including gas hobs, fires and even cigarettes.)

- Chemical lice treatments should be used **only if you have found live lice** (not just nits) by detection combing – so that none is exposed unnecessarily to the noxious chemicals in the lotion and to minimise the build-up of resistance in the lice population. If you use a chemical treatment, it must be re-applied after seven days (whatever the package insert says).

- Two or three days later, perform **detection combing** again – lice eggs can still hatch after treatment.

- Unfortunately, the head lice population is now resistant to many insecticides. **If the first brand you use doesn't work**, you will need to choose another class of insecticide. Ask your pharmacist, who may also know about local resistance patterns.

Heartburn

Heartburn is extremely uncomfortable and it's not always clear what causes it. Some people say 'don't eat so much' or 'don't eat so fast'. Others like to blame spicy foods such as hot curries or Cajun seasonings; others cite grapefruits, oranges and other acidic foods. As a first line of defence, see your pharmacist for over-the-counter antacids or an acid suppressor like ranitidine, omeprazole or cimetidine. But the long-term goal is to pinpoint – and avoid – your personal heartburn triggers.

Douse the flame

- As soon as you feel the telltale flicker of heartburn, drink a large glass of **water**. It will wash the acid back down your oesophagus into your stomach.
- To make a heartburn-easing tea, add a teaspoon of freshly grated **root ginger** to a cup of boiling water, steep for 10 minutes, and drink. Long used to quell the nausea caused by motion sickness, ginger also helps to relax the muscles that line the walls of the oesophagus, so stomach acid doesn't get pushed upwards.
- A tea made from **anise, caraway** or **fennel seed** can also ease the burn, according to herbalists. Add 2 teaspoons of any one of them to a cup of boiling water, allow to infuse for 10 minutes, strain and drink.
- Practitioners of Ayurvedic medicine, the traditional medicine of India, prescribe teas made of crushed **cinnamon** or **cardamom** to cool the heat of heartburn. Add a teaspoon of either crushed or powdered herb to a cup of boiling water, steep, strain and drink.

Don a protective coat

- **Marshmallow root** is one of the oldest remedies known for heartburn. The plant produces a gooey, starchy substance called mucilage, which coats and protects the mucous membranes of your oesophagus – and this may be just what you need if your oesophagus feels as if it's on fire. Stir a teaspoon of powdered marshmallow root into a cup of water and sip it. Drink 3 or 4 cups a day.

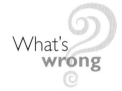

What's wrong

When stomach acid backs up into your oesophagus, you feel a burning pain. A 'trapdoor' of muscular tissue called the lower oesophageal sphincter usually keeps stomach acid where it belongs. With heartburn, it allows acid to leak upwards, a problem known as reflux. Large meals as well as certain foods can lead to heartburn. You're more likely to have heartburn if you're pregnant, over-weight or a smoker, or if you have a condition called hiatus hernia. Some medications, including aspirin, certain antibiotics and some antidepressants and sedatives, may aggravate heartburn.

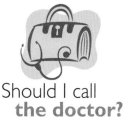

Should I call the doctor?

Occasional heartburn isn't serious. Recurrent heartburn could be a sign of gastroesophageal reflux disease, which can cause or contribute to conditions such as ulcers of the oesophagus and chronic cough. See your doctor if you get heartburn three or four times a week for weeks on end, if you wheeze or become hoarse, find it difficult to swallow or lose weight rapidly. These could be signs of cancer, especially if you are over 40. The symptoms of severe heartburn can be mistaken for a heart attack. If they occur after a meal and are soothed by water or antacids, it's probably heartburn. But if you have a feeling of fullness, tightness or dull pressure or pain in the centre of the chest, shortness of breath or light-headedness and a cold sweat, dial 999 for immediate medical help.

- You can make a similar soothing drink from **slippery elm.** Add a teaspoon of the powdered bark to a cup of hot water and drink a few cups throughout the day.
- A form of **liquorice** called DGL (deglycyrrhizinated liquorice) also provides soothing mucilage. Although it is available in capsule form, it works best when combined with saliva, so it is most effective when taken as chewable wafers. You may need to order these from a health-food shop. Eat two to four 380mg DGL wafers three times a day, 30 minutes before meals. If you cannot get hold of the wafers then buy DGL capsules (up to 1g a day is fine). Some brands contain 250mg with a recommended dose of 2-4 capsules daily.

Put it in neutral

- Saliva helps to neutralize stomach acid. So chew a piece of **sugar-free gum,** suck on a boiled sweet or daydream about juicy steaks or buttery new potatoes – whatever it takes to get you to generate and swallow extra saliva.
- **Bicarbonate of soda** (bicarb) is alkaline, so it neutralizes stomach acid. Mix ½ teaspoon of bicarb and a few drops of **lemon juice** in half a cup of warm water. Don't drink the diluted bicarb on its own: you need the lemon juice to dispel some of the gas which bicarb creates in the stomach when it comes into contact with stomach acid.
- The juices of vegetables like **carrots, cucumbers, radishes** or **beetroot** help to tame the acid in the stomach due to their alkaline nature. Feel free to add a pinch of salt and pepper for flavour. If juicing vegetables is inconvenient or doesn't appeal to you, just eat some raw vegetables.

The power of prevention

- No matter how bad you feel, **stay upright.** If you're standing, gravity helps to keep acid in your stomach. Avoid bending over after a meal, and definitely don't lie down.
- If night time heartburn plagues you, eat meals at least **two to three hours before you go to bed.** The added time will give acid levels a chance to decrease before you lie down.
- You might also **raise the head of your bed** 10-15cm with large wooden blocks or old phone books. When you sleep tilted at an angle, gravity helps to keep acid in the stomach.

- Try **sleeping on your left side.** When you lie on your left side, the stomach hangs down and fluids pool along the greater curvature, away from the lower oesophageal sphincter. Pooled fluids thus stay farther away from the oesophagus.

- Eat **smaller, more frequent meals** to minimize the production of stomach acid. And avoid eating too much in one sitting; doing so can force open the lower oesophageal sphincter, the thick ring of muscle that separates the stomach from the oesophagus and keeps stomach acid where it belongs.

- If you haven't done so already, **give up cigarettes.** Research shows that smoking relaxes the lower oesophageal sphincter. Breathing secondhand smoke is almost as bad, so stay away from smoky pubs, too.

Foods to avoid

If you're prone to heartburn, certain foods and drinks are best avoided. Limit or cut out the following:

Beer, wine and other alcoholic drinks They tend to relax the lower oesophageal sphincter, the important valve between your stomach and lower oesophagus.

Milk It feels soothing as you swallow it, but the fats, proteins and calcium it contains can stimulate the stomach to secrete acid.

Coffee, tea and cola Caffeinated drinks also relax the lower oesophageal sphincter, and can irritate an inflamed oesophagus.

Chocolate It's loaded with two heartburn triggers – fat and caffeine.

Bubbles The carbonation in fizzy drinks can expand your stomach, which has the same effect on the lower oesophageal sphincter as overeating.

Fried and fatty foods They tend to sit in the stomach for a long time, where they can cause excess acid production.

Citrus fruits and juices They are acidic – though the acid is bland in comparison to what your stomach manufactures, and may not be a problem.

Peppermint and spearmint They relax the lower oesophageal sphincter, as do tomatoes.

HEALING YOUR HOME

You've installed smoke detectors. Had your tap water tested for lead. Bought (and always use) a water filter. The bathrooms have antibacterial soap and you put clean towels out every morning. What else can you do to protect your family against illness? Quite a lot, as it turns out – especially if you live in a tightly sealed, energy-efficient home, in which airborne toxins can quickly build up.

Use Mother Nature's cleansers

No doubt you are already aware that you should open windows and turn on extractor fans when using solvents, harsh cleansers and other noxious chemicals. But it's even better if you can replace these products whenever possible with homemade alternatives.

• All-purpose cleaner: Dissolve 4 tablespoons of bicarbonate of soda in a litre of warm water.

• Drain cleaner: Pour ½ cup of bicarbonate of soda down the drain. Add ½ cup of white vinegar. Wait 5 minutes, then flush down with a kettle full of boiling water.

• Toilet bowl cleaner: Make a paste with lemon juice and borax (available from hardware stores). Apply the paste to the bowl, leave it for 2 hours, then scrub and rinse.

• Oven cleaner: Sprinkle water on spills while the oven is still warm, then add salt. When the oven cools, scrape the spill away.

• Window and mirror cleaner: A weak solution of vinegar in water makes an effective cleaner. Apply it using a plant sprayer for maximum efficiency.

• Air freshener: Avoid chemical fresheners. Open the bathroom window, grow a scented plant in the bathroom or hang up bunches of lavender or mint.

Get bold about mould

Many people who blame their coughing and wheezing on animal fur or pollen are actually experiencing a reaction to mould spores in their own homes. Nothing helps mould to flourish like high humidity, so do everything you can to get household moisture under control. Obviously, that means keeping an eye out for leaking roofs or dripping taps. But you should also make sure that all space heaters, wood burning stoves, gas log fires, open fireplaces and so forth are regularly serviced and the rooms in which they are used are well ventilated. Not only can these heaters emit carbon monoxide and other combustion products, they also fill the air with water vapour. You may want to consider buying a dehumidifier to run in the room at the same time.

Consume less chlorine

Most tap water is chlorinated. This is a good thing because chlorine is such an effective germ-killer. Unfortunately, chlorinated water has been linked with some pretty nasty ailments, including cancer of the bladder and rectum.

Bottled water is getting cheaper all the time but if you don't want to keep buying bottled water, you can dechlorinate your tap water by equipping your kitchen tap with an activated charcoal water filter.

Get the lead out

The toxic metal isn't found only in tap water and old paint. Although leaded petrol has been banned for decades, the topsoil in some areas remains contaminated by residues from the exhausts of cars that used to run on leaded petrol. To be safe, dust regularly and, if you live on a busy road, get everyone to take their shoes off before coming indoors.

Give germs the cold shoulder

No matter how carefully you clean, it's impossible to get rid of all the germs in your home. But you can get fewer colds and other viruses simply by insisting that everyone in the household washes his or her hands before each meal and after each trip to the toilet. Try not to touch your eyes or mouth with your hands; if germs have no way into your body, they can't make you ill. Use a disinfectant spray on door handles, telephone receivers and taps to protect the rest of the family when one of you is ill.

• Tame your toothbrush. One place germs lurk is on a damp toothbrush. Many viruses, including those that cause flu, can survive for more than 24 hours on moist bristles. Alternate between three toothbrushes, so you use a dry toothbrush each time. If you do get a bad cold, replace all of them once you recover, just to be safe. If you don't like the idea of so many toothbrushes, use one and rinse it daily with hydrogen peroxide or mouthwash.

• Expunge germs from your sponge. Like toothbrushes, kitchen cloths or sponges are breeding grounds for bacteria. It's also possible to transfer food-borne bugs, such as salmonella and campylobacter, from cloths used to wipe worktops and chopping boards to dishes and saucepans. To be safe, change the cloth or sponge every week and always allow it to air-dry between uses. It's also a good idea regularly to disinfect washing-up sponges, brushes and cloths in a mixture of water and bleach.

Declare war on dust mites

These microscopic creatures feed on shed skin cells and the droppings they leave behind can trigger allergies. How do you get rid of pests you can't even see? Once a week, vacuum rugs and upholstered furniture and wash sheets and towels in hot water – at least a 60°C wash cycle. Duvets and eiderdowns that you don't want to wash that frequently can be put through the tumble dryer once a week to kill mites. If you store these items away at the end of each season, be sure to wash or dry-clean them first.

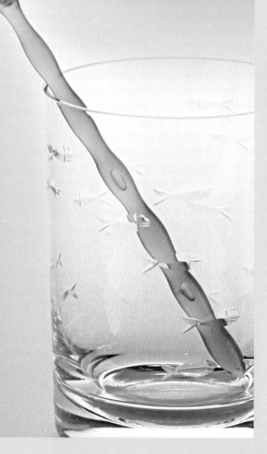

Heat rash

When your skin has been prickled by the heat, a condition known medically as *miliaria rubra*, the first priority is to cool down. For the next few days spend as much time as you can indoors – ideally in an air-conditioned environment. Take plenty of cool baths or showers. Ask your partner, friend or children to fan you – or sit beside an electric fan. And while you're waiting for your skin to chill, try these other remedies.

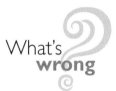

What's wrong

The itchy red bumps dotting your neck, armpits, chest and groin are caused by sweat with nowhere to go. Normally, perspiration evaporates, which cools your skin. But sweat trapped by fabric can't escape. The skin swells, blocks the sweat pores and perspiration leaks into the skin, which erupts into that bumpy rash. As the bumps burst, releasing their sweat, you may feel the stinging sensation that gives heat rash its other name – prickly heat. Hot, humid weather, sweat and tight clothes are a recipe for heat rash. So is skin rubbing against skin – common in people who are overweight.

Pack it with ice
● Anything that cools the temperature of your skin will help to reduce the itching and swelling. So if you don't have time for a bath, put an **ice pack** or a **cool compress** on the rash for 10 minutes every few hours.

Add the magic powder
● Sometimes, it appears that **bicarbonate of soda** is good for pretty well everything – and it's certainly good for relieving heat rash. Add a few tablespoons to a bath and have a long soak. It will help to ease the itching and will make you feel more comfortable while the rash heals. You can also add finely ground **oatmeal**, sold in pharmacists under brand names such as Aveeno.
● Apply bicarbonate of soda or **cornflour** directly to the rash area to absorb sweat and moisture. This is an age-old approach, recommended by many country grandmothers. Some say cornflour is better because it is softer on the skin. Reapply every few hours, rinsing and drying the skin first.

Smooth on a soother
● The cooling gel of the **aloe vera** leaf has long been used to relieve itching and promote healing. Apply the gel to the affected skin two or three times a day, washing the skin before each application. You can use gel from a freshly cut leaf or buy a product that contains it (many aftersun products do).
● Apply **calamine lotion**. A traditional remedy for sunburn, the pink stuff can also ease the itching of heat rash. Ask your pharmacist for oily calamine lotion.

Get out in the open air

• If blisters accompany the rash, **don't cover them up.** Fresh air will speed up their healing.

The power of prevention

• Limit physical activity in extremely hot and humid weather. (The threat of heat rash is a great excuse to avoid a workout.) And to avoid heat rash (rather than to treat it) take as many **tepid baths** or **showers** as needed to cool yourself. Tepid water is better than cold – cold water tends to close down skin blood vessels to conserve heat, so making you even hotter inside.

• Wear **loose cotton** or **linen** clothing. It's more likely to keep your skin dry, making heat rash less likely to plague your tender skin. Avoid all synthetic fabrics and tight clothing in general, especially on warm summer days.

• **Avoid oil-based sunscreens** or products that contain **cocoa butter.** Choose a less greasy sunscreen and one that is also hypoallergenic and blocks both UVA and UVB light.

• On the beach, sit under an **umbrella.** Your place in the shade will be significantly cooler than a seat in the sun.

• If you can manage to **lose a little weight**, do. Overweight people tend to sweat more and generate more body heat, making a rash more likely to erupt.

• Increase your intake of **essential fatty acids** by eating more salmon, tuna, mackerel or other oily fish, and flax seed (linseed) oil. These healthy fats help to inhibit inflammation in the body, making you less susceptible to rashes.

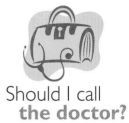

Should I call the doctor?

Simple heat rash is irritating but hardly serious; the itching and inflammation should clear up in a day or two. But see your doctor if the rash doesn't disappear within a few days or if the bumps become infected. You may need medication. Also seek emergency medical treatment if nausea, dryness, thirst, headache and paleness accompany the rash. In severe forms, heat rash can interfere with the body's temperature-regulating mechanism and cause fever and heat exhaustion.

Hiccups

Hiccups can come at the most inconvenient times – just before you have to toast the bridesmaids at a wedding or give a presentation at work, for instance. When you're in public, you might have to use some very subtle methods to control the hiccupping. Some 'cures' involve gentle pressure; others, a glass of water. And, if you have a high threshold of embarrassment – or you can hide somewhere – there are some wonderfully strange contortions that hiccup-prone people have devised to stop the contractions. Do whatever works for you.

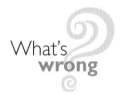

What's wrong

Surprisingly enough, given how common hiccups are, no one really knows what causes them. But we're all hiccup-prone. Even foetuses in the womb. Something prompts your diaphragm to contract, suddenly and involuntarily, producing a spasm that gets released as a sometimes embarrassing 'hiccup' noise. Certain foods can cause these contractions. So can drinking excessive alcohol or swallowing air – such as when you swig down a fizzy drink or get excited.

Emergency action in public places

• Press the palm of your hand with the thumb of your other hand, the harder, the better. Alternatively, you can squeeze the ball of your left thumb between the thumb and forefinger of the right. The discomfort is a distraction that affects your nervous system and may put an end to the hiccups. (And you can do it under the table without anyone staring at you.)

• **Take a deep breath** and hold it. When there's a build-up of carbon dioxide in your lungs, your diaphragm relaxes.

• If you can disappear for a few minutes ('sorry – must pop to the loo'), **stick your fingers in your ears** for 20-30 seconds. Or press the soft areas behind your earlobes, just below the base of the skull. This sends a 'relax' signal through the vagus nerve, which connects to the diaphragm area.

• When no-one's watching, **stick out your tongue**. This exercise is done by singers and actors because it stimulates the opening between the vocal cords (the glottis). You breathe more smoothly, quelling the spasms that cause hiccups.

• **Cup your hands** over your nose and mouth, but continue breathing normally. You'll get hiccup relief from the extra dose of carbon dioxide.

Drinkable cures

• Take nine or ten **quick sips** in a row from a glass. When you gulp a drink, rhythmic contractions of the oesophagus over-ride spasms of the diaphragm.

• If you can **block your ears** when you drink, so much the better. Stick your fingers in your ears and sip through a straw. That way you're pressing on the vagus nerve while also getting the benefits of steady swallowing.

• Place a single layer of **kitchen paper** over the top of the glass, then drink through the towel. You'll have to 'pull' harder with your diaphragm to suck up the water, and concentrated gulping counteracts spasmodic muscle movements.

Remedies to surprise your taste buds

• Put one teaspoon of **sugar** or **honey**, stirred in warm water, on the back of your tongue and swallow it.

• The sharp surprise of something sour can make lips pucker and beat the hiccups. Cut a slice of **lemon** and suck on it.

• Swallow a teaspoon of **cider vinegar.** This is a challenge, but if you cope with the assault on the taste buds, it's a quick cure. (Another vinegary method is to suck on a **pickled gherkin.**)

Take a breather

• Sometimes **relaxation** is the key. Lie on a bed, stomach down, with head turned and arms hanging over the side. Take a deep breath, hold it for 10 to 15 seconds and exhale slowly. After a few repeats, rest for several minutes before you get up.

• If you can elicit the help of your partner, stand with your back against a wall and ask your partner to place a fist lightly in the soft area just under your breastbone. Take a few deep breaths and, on the last one, exhale completely. Your partner should then **press gently but firmly** to help expel air from your lungs.

• **A long, passionate kiss** has been known to work (and if it doesn't, well, no harm done). Just make sure you choose the right partner for this remedy.

Cures from the children's menu

• Offer a big teaspoon of **peanut butter.** In the process of chewing and getting it off the tongue and teeth, swallowing and breathing patterns are interrupted.

• With a scoop of **ice cream**, a cure becomes a treat. The chill of the ice cream, steady swallowing and such a pleasurable distraction all add up to calming the diaphragm.

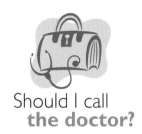

Should I call the doctor?

Believe it or not, some people get hiccups that last for days. If yours continue for a long time, your doctor will want to find out what's causing them. It could be a problem with your nervous system or an intestinal disorder such as ileus (which occurs when intestinal muscles don't contract properly). You might have an ongoing stomach irritation or an infection of some kind. Doctors can prescribe tranquillizers – such as chlorpromazine or haloperidol – for what are called 'intractable hiccups'. The drugs help to relax the diaphragm.

The power of prevention

- **Avoid beer** or **fizzy drinks**, especially if they're cold. The low temperature combined with the bubbles creates a cocktail of irritants that could set off your diaphragm.
- When you **eat, slow down.** Eating quickly makes you swallow more air, and that can cause hiccups as well as burping.
- A few medications such as **diazepam** (Valium) have been known to contribute to more frequent hiccups. If you suspect that a prescription drug is the problem, talk to your doctor about taking an alternative.
- If a baby has hiccups, it could be the result of swallowing too much air while feeding. So perform the same ritual you would for burping: hold the baby against your shoulder and **pat him or her gently on the back.** That can bring up the air and stop the hiccups. Also check the teat of the baby's bottle to see if it's letting the milk flow at the right rate. Turn a full bottle upside down; you should get a regular drip that slows down and eventually stops. If too much or too little liquid comes out, that can contribute to hiccups.

High blood pressure

Half of all the people who have high blood pressure don't know they have it. Of those who do know, about seven out of every ten don't have their blood pressure under control. So if you have no idea what your blood pressure is, ask your doctor to check it. If you've already been diagnosed with hypertension, make sure you follow the advice your doctor has given you. Whilst medication is required in many cases, the cornerstones of any treatment are exercise and diet changes. Even if your doctor has prescribed blood pressure lowering medication, these lifestyle efforts are essential.

Start tackling the problem in the kitchen

- Studies in the USA have shown that a diet known as DASH (short for Dietary Approaches to Stop Hypertension) is very effective at lowering blood pressure. The gist of the diet is this: it's **low in saturated fat** and **cholesterol** and high in **fruit, vegetables, whole grains** and **low-fat dairy foods**. A diet based on these principals can produce positive results – a reduction in blood pressure – in as little as two weeks.

- **Reduce your salt intake.** Eating too much salt causes your body to retain water. The effect is the same as adding more liquid to an overfilled water balloon: pressure rises. In a follow-up to the DASH study, researchers found that the biggest drop in blood pressure came when people followed the DASH diet and also limited themselves to 1500mg of sodium a day. That's less than a teaspoon of salt a day.

- Even if you don't add salt to your food during cooking or at the table, you may still be getting a considerable amount of 'hidden' salt in packaged and processed foods, especially snacks, meat products and tinned soups. So before buying food, **read labels carefully** to find out the sodium or salt content. Look for low-salt soups and biscuits and rinse beans and other foods canned in brine before using them.

- Try **making your own bread**. If you have a bread maker, it takes less than 5 minutes a day to tip in the ingredients and, 2 hours later, there's the bread. Why bother? Because most shop bread contains high levels of salt, and you can control

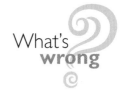

What's wrong

A high blood pressure reading means your heart is working harder than it should to pump blood, and your arteries are stressed. That's risky. If you don't lower your blood pressure, you face an increased risk of stroke, heart attack, kidney disease and other deadly illnesses. You are considered to have high blood pressure (hypertension) when systolic pressure (the top number) is 140 or higher or the diastolic pressure (bottom number) is 90 or higher. But whenever your blood pressure starts to creep up, your doctor will urge you to take measures to control it.

exactly how much salt – and fat – goes into a homemade loaf. And it's delicious and makes the house smell wonderful.

Other dietary do's and don'ts

• Even if you don't follow a special diet, you'll see major benefits if you make sure you eat plenty of **fresh fruit** and **vegetables** – raw or cooked. The goal is to eat five servings of fruit and vegetables a day – more if you can manage it. Fruit and vegetables are important sources of potassium, magnesium and fibre – all of which help to keep your arteries healthy.

• **Porridge** is good in two ways – it helps to lower blood pressure as well as cholesterol levels, as some studies have shown. Its beneficial effect seems to come from a form of soluble fibre known as beta–glucan. If you start every day with a bowl of porridge, your blood pressure will probably fall.

• **Cut back on alcohol.** Heavy drinkers tend to have high blood pressure. If you do drink, limit yourself to one drink a day if you're a woman, two a day if you're a man. One drink is half a pint of standard strength beer, a small glass of wine or a single pub measure of spirits.

Lose some excess baggage

• Carrying extra weight forces the heart to pump harder. That's why blood pressure rises as body weight increases. If you're overweight, **losing as little as 5 kilos** (10lb) can lead to a significant reduction in blood pressure.

Stamp out those cigarettes

• **If you smoke, give it up now.** Compounds in tobacco smoke contribute to hardening of the arteries by causing injury to blood vessels. And the nicotine in cigarettes causes

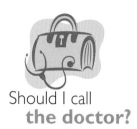

Should I call
the doctor?

If you've been diagnosed with high blood pressure, call your doctor at once if you experience chronic headache, palpitations, shortness of breath, fatigue, nosebleeds, blurred vision, flushed face, frequent urination or ringing in the ears. These symptoms suggest that your blood pressure is not being adequately controlled.

Could the noisy street you live on be to blame?

We all know that driving in heavy traffic is tiring and increases our stress levels. In fact a recent German study suggests that just the *noise* of traffic can send blood pressure soaring. The study of 1,700 people, conducted at the Robert Koch Institute in Berlin, found that people living in areas of heavy traffic were twice as likely to be having treatment for high blood pressure as those living on quiet streets. People who kept their windows open at night, in spite of the racket, were at highest risk.

blood vessels to constrict. That's bad for anyone, but it is especially bad for people who have high blood pressure.

Shake a leg

- At least three times a week – and preferably five – take 30 minutes of **brisk exercise.** This advice might seem unwise as most forms of exercise temporarily *raise* blood pressure. But when you work out regularly, you help to keep your resting blood pressure at a safe level. Running, brisk walking, cycling and swimming are excellent choices.

Seek peace

- Consider **getting a pet.** Whether walking a dog, sitting with a cat on your knee or even gazing at a tankful of fish, interacting with animals has been shown to bring noticeable decreases in blood pressure.
- **Learn to meditate.** This isn't New Age silliness. Research shows that meditation really does affect blood pressure, apparently by lowering levels of stress hormones in your body. To begin, choose a simple word or phrase to focus on. Close your eyes and relax all your muscles. Breathing slowly and naturally, repeat your word or phrase every time you exhale. As you do this, try to assume a passive attitude. Don't try to evaluate whether you're relaxed or 'doing well – just concentrate on your words and your breathing. Do this once or twice a day for 10 to 20 minutes.
- Engrossing **hobbies** such as gardening, playing a musical instrument or tapestry making may be just as beneficial as meditation.

Supplement your efforts

- Take **magnesium.** The mineral helps to relax the smooth muscle tissue that lines blood vessels, allowing them to open wide. Magnesium is especially effective at reducing high blood pressure associated with pregnancy, but always consult your doctor before taking any supplement when you're pregnant. Look for a magnesium supplement in the form of magnesium citrate or magnesium gluconate, which has a gentler effect on the digestive tract. If you take magnesium, be sure to **take calcium as well** – but take the supplements at least 2 hours

Home blood pressure tests

Some people get so nervous when a doctor checks their blood pressure that they experience a temporary rise in blood pressure – known as 'white coat hypertension'. You may be able to get a more accurate picture of your blood pressure by buying a blood pressure monitor and taking your own readings at home. You will find a list of upper arm monitors that have been independently tested for accuracy on the Blood Pressure Association's web site: **www. bpassoc.org.uk/information/bp_monitors.htm** By averaging out the readings, you'll get a true picture of your blood pressure – but you should still have your BP checked by your practice nurse or GP on a regular basis.

apart for maximum absorption. The recommended dose for lowering blood pressure is 400mg magnesium and 1000mg calcium a day.

- Take 100 to 150mg of **hawthorn** extract (standardized to contain at least 1.8% vitexin) a day. Hawthorn has long been known to dilate arteries. It seems to work by interfering with an enzyme (angiotensin-converting enzyme, or ACE) that constricts blood vessels. This is the enzyme targeted by ACE inhibitors – prescription drugs that reduce blood pressure. If you currently take medication for high blood pressure, consult your doctor before taking this herb. Hawthorn may take several weeks or even months to build up in your system and have an effect.

- **Garlic** helps to lower blood pressure, too, although it's not known why. Some experts recommend simply eating a clove of raw garlic a day. Others advise taking dried concentrate equivalent to 4g fresh garlic a day. If you opt for supplements, choose enteric-coated capsules for best results.

- Take **fish-oil supplements** to boost your intake of omega-3 fatty acids. Omega-3s inhibit the body's production of substances, such as prostaglandins, that narrow the arteries. These 'good' fats come from oily fish like mackerel and salmon; a typical supplement contains 1000mg. Taking two doses a day encourages good circulation and can help to reduce high blood pressure. Or take 1 tablespoon of flax seed oil a day, stirred into fruit juice or mixed into salad dressing.

High cholesterol

The top three places you're likely to find unwanted sludge are in your drains, in your car's engine and in your arteries. The first will block your sink, the second your mobility – and the third, your life. To keep your arteries from getting clogged up – or to prevent them from getting any more clogged up – you'll need to lower your levels of cholesterol. But not all cholesterol is harmful. Low density lipoprotein (LDL) cholesterol is the bad stuff; high density lipoprotein (HDL) cholesterol is beneficial, as it helps to remove LDL from the blood. Often, changes in diet and lifestyle are enough to bring cholesterol levels back to a healthy balance.

Cut out the 'bad' fats

- Eliminate as much **saturated fat** as possible from your diet. That means switching to leaner cuts of meats and lower-fat versions of dairy products such as butter, milk, ice cream, cheese and yoghurt. Cut out processed meats – such as salami, corned beef and pork pie – altogether.
- Run screaming from **palm oil** and **coconut oil**, which are very high in saturated fat. These so-called tropical oils are found in many processed foods, particularly biscuits and cakes.
- Another type of fat, called **trans-fatty acids** should be avoided as much as possible. They are produced when plant-based oils are hydrogenated to produce solid spreads, such as margarines. They have the same effect on cholesterol levels as saturated fat. Many shop-bought cakes, biscuits, snack foods – and even breads – contain these fats. To find them, look for the word 'hydrogenated' on the list of ingredients.
- **Eat more fresh fruits, vegetables** and **whole grains.** That is the easiest way to feel full as you cut back on meat and other fatty foods. In addition to being low in fat and cholesterol-free, plant foods contain lots of cholesterol-lowering fibre and vitamins and antioxidants that are good for your heart.
- If you love dark meat, try **venison**. This game meat has a fraction of the fat found in most of the beef that is sold in supermarkets. In fact, it is as low in fat as most fish. Marinate venison to improve its tenderness.

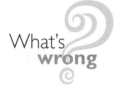

What's **wrong**

Inside your arteries, a dangerous change has taken place in the balance of fatty substances that circulate in your blood-stream. There is too much of the 'bad' type of cholesterol, called low-density lipoprotein (LDL). This is the type that gums up your arteries and raises your risk of heart attack and stroke. Meanwhile, you probably don't have enough 'good' cholesterol, known as high-density lipoprotein (HDL). These are the molecules that act as 'dustcarts', carrying LDL away to the liver for disposal.

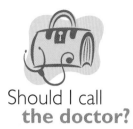

Should I call **the doctor?**

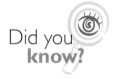

Did you **know?**

Recent research has shown that not all breads are as low in fat as you think. Fat, often in the form of hydrogenated oils, is added to many breads to improve the taste and keep it fresher for longer. As a result, three slices of some brands now provide more fat than a Mars bar. So read the labels and choose loaves that contain less than 1g fat per slice.

Get more good fats

• Numerous studies have shown that **olive oil** not only lowers LDL but also raises HDL. One study found that people who ate about 2 tablespoons of olive oil a day had lower LDL levels in just one week. Use it in garlic bread, salad dressings, in place of margarine and in place of other oils when frying.

• Enjoy **nuts.** They are packed with healthy unsaturated fats, including omega-3s. Walnuts and almonds seem to be especially good at lowering LDL. Eat a small handful a day and watch your cholesterol levels drop. But nuts contain a lot of calories, so make sure you eat them instead of – not as well as – other snacks.

• Have an **avocado** a day and you might lower your LDL by as much as 17 per cent. Like nuts, avocados are very high in fat (and therefore calories), but it's mainly the unsaturated kind.

• Eat **peanut butter.** Yes, peanut butter. It may be high in calories, but most of the fat it contains is unsaturated. Buy a 'natural' brand that contains no hydrogenated oils.

Fish for omega-3s

• **Fish** is much more than a replacement for meat. It contains omega-3 fatty acids, which actually lower LDL cholesterol. Aim to eat fish three times a week – even if it's tinned sardines or pilchards. Your best bets are fresh mackerel, tuna and salmon, all very high in omega-3s. Interestingly, tinned tuna loses almost all its beneficial oils during processing, although tinned sardines and most other tinned fish retain theirs.

• If you really detest fish, take a daily **fish-oil supplement** that contains both EPA and DHA (two types of omega-3 fatty acids). Take 1,000mg twice a day.

• Cook with **onions** – especially red onions. Onions are rich in HDL-raising sulphur compounds plus an antioxidant called quercetin, which fights off LDL cholesterol. The red in red onions is made up of further beneficial antioxidants known as flavonoids.

• **Flax seeds** are great sources of omega-3 fats and soluble fibre. Grind the nutty seeds and add them to your yoghurt or breakfast cereal. One study found that eating two tablespoons of ground flax seeds a day cut LDL cholesterol by 18 per cent.

Health-food shops sell flax seeds (linseed) and their oil, but for high cholesterol you are better off eating the seeds. If you buy whole seeds then **grind them** before you eat them, or they will pass straight through your digestive system without being broken down.

Get your oats

- **Porridge** is a rich source of soluble fibre, which forms a kind of gel in your intestine to reduce your body's absorption of the fat you eat. Eating a bowl of porridge a day has a marked cholesterol lowering effect. Choose quick-cooking or old-fashioned oats rather than instant hot oat cereal.
- Other especially good sources of soluble fibre include **prunes, barley, beans, aubergine** and **asparagus.**
- Add soluble fibre in your diet with **psyllium** seeds (ispaghula). These are sold in health-food shops and pharmacies. One tablespoon of the crushed seed is equivalent to a bowl of high bran cereal. Add it to any food or juice. Or simply ask your pharmacist for a psyllium based laxative, these are usually labelled 'natural' or 'vegetable'. Research has shown that taking about 10 grams of psyllium seeds a day for eight weeks can reduce LDL by up to 7 per cent.

Put the squeeze on cholesterol

- Freshly-squeezed or straight out of the carton, **orange juice** can improve your cholesterol balance. Participants in a recent study who drank three glasses of juice a day for a month increased their HDL levels by 21 per cent and lowered the ratio of bad to good cholesterol (LDL to HDL) by 16 per cent.

Niacin: should you or shouldn't you?

At high doses, the B vitamin niacin can lower cholesterol. But don't take it unless your doctor recommends a specific dose and monitors your health while you're taking it. Niacin has the effect of lowering LDL cholesterol while raising HDL – and in this respect, it resembles prescription drugs.

However, the amount of niacin you need to reap these benefits is very high and when you take excessive doses, you risk many potential side effects. Some people get uncomfortable hot flushes and there's even a risk of liver damage. So it's unwise to take niacin supplements without medical advice.

Give soya a whirl

For a delicious, cholesterol-lowering milk-shake, blend 1 cup of vanilla soya milk with 2 tablespoons of ground flax seeds. Add some fresh or frozen berries and mix it all together in a blender. The soya protein and flax seeds help to lower LDL cholesterol and raise HDL cholesterol, while the berries add cholesterol-lowering fibre.

Why not drink wine?

• **Alcohol** – no matter what kind you drink – **raises levels of 'good' HDL cholesterol.** 'Moderate' means 1 unit a day for a woman, and 2 units a day for a man. If you drink more than that, the damage will far outweigh any benefits. Red wine offers additional goodies in the form of powerful antioxidants that come from the pigments in grape skin. (One unit of alcohol is a pub measure of spirits, 1 small glass of wine or ½ pint of standard strength beer.)

Get into sporting life

• Lace up your **walking shoes**, and stride out briskly for 30 minutes a day. Alternatively, you could visit a gym and climb a stair machine for 30 minutes. Or go swimming or jogging before or after work. The benefits of **regular exercise** are undeniable. Studies show that physical activity will decrease your overall risk of heart disease and stroke. And regular exercise also helps to control diabetes and high blood pressure, both of which are independent risk factors for heart disease.

Of garlic and ginger

• Get your daily dose of **garlic** – either fresh garlic or garlic tablets. Garlic contains a compound called allicin, which is thought to be responsible for the bulb's cholesterol-lowering effect. If you decide on garlic supplements, look for enteric-coated products, to prevent 'garlic breath'. Supplements should supply a total allicin potential of 4,000mcg per tablet.
• Four times a day, take **ginger** capsules. The usual dose is 100 to 200mg. Studies suggest that the compounds in ginger help to reduce the absorption and increase the excretion of LDL cholesterol.

Hives

A simple antihistamine can help to reduce the allergic reaction that causes hives – also known as nettle rash or urticaria (*urtica* is the Latin word for nettle). Ask your pharmacist for a drug that doesn't cause drowsiness. While you let the medicine do its work, try any of the home treatments below for added relief. You will also want to try and identify what triggers your hives so you can avoid flare-ups in future.

Drown them with attention

- Unless you have hives that are triggered by cold (which is rare), have a **cool bath** or apply a **cold compress.** Cold shrinks the blood vessels and blocks further release of histamine. To further relieve itching, add **colloidal oatmeal** (such as Aveeno) to the bathwater and soak in it for 10 to 15 minutes. (Be careful getting out of the bath, however – that finely ground oatmeal makes it very slippery.)

Wipe on relief

- Dab the weals with **calamine lotion** or **witch hazel.** These astringents help to shrink blood vessels, so they don't leak so much histamine.
- Or try **milk of magnesia** or **Pepto-Bismol.** Because they are alkaline, they help to relieve the itching.
- In a small cup, add a few drops of water to **bicarbonate of soda** or **cream of tartar** and stir to make a paste. Spread this on the hives to help stop irritation and relieve the itching.
- If you just have a few small hives and want to temporarily stop the itching, apply an over-the-counter **hydrocortisone cream.** Brands include Dermacort, Eurax Hc, Hc45, Lanacort and Zenoxone. Follow label directions.
- Mix a teaspoon of any kind of **vinegar** with a tablespoon of lukewarm water and apply the liquid to your hives with a cotton wool ball to soothe the itching.
- An old Chinese folk remedy for hives recommends boiling 60g **brown sugar** and 30g **fresh ginger** in 200ml **vinegar** for several minutes. Mix a little of the resulting liquid with warm water and apply several times a day.

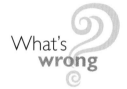

What's **wrong**

As small as Smarties or as large as saucers, hives are an allergic reaction that take the form of itchy reddish or white bumps or weals on the skin. They are the result of cells releasing histamine, a chemical that makes blood vessels leak fluid into the deepest layers of skin. It's not clear why some people get hives, while others don't, and the 'triggers' associated with hives are so numerous, they all fit into the broad category of 'miscellaneous'. Just for starters, hives can be caused by sunlight, heat, cold, pressure, stress, viral infections or medications. Anything that can cause an allergy can also cause hives – including pollen, dust, dander, dust mites, shellfish and other foods.

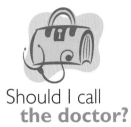

Should I call **the doctor?**

While hives can be uncomfortable, they're usually harmless and disappear within minutes or hours, although sometimes they remain for a few days. If you develop hives around your eyes or in your mouth or experience difficulty breathing, wheezing, light-headedness or dizziness dial 999. You may have a life-threatening condition called anaphylaxis – and the internal tissue swelling can block breathing passages. If you're prone to hives, ask your doctor if you should carry a rapid-injection adrenaline kit in case you develop anaphylaxis. If you have chronic hives that don't respond to milder treatments, your doctor may prescribe oral steroids.

Try a common weed

• Herbalists may recommend **nettle** as an alternative to anti-histamines. Take up to six 400mg capsules a day. Or pick a few handfuls of the weed, steam and eat. Wear gloves, long trousers and long sleeves to guard against nettle's stinging leaves.

Fish and the C

• Take 1,000 milligrams of **fish oil** in capsule form three times a day. These capsules contain essential fatty acids that have anti-inflammatory properties. Oily fish such as salmon, fresh tuna and mackerel are good food sources.

• Take up to 1,000mg of **vitamin C** in three divided doses. At this level, vitamin C has an effect that mimics the action of antihistamines. Don't take more than 1000mg a day or you might experience diarrhoea.

Take steps to stop stress

• Stress can cause hives or make them worse. If your tension needs taming, master a relaxation technique such as **meditation** or **yoga**.

• Brew a cup of **camomile** or **valerian tea**. These herbs have a sedative effect that may soothe stress – and therefore hives. To make the tea, stir a teaspoon of the dried herb into a cup of boiling water, steep for 10 minutes, strain and drink.

The power of prevention

• To avoid hives, you need to work out what causes them. If you don't know, start **keeping a daily diary**. The most likely culprits are things that you eat, drink or swallow – food, drink, supplements and medications. But even if you don't see any obvious connections, continue keeping your diary, noting

Skin graffiti

You probably don't think of your skin as a handy notepad, but if you have a hive condition called dermographia, it could be. People who have dermographia find that whenever they scratch their skin, they raise hive-like weals. That's because histamine and other chemicals are released in a way that causes localized swelling. Often, people who have dermographia have no evidence of allergies and the individual reaction usually disappears without treatment – although the tendency doesn't.

other factors such as weather, stress levels, what you are wearing or how much time that you spend in the sun. With careful tracking, you may be able to link a specific lifestyle factor with the eruption of those itchy weals.

- Foods most likely to trigger hives include **shellfish**, **nuts**, **chocolate**, **fish**, **tomatoes**, **eggs**, **fresh berries** and **milk**. Some people react to preservatives in certain foods and wine, such as sulphites. Once you have identified a food trigger, eliminate it from your diet and see whether you have fewer outbreaks as a result.

- Common **drug triggers** include antibiotics and nonsteroidal anti-inflammatory drugs (NSAIDs) such as aspirin and ibuprofen. But doctors have heard about many other triggers, including sedatives, tranquillizers, diuretics, diet supplements, antacids, arthritis medications, vitamins, eye drops, eardrops, laxatives and douches.

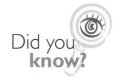

Did you know?

In their relentless hunt for causes of hives, doctors have discovered some very peculiar triggers. Some people get hives immediately after their skin is exposed to water. Weirder still, hives can be triggered by exposure to something that's vibrating – such as the grip of a vacuum cleaner or the rapid vibration of an electric foot massager.

Impotence

As most men know, numerous mental and physical factors influence the ability to achieve an erection. Once you've seen your doctor and ruled out the possibility of more serious health problems, you might want to take a multi-faceted approach to dealing with erectile dysfunction. So take up regular exercise and, at the same time, look at some of the mental factors that might be getting in the way – including boredom or anxiety in the bedroom. There are also some well known herbs and supplements that might prove to be your key to more reliable arousal.

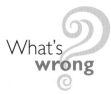

What's wrong

An erection is the end result of a complex chain of events. The brain sends signals to the genitals, blood vessels dilate and the penis gets engorged. Meanwhile, the veins that normally drain away blood get blocked. When a man cannot get or keep an erection, the problem is called impotence or erectile dysfunction (ED). Common causes include blocked arteries, diabetes and nerve problems. Depression, anxiety and alcoholism can also be factors – in fact, roughly 30 per cent of ED cases have psychological causes. Some medicines are also to blame, especially those used for high blood pressure and depression.

Diagnose your own problem

- Healthy men normally have several erections during a night's sleep. Doctors have devices to test this, but here's a simple way to test on your own. Before going to sleep, take a **single-ply tissue**, cut a strip and wrap it relatively tightly around your penis. Tape the end. If in the morning the tissue is torn, the chances are you had a nocturnal erection. That's good news – it means you probably don't have an underlying physical problem to solve but, instead, psychological matters to deal with.

Stoke the fire with herbs

- Take **ginkgo biloba.** It can improve bloodflow in vessels throughout your body, including your penis. In one study, the herb helped men to have erections even after a prescription injection didn't work. Use supplements that contain ginkgo biloba extract, or GBE, the concentrated form of the herb. Take up to 240mg of GBE a day divided into two or three doses. You should notice a difference in four to six weeks.
- Try **panax ginseng**, sometimes called Asian, Korean or Chinese ginseng. It's long been used to bolster male virility, as it can improve bloodflow to the penis, reduce fatigue and improve energy. Take 100–250mg twice a day. Start at the lower dose and increase it gradually. (*Alert* Do not use if you have hypertension, uncontrolled or otherwise, except under the supervision of a doctor or if you have a heart beat irregularity, or if you take MAOI antidepressants such as Nardil.)

Supplement your efforts

- Buy **zinc** supplements and take 15mg to 30mg a day. This mineral has beneficial effects on the production of various hormones including the male sex hormone, testosterone. Take zinc an hour before or two hours after a meal.
- Take **vitamin C.** It helps blood vessels stay flexible, allowing them to widen when you need more bloodflow. Take 500mg twice a day. Cut back the dose if you develop diarrhoea.
- Omega-3 fatty acids from **fish oils** or **flax seed oil** also improve bloodflow. In the long term they can help lower cholesterol and prevent blood vessels from narrowing. Take 2 teaspoons of fish oil or 1 tablespoon of flax seed oil a day.
- Take a supplement containing 1000mg **evening primrose oil** three times a day. The oil contains essential fatty acids that promote good blood vessel health. Take with meals to enhance absorption.
- The amino acid **arginine** can improve bloodflow to the penis by increasing the production of nitric oxide in the blood vessel walls, making arteries more flexible and helping blood vessels to dilate. The best form is L-arginine. Take two 750mg capsules twice a day between meals.

Watch your weight

- Exercise helps keep off excess weight, improves bloodflow throughout the body (including to the vessels that keep your penis working properly), boosts energy and reduces stress. Get 30 minutes of aerobic activity – such as walking, jogging, swimming or playing tennis – several times a week.

Get out of the saddle

- **If you're a cyclist, be careful.** Too much riding, or riding on the wrong saddle, can damage the delicate nerves and blood vessels in the areas you sit on. Make sure you buy a saddle that has a groove running down the centre. You should also make sure that your knees are slightly bent when your feet are at the bottom of each pedal cycle – this puts more of your weight *on* your legs instead of *between* them. Stand up at least every 10 minutes to let blood circulate to the genital area, and also level the pedals and stand up when you go over bumps to reduce jarring to your crotch.

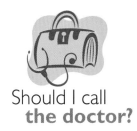

Should I call the doctor?

If your inability to have an erection lasts for more than two months or recurs frequently, talk to your doctor. You might be a good candidate for Viagra (or similar medication) and your doctor can outline the benefits and possible side effects. Also, by reviewing the medications that you take, your doctor might be able to identify one that contributes to erectile dysfunction. And a physical examination might indicate that the erection problem is a sign of another condition, such as diabetes or a circulatory disorder.

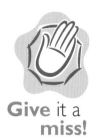

Give it a miss!

Alcohol helps to relax you and stoke the fires of your desire, but it makes you less likely to be able to perform. Limit your consumption to two drinks a day or fewer.

Give up smoking

- If you use tobacco in any form, **give up now.** Nicotine causes blood vessels to clamp down, impairing circulation. That means less blood can get to your penis.
- Smoking marijuana has a detrimental effect on performance, too, as do other **recreational drugs**, such as cocaine and amphetamines.

Do things differently in the bedroom

- If your erectile problems are due to stress and emotions rather than something physical, there are lots of ways to get yourself back in the game. For example, enjoy bedroom intimacy **without having intercourse.** This takes the pressure off, relieving performance anxiety. Just get into bed and cuddle, massage each other or think of fun things to do that don't require an erection.
- Keep **variety in your activities.** Boredom with the same old routine can hinder your ability to have an erection. Try new positions or make love somewhere other than the bedroom.
- **Have sex in the morning.** You may have more spark since your testosterone level is higher at this time of day. Plus you shouldn't be as fatigued and frazzled as at the end of a long day.

Talk to each other

- If you keep the problem to yourself, you might be making it worse. Instead, **talk about it** with your partner. You can both work through possible reasons why this may be happening – perhaps a niggling disagreement or a preoccupation with money worries is stopping you from performing properly. Not only will you find out your partner's point of view, you also benefit from having two people thinking of possible solutions.
- Let it go. Worrying about it too much will only make it worse. **Focus on other parts of your life** for a while, such as your hobbies or your children.

Look at your medicines

- Some blood-pressure drugs can contribute to erectile dysfunction, especially **calcium channel blockers** such as **nifedipine (Adalat)** and **beta-blockers** such as **metoprolol**

(Lopressor). If you take these drugs, ask your doctor if you can be prescribed something else that won't produce the same side effects.

- Digitalis medicines for heart ailments, such as **digoxin (Lanoxin)**, can also present problems. But don't stop the drug or change the dosage without first consulting your doctor.
- Men taking certain **antidepressant** medications frequently report erection problems. Since side effects are not predictable, your doctor may be able to let you try a different kind of anti-depressant to see if that improves matters.
- If you take the stomach ulcer drug **cimetidine** and are also experiencing erectile dysfunction, be sure to let your doctor know. This, too, is a common culprit.

Get plenty of rest and relaxation

- Try to get at least **6 to 8 hours'** sleep a night. Being fatigued definitely puts a damper on your ability to have an erection.
- **Reduce your stress levels.** Anxiety and anger are not conducive to the frame of mind needed for sex – and worse still, anxiety causes your body to make a form of adrenaline that interferes with the physical process behind an erection.
- If you have trouble unwinding, practise some form of relaxation technique, such as **yoga** or **meditation**. This can be as simple as spending a few minutes each day doing deep-breathing exercises – just focusing on breathing in and out.

Is it all in your mind – or further south?

Knowing whether your erectile dysfunction is rooted in your mind or body will help you to work out how to solve it.

The problem is probably psychological if you still have erections sometimes – for example, when you wake up in the morning.

It's probably physical if the problem came on gradually and you have other problems in your genital area, such as difficulty urinating or numbness in your penis.

Incontinence

Any programme designed to curb incontinence will involve pelvic floor or 'Kegel' exercises. These are named after Arnold Kegel, the doctor who first advocated the technique. Kegel exercises are an easy way to strengthen the muscles that retain your urine. They are not a cure-all, but they can help both women and men to overcome mild incontinence. You will also need to watch what you drink and when, be aware of what medicines you take – and be prepared to be patient in the loo.

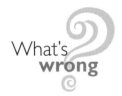

What's wrong

There are two types of urinary incontinence. In stress incontinence, urine leaks out as you bear down while laughing, sneezing, coughing or lifting something heavy. In urge incontinence, you feel the need to urinate but can't get to the loo in time. Incontinence is more common in women, as childbirth can damage the structures that help to retain urine and can also damage the nerves that tell the neck of the bladder to contract. In men, incontinence is often caused by an enlarged prostate. Other causes of incontinence include muscle relaxant drugs, urinary tract infections, Parkinson's disease and multiple sclerosis.

Imitate a cricket

• If you suddenly get the urge to go, sit down at once and rub your right **ankle down the shin** of your left leg (or vice versa). Keep steady pressure all the way. Rubbing your legs together like this inhibits bladder contractions by putting pressure on a sensory nerve (called the dermatome L5) that affects the need to urinate.

Learn the number one exercise

• Do **Kegel exercises** regularly to strengthen the pelvic floor muscles that support the bladder. To pinpoint these muscles, stop your flow while urinating; the muscles you use to do this are the ones you want to strengthen. (Do this just once for identification purposes only. Repeatedly stopping urine flow is bad for the bladder.)

• Squeeze the muscles for a second or two, then relax them. Repeat ten times, three to five times a day. Since all of the action is internal, and imperceptible to anyone else, you can do Kegels while **waiting in a queue** at the checkout, sitting in a traffic jam, having a shower, watching television and so forth.

• As your pelvic floor muscles get stronger, start holding the contraction for 5 seconds. Gradually work your way up to **15 seconds**.

• If you feel that you're about to laugh, cough, sneeze or do anything else that could put pressure on your bladder, quickly do a Kegel exercise to help keep you from having an accident.

Drinking lessons

- If you've been bothered by urge incontinence, **cut back on caffeinated drinks** or avoid them altogether. Caffeine, a diuretic, makes your body produce more urine. It can also make bladder muscles contract, causing accidents. Have no more than 200mg of caffeine a day. That's a little less than the amount in two cups of coffee.
- **Avoid alcohol.** Like caffeine, alcohol increases your body's production of urine. Have no more than one beer, glass of wine or mixed drink a day.
- **Don't go without** drinking fluids in an effort to produce less urine. You can become dehydrated and increase your risk of bladder infection and of kidney stones. Doctors advise everyone to drink the equivalent of eight 250ml glasses of water a day.

Avoid bladder irritants

- Cut **strawberries, rhubarb** and **spinach** from your diet and see if it makes any difference. These foods are high in bladder-irritating compounds called oxalates.
- Avoid **artificial sweeteners** and **colourings**. They, too, can irritate the bladder.

Have a routine

- If you've been troubled by urge incontinence, **urinate every 3 hours**, whether you need to or not. Wear a digital watch and set the alarm if you need a reminder. Some people go too long without urinating, failing to realize that their bladder has filled up. Urinating regularly helps you to avoid this problem.
- If you can't manage 3 hours without urinating then go at the **beginning of each hour**. Every few days, try holding off for few more minutes before going to the toilet. You should eventually be able to manage the full 3 hours between bathroom breaks.

Spend a bit more time here

- Once in the toilet, **don't rush to empty your bladder.** If you're a woman, stay sitting down until you feel that your urine is fully drained. Then sit a while longer. Or stand up and sit down again. If you do, the bladder will spontaneously

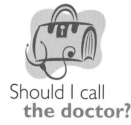

Should I call the doctor?

If there's blood in your urine, or it looks cloudy, or if urination causes pain or a burning sensation, see your doctor. These may be signs of a bacterial infection, kidney stones or a bladder tumour. You should also check with your doctor if your incontinence makes it hard to live a normal life, or if you suspect that a medicine you take might be causing your problem.

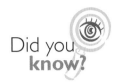

contract, emptying out any remaining urine. For men, you'll get all the urine out if you just stand for a while, relax and wait. Some men find it easier to sit on the toilet. Spending a bit more time in the toilet to make sure your bladder is completely empty, will help to prevent accidents later.

For women only

• If you have mild stress incontinence, place an **extra-absorbent tampon** in your vagina. The tampon presses against the urethra, helping it to stay closed. To ease insertion, dampen the tampon with a little water. Be sure to remove it before going to bed. Wear a tampon only for exercising if that's when your stress incontinence usually occurs.

• Another option is to consider vaginal **muscle weight training** with the help of a cone-shaped weight that you insert and hold in the vagina. They come in different weights (from 5g to 60g, either as a set of cones or as one holder into which you insert different weights), the idea being that the vaginal muscles have to contract to hold the cone in place, and you progress to increasingly heavy weights as the vaginal/pelvic muscles increase in strength. One make, called Aquaflex, is available from the larger branches of Boots.

• You can also buy a device called a **pelvic toner** – described as a 'progressive resistance vaginal trainer' and claimed to work better than cones or Kegel exercises. It is available online.

Get some exercise

• Being overweight puts pressure on the bladder. Exercise will help you to **shed unwanted pounds.** (Of course, so will watching what you eat.)

Indigestion

Our great grandparents soothed their stomach pains with some of these comforting cures, and you may be lucky with them as well. But no matter which of these remedies you choose, you will also need to take a careful and critical look at the foods you eat – as well as how often you eat and how much. You might want to look at what you wear, too: clothes that are tight around the middle put pressure on the abdomen, forcing stomach contents upwards.

Well-rooted in tradition

- **Ginger** has long been used for settling stomach upsets and quelling nausea. No one is quite sure how it works, but it has been shown to improve digestion and it has antispasmodic properties, which makes it a helpful remedy for stomach cramps. Ginger is easily taken in capsule form: take two 250mg capsules after food. Or follow a meal with a few pieces of candied root ginger or a tummy-warming cup of ginger tea. To make the tea, stir a teaspoon of fresh grated ginger root into a cup of boiling water, steep for 10 minutes and strain.
- **Camomile** is an age-old treatment for indigestion. The herb is best taken as a soothing tea – widely available in sachets from health food stores and supermarkets. Drink 3 cups of camomile tea a day, before meals.

Pamper yourself with peppermint

- **Peppermint oil** soothes intestinal cramps and helps to relieve abdominal bloating. It is best taken as slow release capsules such as Colpermin or Mintec. Take 1 or 2 capsules three times a day after food. Or you could try Obbekjaers peppermint oil capsules, available from health food stores or online. Take 1 capsule three times a day, with a little water, before meals. (*Alert* If you have heartburn, peppermint is *not* the best cure for you – it can make acid reflux problems worse. Avoid taking indigestion remedies at the same time of day as peppermint oil. If you take cyclosporine (a drug for rheumatoid arthritis), check with your doctor before taking peppermint oil.)

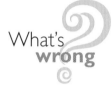

What's **wrong**

Also known as dyspepsia, the term 'indigestion' covers a wide range of unpleasant symptoms, largely as a result of food not passing through your digestive tract as smoothly and comfortably as it should. Sufferers can experience nausea or heartburn as stomach acid flows back up into the oesophagus. Or maybe the problem is abdominal pain or bloating. There are many possible causes of indigestion, including eating too much or too quickly, eating foods that don't agree with you and having too much or too little acid in your stomach.

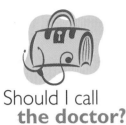

Should I call the doctor?

• Instead of taking capsules, you could try rounding off meals with a refreshing cup of **peppermint tea**. Place one dessert-spoon of dried leaves or a peppermint tea bag into a cup of boiling water, leave to infuse for 10 minutes and strain.

Chewable resources

• Chew and swallow a teaspoon of **fennel** or **caraway seeds** when you have indigestion (or after you've eaten a big or especially spicy meal that might cause indigestion). These seeds contain oils that soothe spasms in the gut, relieve nausea and help to control flatulence.

• Make a **seed infusion**. Steep 1 teaspoon of a mixture made up of equal parts caraway, fennel and anise seeds in 250ml of boiling water for 2 or 3 minutes. Strain and divide into two or three servings. Drink over the course of one day before meals.

• The ancient Greeks relied on **liquorice** to ease tummy pains, and research has found this herb to have all sorts of benefits. The root is used to treat a range of ailments from menstrual problems to respiratory infections. Another form, known as DGL (deglycyrrhizinated liquorice) has a beneficial effect on the digestive tract, soothing stomach upset and indigestion by coating the lining of the oesophagus and stomach. Although DGL is available as capsules, it is more effective when taken as a **chewable wafer** as it only works when mixed with saliva. Chew two to four 380mg wafers three times a day about 30 minutes before a meal. (*Alert* Don't take *pure* liquorice that contains glycyrrhizine – as opposed to DGL – if you have high blood pressure: it can raise blood pressure and can also be dangerous if it is taken with certain diuretics prescribed for the condition.)

The soda solution

• Stir a teaspoon of **bicarbonate of soda** (bicarb) into a glass of water and drink it. This will neutralize stomach acid and help to relieve painful wind. Bicarb can produce quantities of gas in the stomach, so some experts suggest adding a few drops of **lemon juice** to dispel some of the gas before it hits your stomach. This bicarb treatment should not be used more than three or four times in a year. (*Alert* Do not take bicarb if you are on a low-sodium diet as it is high in sodium.)

Sour solution

● Try drinking a teaspoon of **cider vinegar** stirred into half a glass of water, especially after a large or rich meal. It will help you to digest the food if you don't have enough acid in your stomach. Add a little honey if you wish to sweeten the taste.

Sip this

● Some people claim that drinking a simple cup of **hot water** eases indigestion.

● Warm **ginger ale** or **lemonade** or **flat cola** are also said to soothe an upset stomach. If there are any gassy bubbles, get rid of them by stirring the drink briskly first.

Beware of juice and dairy produce

● While it may be healthy, fruit juice can actually cause abdominal pain and wind. It contains fructose, a sugar that passes undigested into the colon. When bacteria in the colon finally break down the sugar, you're likely to get bloating and wind. If drinking juice, have **no more than 150ml** at a time and drink it **with food** so you can digest it better.

● If dairy foods make you feel gassy and bloated, the problem could be lactose intolerance – an inability to digest lactose, a sugar found in milk. To find out for sure, try this simple test. Drink 2 glasses of milk and see if this triggers the symptoms that have been bothering you. If so, try cutting dairy foods from your diet or look for **lactose-free products**. If you don't want to give up milk, buy liquid lactase from your pharmacy and add it to milk before you drink it, or switch to soya milk.

Eat slowly, finish early

● **Eat slowly** and deliberately. Wolfing down your food puts big chunks of material into your digestive system and you also swallow air, which can contribute to bloating and flatulence. Furthermore, when you eat too fast, food doesn't get fully coated with saliva. That interferes with the digestive process.

● Eat your last big meal of the day at least **three hours before bedtime.** Your digestive system works best when you're up and moving about, not while you're asleep.

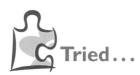

Tried...

Rubbing your tummy can help to relieve indigestion.

...& true

When you massage your lower abdomen, you push trapped wind and digestive products towards their natural exit. This can help to dispel bloating and constipation.

Infant Colic

The plaintive cries of a colicky baby can put parents under enormous stress and even send them into a total panic if they can't find a way to stop the heart-wrenching screaming. So the first thing on the agenda is to relax. Take a break. If there are two of you, take it in turns. If not, ask a supportive friend to stand in for you now and then. To calm the crying, first check the most obvious causes of distress – hunger, a wet nappy, excessive heat or cold or simply wanting to be held. Then try the parent-tested strategies below.

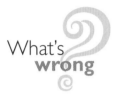

What's
wrong

Your baby is crying … and crying … and crying – and nothing you do seems to help. The baby may clench its hands into fists and draw up its legs against its tummy, which can feel as tight as a drum. The baby may also pass wind or have a bowel movement immediately before or after the screaming bout. A baby who cries for more than 3 hours a day, three days a week, for at least three weeks – when there is no underlying health problem – is said to have colic. Colic tends to be worst at four to six weeks and subsides, for no discernible reason, at three or four months.

Tummy-down is best

- Hold the baby in a **tummy-down** position. For some reason, a colicky baby seems to be more comfortable when lying on its stomach. If you're in a rocking chair, hold the baby along your forearm, face down, as you gently rock back and forth. The head should be cradled in one hand. (An infant at this age always needs head support.)
- When you want to **walk around**, continue holding the baby on your forearm, with the head in your hand. But bring the baby close to your chest, supporting with your other hand.
- Put the baby in a **chest carrier** like a **Snugli**. Just being nestled against your warm chest is comforting and so is your heartbeat. With your hands free, you can take a nice, long walk, which may help to console your child. If carrying a screaming baby in a sling, parental sanity (and future hearing) may be salvaged by a pair of **earplugs**.
- Your baby might settle down in its crib if **wrapped tightly** and lying on its side. But stay nearby and keep watch. If the baby rolls onto its front, roll it onto its back. The Foundation for the Study of Infant Deaths says that placing a baby on its back to sleep is key to cutting the risk of cot death.

Swaddle snugly

- Swaddling **mimics the pressure** a baby would have felt in the womb. The idea is to make the baby feel **secure** rather than just keep it warm. Swaddling has also been reported to cut the risk of cot death. Spread out a cotton cot sheet, with one corner folded over. Lay your baby face up on the sheet with the fold behind its neck. Wrap the left corner of the sheet over its arms and body and tuck it beneath the baby. Bring the bottom corner over its feet, and then wrap the right corner around the baby, leaving only the head and neck uncovered. **Don't use a cosy blanket** to swaddle the child – the infant may overheat – and don't wrap too tightly, or you risk cutting off your baby's circulation.

- For extra comfort, soothe a baby that stays resolutely awake by **warming its tummy** with a warm (not hot) hot-water bottle. Choose a hottie with a cover or wrap one in a soft towel, and rest it on the baby's tummy while he or she sits on your knee. Do not leave a baby wrapped up in bed with a hot-water bottle, however, in case it leaks or burns.

Swing the baby

- Place your infant in a mechanical **baby swing**. For some reason, the back-and-forth motion has calmed many a squawking child. Continual, steady movement is the key.

Let appliances hush-a-bye baby

- Run the **vacuum cleaner.** The sound is a lullaby to the ears of some colicky infants. As an added bonus, you'll get a clean rug. If the vacuum cleaner doesn't work, try the hair-dryer.
- Find a **radio station that's all static**, and leave the radio on with the volume turned low. The steady 'white noise' helps some babies settle down. Or **buy a CD** featuring sounds that babies find comforting, such as a mother's heartbeat, a waterfall, a distant lawn mower or a whirring fan.
- Some colicky babies respond to the sound and vibrations of a **tumble dryer**. If you're in the kitchen or utility room, put your baby in a seat that touches the side of the dryer.

Offer your little finger

- Even when the baby's not ready for a feed, it draws comfort from **oral stimulation**. Let your baby suck on your little finger. As long as the finger is clean, the nail is well-trimmed and you're not wearing nail varnish, it's just as good as a soother – even better, in fact, as it doesn't keep falling out.

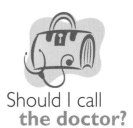

Should I call the doctor?

Your doctor can help you to ascertain whether your baby's crying is a symptom of an underlying infection or illness. If a one-week-old baby cries endlessly, for example, it means the infant has a health problem more serious than colic. But if your GP concludes that your baby has colic, the challenge is to deal with the crying. Take comfort from the knowledge that it will subside at three or four months. See your doctor urgently if any episode lasts for longer than 4 hours, if the baby seems ill and in pain between crying bouts – especially if there is projectile vomiting, if he or she is constipated or has diarrhoea, if he or she has a fever, or is reluctant to feed. You should also see your doctor if you are finding your baby's crying too hard to handle. Seek help if you feel excessively anxious or miserable, or if you fear you might harm the baby.

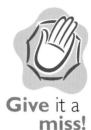

Give it a miss!

Cut out the dairy produce

- Some experts have suggested that crying might be caused by the mother-to-baby transmission of **cow's milk**. If you breast-feed your baby and you've been drinking milk or eating milk products (such as cheese), try going without any dairy produce for a week. If this doesn't solve the problem, you can go back to your usual diet.
- **Avoid** foods and drinks that contain **caffeine**, such as tea, coffee, colas and chocolate. Try this plan for a few days to see if it helps.
- **Monitor other 'trigger foods'** that could be affecting your baby through your breastmilk. Common ones are beans, eggs, onions, garlic, grapes, tomatoes, bananas, oranges, strawberries and anything spicy. Of course, if you find that eliminating these foods for a week makes little or no difference, then you can go ahead and eat them again.

Cut down external stimuli

- Sometimes the more you try to calm a colicky baby, the more it seems to cry. That may be because the baby's nervous system is too immature to handle any noise – or even gentle movement like rocking or swinging. Even the sound of your singing voice, softly crooning, may be too much noise for its sensitive ears. To **minimize stimulation**, try letting the baby cry for 10 to 15 minutes. Put the baby down during this time or hold it passively in your arms. Avoid direct eye contact, which is a form of stimulation.

Sit your baby up and wind frequently

- **Keep your baby upright,** when feeding, not horizontal, and **burp the infant frequently.** When you bottle-feed, burp the baby after every ounce and try different teats. Some are specially designed to reduce the amount of air swallowed.
- **Don't let a baby suck on an empty bottle**; it can cause the infant to swallow air, leading to a tummy full of wind. For the same reason, don't let the baby suck on a teat that has a hole that's too large. Although trapped wind is not the cause of colic, it can sometimes lead to just as much crying.

Infertility

When nature takes its course, eventually a baby results. Except that sometimes it doesn't. Doctors now know that men and women are equally likely to be infertile – defined as the inability to conceive a child within a year. The home remedy 'homework' below is divided by sex. But no matter whether the problem lies with one or other or both of you, you must work together to find a solution. Making a baby is, after all, a joint undertaking. Here are some ways to help make it successful.

FOR WOMEN
Know when your egg is ready

- Check your **cervical mucus.** You are most fertile five days before and one day after ovulation. When your cervical mucus turns thin and clear, ovulation is about to begin. (Thin mucus makes it easier for sperm to reach the egg.) Periodically wipe your vaginal area with a tissue: If the secretion is stretchy and looks like egg white, the going is good for getting pregnant.
- Make sure that you're actually ovulating. Buy an **ovulation testing kit** at the pharmacy. Some work like a pregnancy test kit, requiring a urine sample; others test your saliva. If, after three months, the test kit fails to indicate ovulation, see your doctor.

Slim down – or build up

- If you need to **lose weight**, your wish to conceive should be a real motivator. Body fat can produce oestrogen, and too much oestrogen can impair your ability to conceive.
- **Being too thin** is another cause of infertility in women. Without enough body fat, you may not ovulate normally, or your uterus may be unable to accept implantation of a fertilized egg. If you are worried that you might be too thin to conceive, add more healthy calories to your diet – lean protein, whole-grain foods and beneficial fats such as olive oil.

Take things easy

- If you're already making lots of physical demands on your body, it may be less capable of 'accepting' the demands of pregnancy. In particular, **exercising for more than an hour a**

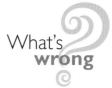

What's **wrong**

Infertility is defined as an inability to become pregnant after having unprotected sex for a full year. In women, infertility has many possible causes, including sexually transmitted diseases, endometriosis, uterine fibroids, irregular menstruation, a deficit of healthy eggs and hormone trouble. Some women are infertile because of a hidden birth defect affecting the uterus or Fallopian tubes. Others experience irregular ovulation. In men, a low sperm count is just one possible cause of infertility. The sperm might be misshapen or unable to swim properly to the egg.

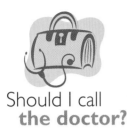

Should I call the doctor?

If you're a woman over 35, you should let your doctor know you're trying to conceive. If after six months you're still not pregnant, it's time to begin doing what you can to improve your chances. If you're under 35 and trying to get pregnant, you might prefer to wait for up to a year before seeking medical help. A man should also see his doctor at the same time as his partner to rule out problems such as a low sperm count.

day can interfere with ovulation; this problem is sometimes experienced by female athletes and ballerinas. If you usually exercise strenuously, take it down a notch.

• Take it a bit easier at work. Research shows that women who work at a hectic pace in **stressful jobs** can have trouble getting pregnant. Set reasonable work goals and try to leave office stress behind when you go home. Consider **meditation** or **yoga** as a way of keeping stress in check.

Check your medicine cabinet

• Try to **avoid antihistamines** and **decongestants.** These drugs are designed to reduce the amount of mucus in your sinuses, but they affect your cervical mucus as well. And you need that mucus to help sperm reach the egg.

• Also **don't take ibuprofen** or **aspirin** when you're trying to get pregnant. These anti-inflammatories can interfere with ovulation and prevent a fertilized egg from attaching to the wall of your uterus. For pain relief, try paracetamol instead.

FOR MEN
Stock up on sperm

• **Say no to sex** for a few days before your partner begins to ovulate. You want to inseminate her with the maximum possible number of sperm; the longer it's been since your last ejaculation, the greater that number will be.

• Wear **boxer shorts** instead of briefs. Snug-fitting underwear traps heat, and too much heat reduces the number of healthy sperm produced by the testicles. The same applies to tight denim. So if you've got fatherhood in mind, keep things loose. And avoid hot baths and saunas, too.

Take baby-making supplements

• Each day, take 30mg **zinc.** The mineral boosts your testosterone level, increases your sperm count and helps to give sperm a little extra oomph. Because zinc interferes with your body's absorption of copper, also take 2mg of copper a day while you're taking zinc.

• Protect your sperm with antioxidants in the form of 1000mg **vitamin C** a day and 250mg **vitamin E** (with food) twice a day. Vitamins C and E help to protect sperm by blocking the action of free radicals, rogue oxygen molecules that cause cell damage throughout the body. If you're taking an anticoagulant or another drug that interferes with blood clotting, talk to your doctor before taking vitamin E.

- Take **selenium.** Studies suggest that men who take 100mcg a day for three months experience a marked increase in sperm motility (swimming ability), although there seems to be no effect on sperm count.

- Try **pycnogenol,** an extract from the bark of a pine tree that grows along the coast of south-western France. A potent antioxidant, it may improve the health of sperm in men with fertility problems. One recent study found that men with fertility problems who took 200mg of pycnogenol a day for three months significantly improved the quality and function of their sperm. Pycnogenol is sold over-the-counter in some health-food shops and online.

- Consider taking a daily dose of **flax seed oil.** There's some preliminary evidence that this oil, which is an excellent source of essential fatty acids, can help to keep sperm healthy. Even if it doesn't boost your fertility, it will work to lower your cholesterol and help to protect you against heart disease. Take one tablespoon a day with food. You can mix it into juice, yoghurt, salad dressing – or anything else.

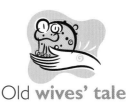

Old **wives' tale**

Some women have been told that douching helps to clean the vagina, creating better conditions for egg fertilization. In fact, douching changes the vagina's acid-alkali balance, and that makes the environment less hospitable for sperm.

FOR WOMEN AND MEN
Steer clear of smoke

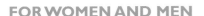

- Smoking not only **decreases fertility** in both sexes but also increases the **risk of miscarriage.** The number of healthy eggs in the ovaries dwindles more quickly in smokers than among non-smokers. In men, sperm counts decrease, and there are more damaged sperm.

Lose booze and cut caffeine

- **Avoid alcohol.** In men, alcohol can impair ejaculation. There is no evidence that moderate alcohol consumption in women causes problems – but it might be easier for your partner to keep off the booze if you join him.

- Avoiding **coffee,** drinks containing caffeine, and medicines can help to boost fertility in both sexes.

Timing is everything

- When ovulation is imminent, **have sex** at least once a day for three days.
- If you've chosen not to track your ovulation – either by examining cervical mucus or using an ovulation test kit – **make love every other day** from day eight to day twenty (counting from the first day of your last period). Sperm have a three-day lifespan. By having sex with your partner that often, you improve the chances that sperm will be ready and waiting when ovulation occurs.

Inflammatory bowel disease

Doctors tend to treat inflammatory bowel disease (IBD) with powerful steroids and other prescription medications, and these drugs can be very helpful, especially during flare-ups. But there are steps you can take on your own to reduce the severity of your symptoms, such as choosing foods that are kind to your bowels, taking vitamin supplements and soothing herbs and doing what you can to lessen stress.

Boost beneficial bacteria

- Boost the population of beneficial bacteria in your gut. You can do this by taking an over-the-counter bacteria supplement known as a **probiotic.** In healthy people, the colon is home to 'good' bacteria (such as *Lactobacillus acidophilus* and *Bifidobacteria bifidum*) that prevent overgrowth of harmful bacteria. But when these bacteria are killed off – often, by antibiotics – the resulting overgrowth of 'bad' bacteria and yeast can cause inflammation. Probiotics help maintain an optimal balance. Take 2 capsules three times a day on an empty stomach or, if you don't want to take a supplement, eat two or three pots of bio-yoghurt a day.

Fuel your body with care

- Favour bland foods – **cooked carrots, white rice** and **stewed apple**, for example. If you're already suffering from diarrhoea and abdominal pain, eating lots of spicy foods will only make matters worse.
- **Cut back on dietary fat.** Fried foods, fatty meats and other sources of fat can trigger contractions in your intestine, which can exacerbate diarrhoea.
- **Eat less dietary fibre** during flare-ups. Ordinarily, high-fibre foods like bran, whole grains and broccoli are good for the digestive system. But during inflammatory bowel disease flare-ups they increase your risk of painful gas. Once you feel better, resume a normal fibre intake.
- Many people with Crohn's disease are unable to digest lactose, a form of sugar found in dairy foods. If you feel gassy and bloated, try **avoiding milk** and all other dairy foods for a

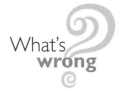

What's **wrong**

The term inflammatory bowel disease, or IBD, encompasses several conditions. The two most common ones are ulcerative colitis and Crohn's disease. Ulcerative colitis causes sores on the lining of the colon and rectum. Crohn's disease is more extensive – sometimes affecting the intestines, stomach, oesophagus and mouth – and tissues can become much more deeply inflamed. Symptoms are similar for both colitis and Crohn's: diarrhoea, abdominal pain and blood or mucus in the stool. These problems can flare up, then go away, with remissions sometimes lasting years.

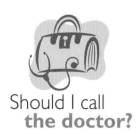

Should I call the doctor?

few days. If your symptoms go away, you may have lactose intolerance. Switch to lactose-free dairy products, take pills containing lactase (the enzyme needed to digest milk) or avoid milk products altogether.

- Take a daily **multivitamin/mineral supplement.** This will help to restore the nutrients that can be depleted by persistent diarrhoea.

Record what you eat

- Keep a **food diary.** Record everything you eat throughout the day (including snacks), what reactions you have and the severity of your discomfort. At the end of a month, review your diary to get a sense of how well you tolerate dietary fibre and potentially troublesome foods, such as dairy products. You'll also find out whether you need to avoid any particular foods altogether.

Lessen stress to digest best

- Stress can trigger IBD symptoms. So every day, practise **yoga, meditation, deep breathing, visualization** or any other relaxation technique. For example, you might sit in a quiet spot for 20 minutes or so and visualize a healing blue light slowly pouring down the length of your digestive tract, soothing the inflammation. Imagine that as this blue light travels through you, it leaves healthy tissue behind.

Natural healers

- A folk remedy was to **drink cabbage juice** for intestinal inflammation, as it is rich in the amino acid **L-glutamine**. But if that doesn't sound particularly appetizing, you can simply take L-glutamine pills (500mg a day). L-glutamine helps to heal ulcers in the gut.
- Because it combats inflammation, a **liquorice** extract called **DGL** (deglycyrrhizinated liquorice) may help to ease symptoms of inflammatory bowel disease. Chew two wafers (380mg) three times a day between meals whenever you have a flare-up. Don't try to substitute liquorice confectionery; most liquorice sweets contain no real liquorice. And unlike DGL, 'real' liquorice can raise your blood pressure.

Pour oil on troubled intestines

- Omega-3 fatty acids are essential for good digestion. Good sources include **flax seed oil** (1 tablespoon a day taken straight from the spoon or mixed into salad dressing or cereal) and **fish oil** (take 2 teaspoons to provide 2g omega-3 fatty acids a day). One Italian study found that fish oil reduced the frequency of intestinal attacks in people with Crohn's disease. (*Alert* Don't take fish oil if you take anticoagulant drugs.)

Time for tea

- Both **peppermint** and **camomile** contain antispasmodic compounds that help to curb cramps and ease pain caused by abdominal wind. To make a tea, put a teaspoon of either dried herb into a cup of boiling water and let it steep for 10 minutes. Strain and drink. If you're susceptible to heartburn, choose camomile over peppermint.
- **Marshmallow tea** also soothes by coating the mucous membranes in the digestive tract. Use 1 to 2 teaspoons of dried herb per cup of hot water. Steep for 10 to 15 minutes, strain and drink.

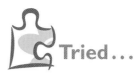

Tried...

People with IBD used to be advised to eat onion skins.

...& true

Onion skins contain quercetin, a naturally occurring antihistamine that helps to block the allergy-like reactions that IBD sufferers have to certain foods. When cooking soup, you can add a whole onion to the pan; the quercetin will seep out of the skin. Remove the skin before eating the onion. If you don't like onions, you can buy quercetin supplements over the counter at pharmacies. Follow instructions on the label.

Ingrowing toenails

Toenail care is probably not high on your list of skills to master but, when an ingrowing nail is bothering you, it's amazing how quickly you can develop an interest in the subject. Of all the minor ills in our lives, this is among the most preventable. But once an ingrowing nail begins to cause you pain, you will try anything to make it better. Try these steps to put it in its place.

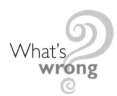

What's wrong

Ingrowing toenails are usually a big-toe problem. A thick, sharp nail starts growing into the tender skin at the corner of the nail, cutting the skin as it grows. The incised area becomes red, painful and vulnerable to infection. Some people have toenails that just naturally grow in ways that set the stage for this problem. But there are other contributing factors – wearing tight shoes or socks, for instance, or cutting toenails improperly. And you're more likely to have ingrowing toenails if you have structural irregularities known as bunions or hammertoes.

Soak your feet
- Half-fill a large bucket with **hot water.** Add several table-spoons of **salt** and stir until the salt dissolves. Soak your problem foot for 15 to 20 minutes each day. Hot water softens the skin around the ingrowing nail while the salt helps to combat infection and reduces swelling.

Try this cotton trick
- After you've soaked your feet, wash off the salt with **warm, soapy water**, rinse and let your feet dry.
- Slip a small piece of **cotton** gauze between the sharp edge of the nail and the tender skin that it's cutting into. You may need a tool to help you to do this. Dip a clean **toothpick** into **surgical spirit** to sterilize it. Then, use the toothpick to carefully push the cotton underneath the cutting edge of your toenail. With the edge of your nail cushioned by the gauze instead of cutting into your skin, you should feel less pain. Also, the nail should now be able to grow past the flesh it's been burrowing into.
- Dab on some antiseptic to prevent infection and repeat the procedure with a clean piece of gauze every day.

Keep your feet clean
- Put on a **clean pair of socks** every day. While you can't keep feet completely germ-free, you will reduce the risk of infection if you keep them as clean as possible.
- Whenever you take a bath or shower, be sure to scrub your feet well with a **soapy flannel**. Afterwards, put some **antiseptic ointment** onto your toe.

Display your toes

- At home and in warm weather, wear shoes that are **open at the end**, such as sandals. Tight shoes only exacerbate the problem because you're jamming the nail ever deeper into skin that already hurts.
- In winter, make sure closed-in shoes are **broad at the toe**. Pointed shoes are a disaster for ingrowing toenails.

The power of prevention

- Before cutting your nails, soak your feet in warm water for a few minutes to **soften the nail**. When you cut toenails, always **cut them straight across**, leaving a little extra nail on each side. Then **file the corners** very slightly – just so they're not sharp. While you should cut all your toenails like this, pay special attention to the big toenail, as it's the most vulnerable.
- **Don't pick** at your toenails. You're more likely to tear off the corners, and the remaining edge of the nail can grow into your toe.
- To make sure you buy shoes that fit properly, have your **feet measured** whenever you buy new shoes. Your feet get longer and wider as you age, and shoes that fitted you once upon a time might be real toe-squeezers now.
- **Buy your shoes** at the end of the day. Your feet often swell from the day's pounding and they will be at their largest during the late afternoon.
- Pay attention to how you **lace up your shoes**. The point is to keep your foot from sliding inside the shoe, so that your toes don't keep running into the end of the toe box. To best achieve that, make sure the laces are tightest (but not uncomfortably so) near the top of your midfoot.
- Believe it or not, tight socks or tights can affect toenails too, even if the shoe is loose and comfortable. Pick **socks or tights that don't squeeze** your toes together.

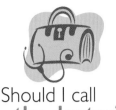

Should I call the doctor?

See your doctor if your toe is oozing pus, a sign of infection. You also need medical attention if an injury to the nail bed is making the nail grow crookedly. Redness, particularly streaks running up the foot, can be a sign of serious infection, whether or not it's accompanied by fever. If you have diabetes, see a doctor or chiropodist if ever you have an ingrowing toenail: like any foot problem, it could lead to serious complications.

Give it a miss!

Don't wrap a bandage or gauze tightly around the wounded toe. That will just press the sharp nail harder into the skin.

Insomnia

Insomnia can become a real nightmare as the clock ticks on into the night and you're awake to notice. But you're not alone. At any one time, the problem affects around 15 per cent of the UK population. So what can you do? Try counting sheep; it really can work. Better still, try some of the approaches listed below. A relaxing tea, a whiff of lavender oil, creating a sleep routine and various other tactics will help you to drop off more easily and wake up less tired and irritable in the morning.

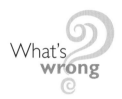

What's wrong

Insomnia can take three forms: (1) you toss and turn instead of falling asleep; (2) you fall asleep okay, but then wake up repeatedly during the night; or (3) you wake up much too early and can't get back to sleep again. Whatever the form of sleep deprivation, you will feel groggy and irritable the next day. The most common causes of insomnia are emotional stress and depression. Other reasons for poor sleep include pain or illness, medications (such as decongestants, diuretics, some antidepressants, steroids and beta-blockers), eating a heavy meal late at night, drinking caffeine or alcohol too near bedtime or simply trying to sleep in an unfamiliar bed.

Bedtime snacks

- Have a slice of **turkey** or **chicken** or a **banana** before going to bed. These foods contain tryptophan, an amino acid that the body uses to make serotonin. And serotonin is a brain chemical that helps you to sleep. Keep the helping small, though, or your full tummy may keep you awake.
- Carbohydrates help trytophan to enter the brain. Try a glass of **warm milk** (milk contains tryptophan) and a **biscuit**, or warm milk with a spoonful of **honey**. A sprinkling of **cinnamon** won't hurt and might add mild sedative properties of its own.
- **Avoid large meals** late in the evening. You need three to four hours to digest a big meal, so if you eat a lot within three hours of your bedtime, don't be surprised if intestinal grumblings and groanings keep you awake.
- Spicy or sugary food, even at suppertime, is usually a bad idea. **Spices can irritate your stomach**, and when it tosses and turns, so will you. Having a lot of sugary food – especially chocolate, which contains caffeine – can make you feel jumpy.

Call on herbs for help

- **Valerian** can help people to fall asleep faster without the 'hangover' effect of some sleeping pills. It binds to the same receptors in the brain that tranquillizers such as valium bind to. The herb itself stinks (think of sweaty old socks), so we don't advise trying to make it into a tea. Instead, take ½ to 1 teaspoon of valerian tincture or 2 valerian root capsules an hour before going to bed.

• Make **passionflower** tea. Put 1 teaspoon of the dried herb into a cup of boiling water, leave to infuse for 5 to 10 minutes, strain and drink before bed. Passionflower is widely used as a mild herbal sedative.

• Or you can combine forces, taking a supplement that includes both **passionflower** and **valerian**. 'Natural' sleep remedies often include other herbal ingredients as well, such as **hops**. Whatever the formulation, follow package directions.

A sweet way to scented sleep

• **Lavender** has a reputation as a mild tranquillizer. Dilute lavender oil in a carrier oil (5 drops per 10ml) and dab a little on to your temples and forehead before you hit the pillow. The aroma should help to send you off to sleep. You can also add lavender oil to a diffuser or vapourizer to scent your bedroom. Or place a lavender sachet near your pillow.

• Put a drop of **jasmine** essential oil on each wrist just before you go to bed. One US study discovered that people who spent the night in jasmine-scented rooms slept more peacefully than people who stayed in unscented – or even in lavender-scented – rooms.

• Try a soothing aromatic **bath** before bedtime. Add 5 drops of **lavender oil** and 3 drops of **ylang-ylang oil** to warm bath-water and enjoy a nice soak.

Adopt a rigid routine

• **Wake up at the same time each day**, no matter how little sleep you had the night before. At weekends, don't have a lie-in. Follow the same routine so your body adheres to the same pattern all week. You'll fall asleep faster.

• Every morning, **go for a walk**. It doesn't have to be long but it should be outdoors. The presence of natural light tells your sleepy body it's time to wake up for the day. With your body clock set to natural daylight, you'll sleep better at night.

• **Try not to nap** during the day, no matter how tired you feel. People who don't have insomnia often benefit from a short afternoon nap. However, if you nap during the day only to turn into a wide-eyed zombie at night, there's a good chance that that afternoon snooze is disrupting your body clock. If you must nap, limit it to half-an-hour at the most.

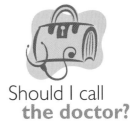

Should I call the doctor?

If you've tried self-help strategies and still can't get a good night's sleep, talk to your doctor. This is especially important if sleep deprivation is harming your relationships, your work performance or endangering your life – as in causing you to fall asleep at the wheel. You may need to be evaluated overnight at a sleep clinic.

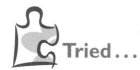

Tried...

A hop-filled pillow can help to relieve insomnia.

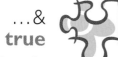

...& **true**

Hops – flowers of a plant used in beer-making – release a mild sedative into the air. To make your own pillow, sew two 30cm (1ft) squares of fabric together along three sides to form a pocket. Stuff it full of dried hops and sew the fourth side shut. Put the pillow near your head so you can smell it at night.

Pillow tricks

• Once you get into bed, imagine your feet becoming heavy and numb. Feel them sinking into the mattress. Then do the same with your calves and slowly work your way up your body, letting it all grow heavy and relaxed. The idea is to **let yourself go**, in gradual phases, all the way from head to toe.

• If you're still awake after this progressive relaxation exercise, **count sheep**. It may sound like an old wives' tale, but the whole point is to occupy your brain with mind-numbing repetition and, while not wanting to insult sheep, there's nothing more boring or repetitive than counting a flock of them. Any repetitive counting activity will lull you.

• If you prefer lullabies, listen to **calming, relaxing tapes** as you drift off.

• If you simply can't sleep, **don't lie in bed worrying about it**. That will only make getting to sleep harder. Get up, leave the bedroom and grab a book, some knitting, a jigsaw puzzle or watch television. Don't read or watch anything too exciting, though, or you'll become engrossed and your mind will be even more wakeful.

Prepare your bedroom for rest

• If you find yourself tossing and turning as you try to get comfortable, consider buying a special **neck-supporting pillow**. They are specially designed for people who have neck pain or tension that prevents sleep.

• **Turn your alarm clock** so that you **can't see it** from your bed. If you're glancing at the clock when you wake up – and it's almost impossible not to – you'll soon start wondering how you can possibly function tomorrow on so little sleep tonight. For truly accomplished insomniacs, just one glance at a glowing digital clock is enough to set a whole anxiety train in motion.

• **Turn the central heating off** (or at least right down) before going to bed. Most people sleep better when the air around them is cool and their bedding is snug.

• If you share a bed, consider buying a **queen or king-size bed** so that you don't keep each other awake. Some mattresses are designed so that when your partner moves – or even if something as heavy as a bowling ball dropped on his or her side of the bed – you feel nothing. Or consider sleeping in separate beds. (If you value your relationship, then reassure your loved one that the suggestion is based on pragmatism rather than preference.)

Check the label
- Be cautious about taking any over-the-counter painkillers before bed. Some of them, like Anadin Extra, contain **caffeine** – a stimulant. Read the label first.
- Check labels of decongestants and cold remedies too. In addition to caffeine, medications like Sudafed may contain ingredients, such as pseudoephedrine, that rev up your nervous system and leave you unable to fall asleep. Look for a **night-time formula**.

Don'ts and more don'ts
- **Avoid exercising** within four hours of bedtime – it's too stimulating. Instead, exercise in the morning or after work. An exception is **yoga**. A number of yoga postures are designed to calm your body and prepare you for sleep.
- **Avoid caffeinated drinks**, particularly within four hours of bedtime. Though people have varying ranges of sensitivity to caffeine, the stimulating effects can be long-lasting.
- Also **avoid alcohol** in the evenings. While a tot of whisky might help you to fall asleep a bit faster than usual, the effects soon wear off and you're much more likely to wake up during the night.
- If you **smoke** within four hours of going to bed, look no further for the **cause of your insomnia**. Nicotine stimulates the central nervous system, interfering with your ability to fall asleep and stay asleep.

Irritable bowel syndrome

There's no cure for irritable bowel syndrome (IBS), and doctors aren't sure what causes it either. Anyone who suffers from IBS develops his or her own ways of living with the condition. The key is not to become discouraged. Dietary changes and stress-management tactics should provide significant relief. For more protection, combine them with one of the alternative therapies described below. Once you have a system for controlling your symptoms, IBS should cramp your style a little less.

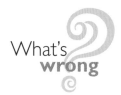

What's wrong

Normally, food travels through your digestive system propelled by wavelike contractions of the intestinal muscles. But if you have irritable bowel syndrome, or IBS, the contractions are irregular – fast and erratic, causing diarrhoea, or slow and weak, causing constipation. Other symptoms include abdominal pain and wind. The exact causes are unknown, but doctors have discovered that raised stress levels, along with certain foods, aggravate IBS. Women are twice as likely as men to be affected by IBS.

Cut the stress circuit

• Since stress is one of the factors known to trigger an IBS flare-up, learn to short-circuit it with **meditation**, **yoga** or a **simple breathing exercise** like this one. Sit comfortably or lie down. Fix your attention on the air going in and out of your body. When upsetting or anxiety-producing thoughts intrude, focus completely on your breathing. Practise this every day. Then, whenever you feel yourself becoming tense and anxious, use it to calm yourself.

• **Keep a diary** of your IBS symptoms, noting what types of problems you have and how severe they are. In this diary, also jot down any stressful events in your day. Occasionally look back at your diary. If you see more IBS symptoms just before aeroplane flights or meetings with your boss, for instance, there's probably a connection. Once you've identified the situations that seem to trigger IBS symptoms, look for ways – such as breathing techniques – to cope with them better.

Be gentle on your intestines

• **Minimize fried foods**, meats, oils, margarine, dairy foods and other fatty foods. They cause your colon to contract violently, which can lead to diarrhoea and abdominal pain.

• **Stay away from spicy foods.** The capsaicin in hot peppers, for example, makes your large intestine go into spasms, which can cause diarrhoea.

• **Cut down on caffeine.** It can worsen IBS.

• Avoid foods known to cause flatulence, including **cabbage, Brussels sprouts** and **broccoli.**

• Don't chew gum or eat sweets that contain artificial sweeteners. Common sweeteners include **sorbitol** and **mannitol**, which can have a laxative effect as they are very difficult to digest. When bacteria in your colon eventually break down these non-absorbed sugars, you get wind and diarrhoea.

• **Stop smoking**. Nicotine contributes to IBS flare-ups. Also, when you smoke, you swallow air and people with IBS are very sensitive to having air in their digestive tract.

Fit in more fibre

Recent thinking on fibre and IBS has changed. It seems that both soluble and insoluble fibre are likely to benefit IBS patients with **constipation, hard stools and urgency**, but are unlikely to help those with abdominal distension, diarrhoea or flatulence and may make such symptoms worse. So consider the following advice if constipation is your main complaint.

• Eat plenty of **insoluble fibre**, which is found in whole wheat and other whole grains, bran, greens, beans and pulses. Insoluble fibre bulks up faecal matter, which speeds its passage through the intestines.

• **Soluble fibre** also helps your intestines to work more efficiently, and has the added bonus of lowering cholesterol levels. Good sources are **beans, porridge** and some **fruits**, such as **apples, strawberries** and **grapefruit**.

• An easy way to add soluble fibre to your diet is to take a daily dose of **psyllium**, the main ingredient in dietary fibre supplements like Metamucil. Psyllium is safe to take in the long term, unlike chemical laxatives. Follow label directions.

• If you haven't had much fibre in your diet up till now, **increase the amount you eat gradually**. Adding too much fibre all at once can actually cause wind and bloating. Start

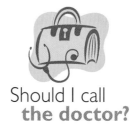

Should I call the doctor?

Call your doctor if you notice blood in your stool, you start losing weight when you're not trying to, or your IBS symptoms are so severe that you can't even leave your home. You should also see a doctor if you're over 50 and start to have IBS symptoms for the first time; and if you've had IBS for many years but notice a change in a previous pattern. Among other things, the doctor will look at your prescription or OTC medications to find out whether a change in bowel habits is related to drug side effects. If food intolerances are suspected, you may be referred to a dietician for advice.

Is it lactose intolerance?

Many people who think they have IBS actually have lactose intolerance, a problem in which the body can't properly digest the lactose sugar in dairy foods. An easy way to self-diagnose this is to drink two 250ml glasses of milk. If you are lactose intolerant, you will get cramps, wind and diarrhoea. If you get these symptoms, you know it's time to drop some dairy foods – especially milk – from your diet. You may find that you can still eat yoghurt and hard cheeses such as Cheddar. (See also page 378.)

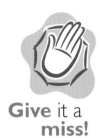

Give it a miss!

If you have IBS, avoid using medications to affect your bowel habits – either laxatives for constipation or drugs to fight diarrhoea. These can make you swing wildly back and forth between constipation and diarrhoea.

with 8g of fibre a day – about what you'd find in two pears – and increase your intake by 3g to 4g a day until you're up to 30g daily.

- Drink at least 6 to 8 glasses of **water** each day to keep fibre moving smoothly through your system.

Graze, don't gorge

- Eat **smaller, more frequent meals.** Taking in too much food at once can overstimulate your digestive system.
- If you usually bolt down your meals, **eat more slowly** and pay more attention to chewing your food. Fast eaters often swallow too much air, which turns into bothersome intestinal wind.

Eat yoghurt

- Having diarrhoea can drain away the good bacteria that help to prevent harmful bacteria from growing out of control. When you're suffering from IBS-related diarrhoea (and you are not lactose intolerant) eat plenty of **bio-yoghurt** containing active bacteria, such as *acidophilus*. Or take **probiotics** supplements. The usual dose is 2 capsules three times a day on an empty stomach.

Peppermint and ginger

- Every day, drink 1 to 2 cups of **peppermint tea**, which relaxes intestines, reduces spasms and relieves painful wind. Buy a tea that contains real peppermint rather than one with peppermint flavouring. Or take enteric-coated **peppermint-oil** capsules. The coating ensures that the oil reaches the intestine instead of breaking down in the stomach. Take 1 or 2 capsules three times a day, between meals. (*Alert* Avoid peppermint if you have heartburn.)
- Drink soothing **ginger tea**. For the very freshest tea, grate ½ teaspoon of fresh root ginger into a cup, then pour in hot water, let it steep for 10 minutes, strain and drink. Ginger tea bags are also available. Drink four to six cups a day.

Exorcise with exercise

- Whenever you possibly can, take at least 30 minutes of non-competitive **exercise** such as walking. Exercise helps to relieve stress, releases natural painkilling endorphins and keeps your body – including your digestive system – working smoothly.

Itching

Just the thought of certain forms of itching is enough to make you stir in your seat – literally. Some types of itching – specifically the one men get in the groin area – are easily treated with over-the-counter antifungal remedies plus a bit of extra hygiene. Anal irritation can be eased with creams and soaks, as well as a rather surprising compress and some new ways to cleanse and wipe. Take note of what you eat too. Though it's only passing through, food can influence how comfortably you're sitting a few hours later.

GROIN ITCHING

Try herbal antifungal wipes

- Soak a cotton wool ball in **thyme tea**, and apply it to your groin. Thyme contains thymol, a potent fungus fighter. To make the tea, stir 2 teaspoons fresh or dried thyme into a cup of boiled water and let it steep for 20 minutes. Cool and apply.
- Another good herb for chasing away fungus is **ginger**. It contains a total of 23 antifungal compounds. Grate 30g root ginger, stir it into a cup of boiled water and then steep for 20 minutes. When cool, apply the tea using a cotton wool ball.
- Liquorice also contains antifungal components and has long been used in traditional Chinese medicine as a remedy for groin itching. Stir 6 teaspoons powdered **liquorice root** into a cup of boiled water and let it steep for 20 minutes. As soon as it's cool, dab it on the affected area.
- **Tea tree oil** is a germ and fungus-fighting antiseptic. Rub a thin layer of the oil onto your skin three times a day and continue using it for two weeks after the itching clears up. If the pure oil irritates your skin, dilute it first; mix 10 drops into 2 tablespoons **calendula cream**. Apply it to the affected site twice a day. Never take tea tree oil by mouth.

What to wear

- Wear **loose, breathable clothing**. Body-hugging clothes heat up your groin, making itching more likely.
- For men who wear a jock strap for sport or exercise, it's a good idea to wear **cotton underwear** underneath the jock strap. The cotton absorbs sweat and protects tender skin.

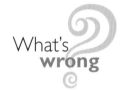

What's wrong

This annoying itch can affect sedentary office workers as well as serious athletes. Usually, the red, itchy, chafed area in the groin is caused by the fungal infection *tinea cruris*. But it can also be caused by the athlete's foot fungus (*tinea pedis*) spreading to the groin. Other causes include yeast or bacteria, or it might be simply skin irritation: the groin is a hot, sweaty place where a lot of friction occurs, so skin problems there are almost inevitable.

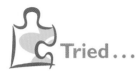

Tried...

Cider vinegar is a useful remedy for groin itching.

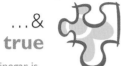

...& true

Vinegar is acidic, and fungi cannot thrive in an acidic environment. Using a fresh cotton wool ball, apply vinegar to the affected area once a day. Only use this treatment on unbroken skin.

Should I call the doctor?

If an itchy groin has blisters or doesn't clear up after a few weeks of self-treatment, talk to your doctor. You might have an allergic reaction to some irritant in your clothing (latex in pants elastic is a common allergen) or the washing powder you use. In rare cases, groin itching is associated with serious conditions such as diabetes or cancer.

If you have anal itching and you notice blood or discharge, or feel a lump, you must consult your doctor as it may signal a serious condition.

Keep the area clean and dry

- After any other activity that leaves you hot and sweaty, **don't hang about in damp kit**. Shower promptly, then put on fresh underwear and clean clothes. You want to wash fungus-nourishing sweat off your skin as soon as possible. Likewise, don't stay in a wet bathing suit any longer than necessary.
- Always **wash sports kit** before wearing it again.
- If you have athlete's foot, **put your socks on before your underwear**. If your pants touch your bare feet as you pull them on, they might spread the fungus to your groin.
- Don't dig a **used towel** out of the laundry basket and use it again. Fungus thrives in moist, dark conditions, and you're likely to get another infection.
- After bathing, dry your groin area using a **hair dryer** set on its coolest setting.
- Apply **Listerine** or another antiseptic mouthwash on a cotton wool ball to kill fungus.

Dust with talc

- When you get dressed or change your underwear, dust your groin with **talc or baby powder**. It will absorb moisture and help to keep the skin dry.

Lose some weight

- If you're overweight, **shed some pounds**. Folds of skin tend to be warm and damp, providing more areas for fungus to set in.

ANAL ITCHING
Instant itch soothers

- If anal fissures (a tear or cut in the skin lining the anus) or haemorrhoids are the problem, **buy an ointment** or suppositories designed for the purpose. Pharmacies sell a range of products that contain a combination of local anaesthetic, anti-inflammatory and a mild steroid. Use night and morning and after every bowel movement. These can stop the swelling – the main source of discomfort – as well as itching. Don't use these products for more than seven days at a time.
- In the bath, dissolve 3 or 4 tablespoons of **bicarbonate of soda** in a few inches of warm water. Sit in the bath for about 15 minutes. Bicarb can help to soothe skin irritation.

• **Witch hazel** is a skin cleanser and can remove irritants that cause an itchy bottom. More important, its astringent action can help to reduce the swelling responsible for the itching. Soak a cotton wool pad and apply it to the irritated area. This may sting for a few minutes after application.

• Use a **warm tea bag** as an astringent compress to ease itching and swelling. Just put boiling water on the tea bag as you would to make a cup of tea to release the chemicals in the leaves, let it cool down to a comfortable temperature, then hold it against the problem area for several minutes.

The power of prevention

• Keep clean. Wipe more than once to remove all traces of stool. To avoid irritating your skin, use moistened white, unscented toilet paper or buy special **moisturizing toilet wipes** from the supermarket or pharmacy.

• Keep your groin and behind dry and sweat-free. Use a **hair-dryer** set on low for 30 seconds to dry yourself. Then sprinkle the area generously with **baby powder** or **cornflour**. If you use baby powder, look for a brand that doesn't contain perfume, which causes skin irritation in some people.

• Choose loose **cotton underwear**, and avoid tights.

• If you have anal itching, temporarily avoid acidic foods such as citrus fruits; and keep off spicy foods like chilli peppers or hot sauces. Both can cause irritation.

• The oils in **coffee** beans are irritants, too. Limit yourself to one or two 200ml cups of coffee a day, or give up coffee altogether, and see if the itch subsides.

• Use **fragrance-free washing powder**, fabric softeners and soap. Avoid scented bath products, too

(See also *Allergies*, page 34; *Dry skin*, page 153;
Eczema, page 162; *Fungal infections*, page 183;
Head lice, page 203; *Hives* page 223 and *Psoriasis*, page 323)

THERAPEUTIC BATHS

From ancient times, in cultures all around the world, baths have been used to treat everything from kidney stones to snake bites. Now we have more reliable means of treating serious ailments but, for a host of minor discomforts (including itchy skin, sore muscles, aching joints, insomnia and anxiety), it's hard to beat a relaxing soak. Baths can do more than make you feel good, especially if you add healing substances.

The warm water of a relaxing bath subtly massages tired muscles and stimulates blood circulation, speeding up delivery of healing nutrients to the tissues while helping to remove lactic acid and other waste products that contribute to soreness. A hot bath can even help you to burn a few extra calories by temporarily boosting your metabolism a little. Avoid prolonged soaks in very hot baths, though. While the heat may feel good, it can promote inflammation.

A technique that has been practised around the world for centuries is contrast hydrotherapy. Alternating between hot and cold water causes blood vessels to alternately dilate and constrict. This translates into a sort of pumping action that increases blood circulation and is said to reduce congestion and inflammation, enhance digestion and stimulate activity of the organs. Natural healers believe that it also boosts immune function. To try this at home, you need a large basin to act as the second bath, or you can simply sit in a warm bath and use a handheld shower nozzle to douse yourself now and then with cold water. Always start with hot water and finish with cold.

Relieve itching

If itching is your problem, a bath – with certain ingredients added – may be just what the doctor ordered. Here are some soothers to add to the water.

• **Bicarbonate of soda** Bicarb is an excellent remedy for itchy skin, as you may already know. If your child has chickenpox, add ½ cup of bicarb to a shallow bath or one full cup to a deep bath to soothe itching.
• **Oatmeal** For relief from skin rashes or itchy sunburn, run a lukewarm bath and add a few tablespoons of colloidal oatmeal (which is finely powdered so it remains suspended in the water), such as Aveeno, sold in pharmacies. If you don't have colloidal oatmeal to hand, simply tip a cupful or so of plain porridge oatmeal in an old nylon stocking, tie the top, and float it in the bathwater while you soak. Oatmeal makes the bath very slippery, so be extra careful when getting out.
• **Vinegar** Vinegar is another substance that can tame itching. It works by acidifying the skin. To relieve itchy sunburn or psoriasis, have a cool bath, to which you have added about 2 cups of vinegar before getting in.

Aches and sprains

For minor sprains, a bath with Epsom salts added can bring rapid relief. The salts draw fluid out of the body and help to shrink swollen tissues. Add 2 cups to a warm bath, and soak. An Epsom salts bath also draws out lactic acid, the build-up of which contributes to muscle aches. After a vigorous exercise session, add 1 or 2 cups of the salts to a hot bath and enjoy a relaxing soak.

Adding essential oils

A wonderful way to enhance the medicinal value of a bath is to add essential oils, which are available from chemists and health stores. Each has its own healing profile. After a long, hard day, a few drops of pine oil added to the water can be wonderfully invigorating. Eucalyptus oil promotes alertness and breaks up congestion. Geranium oil reduces anxiety. Lavender fights depression. Rosemary is said to stimulate memory. Essential oil combinations can also be beneficial.

If prone to allergies, test your reaction to essential oils before using them. Dab a little of the diluted oil on the inside of your arm. If you don't have a reaction within 12 hours, it's safe to add them to your bath.

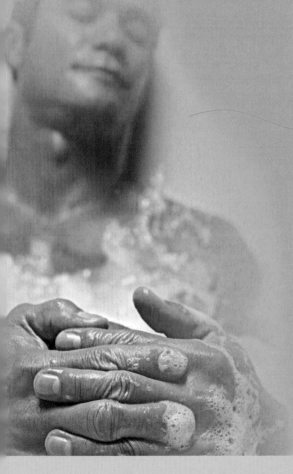

• **Arthritis treatment bath** Try combining 4 drops of juniper oil and 2 drops each of lavender oil, cypress oil and rosemary oil, along with half a cup of Epsom salts. For a simpler soak, use 3 drops of lavender oil and 3 drops of cypress oil.

• **Soothing-sleep soak** Use 2 to 4 tablespoons of sea salt, 4 drops of lavender oil, 3 drops of marjoram oil and 3 drops of lemon oil. Other oils that help to promote sleep include lime tree flower, Roman camomile, frankincense, neroli and rose.

• **Tension-easing bath** Add 3 drops of ylang-ylang oil, 5 drops of lavender oil, 2 drops of bergamot oil and ½ cup of Epsom salts.

You can also use dried herbs, instead. Add camomile – along with other calming herbs, such as lavender and valerian – to bathwater for an anxiety-soothing soak. For maximum benefit, tie them in a piece of muslin or cheesecloth and hold this under the running tap while you fill the bath.

Basin baths

You don't have to immerse your whole body in the water to reap the benefits of a bath. A footbath or sitz bath (a bath or basin you sit in) can provide a fast, simple solution to everything from headaches to haemorrhoids.

• For fever, congestion or headache, soak your feet in warm water plus a sprinkling of **mustard powder**. This draws blood to the feet, which boosts circulation and also eases pressure on the blood vessels in your head.

• For haemorrhoid pain and itching, prepare a bath or basin with warm water and a handful of **Epsom salts** and have a seat.

• For a soothing foot soak, add 2 drops of **peppermint oil** and 4 drops of **rosemary oil** to warm water.

Jaw problems

The most common jaw problems are night-time teeth grinding and a painful condition known as temporo-mandibular joint – or TMJ – disorder. Teeth grinding (also called bruxism) occurs when you're asleep, usually after a stressful day. It often causes a headache or facial pain the next day. If it hurts to chew or yawn – or even to say 'temporo-mandibular' – you know the discomfort of TMJ pain. Over-the-counter painkillers can help but that doesn't get to the root of the problem. For that you'll need to see your dentist. In the meantime, here are some helpful approaches.

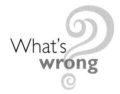

What's **wrong**

You may respond to stressful situations during the day by clenching or grinding your teeth at night, without even realizing you're doing it. This is a problem, as teeth are designed to touch briefly when we chew and swallow. They aren't built for the punishment of constant grinding. Common triggers are tension and anger. Night-time grinding can lead to cracked teeth and headaches, as well as TMJ (temporo-mandibular joint) pain.

IF YOU GRIND YOUR TEETH...
Relax into bedtime

- **Avoid stressful thoughts, activities or videos** in the hours before bedtime. You probably don't realize it but just before bed is the worst time to pay bills, watch films like *Die Hard* or discuss your in-laws. Tackle finances, watch violent movies and talk about sensitive subjects earlier in the evening. If you are bothered by worries, jot down things that you need to address the next day. Then take a **long, warm bath** before you go to bed.
- While you're in the bath – or even when you're lying in bed – cover your jaw with a flannel that's been soaked in hot water. The extra warmth will relax your jaw muscles.
- Practise **progressive muscle relaxation** before you go to sleep, so tension doesn't lead you to grind at night. When you're lying in bed, tense, then relax the muscles in your feet. Repeat with your calf muscles, then thigh muscles and so on, progressively tensing and relaxing each set of muscles all the way up your body. By the time you tense and relax your neck and jaw muscles, you should feel as limp as a rag doll.
- **Avoid eating within an hour of bedtime.** Digesting food while you sleep makes you more likely to grind your teeth.

Watch what you drink

- **Keep alcohol consumption to a minimum** – or better still, stop drinking altogether – especially in the evening. Though sleep experts aren't sure why, people who drink heavily at night are more likely to grind their teeth when they sleep.

IF YOU HAVE TMJ PAIN...
Try cooling and warming

- When you feel occasional sharp pain in your jaw joints, apply a pair of **cold packs**. The cold numbs your nerves, dulling pain messages that go to your brain. Wrap a couple of soft packs in tea towels and hold them on both sides of your face for about 10 minutes or so (not longer than 20 minutes, though, or you could cause mild frostbite). Repeat every two hours as needed.
- If you feel a dull, steady ache rather than sharp pain, **heat** is better than cold. It increases blood circulation to the area and relaxes jaw muscles. Soak a couple of flannels in warm water and hold them to your face for 20 minutes or so. (Run them under hot water every couple of minutes to keep them hot.)

Mandibular massage

- **Massage** the areas around your jaws to relieve muscle tightness and enhance bloodflow to the area. Several times a day, open your mouth, then rub the muscles by the ears near your temporo-mandibular joints. Place your forefingers on the sore areas, and swirl them around, pressing gently, until the muscle relaxes. Close your mouth and repeat the massage.
- With a clean **forefinger**, reach into your mouth until you can feel the sore muscles inside. Pressing firmly with your forefinger, massage one side, then the other, getting as close to the joints as you can.
- Finally, **massage** the muscles on the sides of your neck. Those muscles don't directly control your jaw, but massaging them helps to reduce tension that contributes to jaw pain.

Don't lean forwards

- When you're sitting in a chair most of the day, it's especially important to **sit up straight** rather than lean forwards. Your back should be well supported. Make sure your chin doesn't jut out in front of your body. If you are angled forward, you're putting strain on your neck and back – and that creates jaw pain.
- Use a **document holder** when you type so that you don't have to crane your neck or lean forwards to read the text.
- If you spend a lot of time on the telephone while you're using your hands for other tasks, get a **headset**. Cradling the

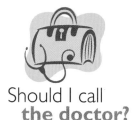

Should I call the doctor?

If you often wake up with pain in your jaw, neck or shoulder, or have morning headaches, talk to your dentist or doctor. This is particularly important if your bedmate says that you grind your teeth at night. And you need to see a dentist immediately if you have a broken tooth from the grinding.

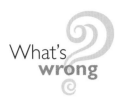

What's wrong

A pair of hinges – temporo-mandibular joints – attach your jawbone to your skull. These structures are surrounded by muscles and ligaments. In temporo-mandibular joint (TMJ) disorder, the muscles around the joints become tight and inflamed. TMJ disorder is marked by pain in the joints, a clicking or popping noise when using your mouth, headaches and aching in your neck and shoulders. Common triggers include emotional stress, chewing tough foods and jaw clenching or teeth grinding. Less often, people have TMJ pain as a result of arthritis or a blow to the jaw.

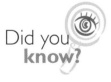

Did you know?

The temporo-mandibular joint is so named because it connects the mandible (or lower jaw) to the temporal bone at the side of the head.

telephone receiver between your shoulder and cheek puts a lot of strain on your neck and jaw.

• **Sleep on your back or side**. If you lie on your stomach, with your head turned to one side, the misalignment produces neck strain that's transferred to your jaw.

• If you spend a lot of time at a desk, disappear for a few minutes to **meditate**. Focus on the muscles in your face and neck, allowing them to relax and grow slack.

• Take 20 to 30 minutes of **aerobic exercise** at least three or four times a week. Not only does exercise reduce stress, it helps your body to produce endorphins, which are its natural painkilling chemicals.

• If you often carry a large bag or briefcase on one shoulder, **lighten your load**. The weight throws your spine and neck out of alignment – indirectly contributing to jaw pain. If you absolutely need to cart a lot of stuff around, buy a rucksack and use *both* straps, or move a heavy bag from shoulder to shoulder as you walk.

A yawning trap

• If you see someone yawning, resist the temptation to join in. Under those circumstances, it's extremely difficult to stifle a yawn, but that's exactly what you want to do, as a **big, wide yawn is bound to cause pain**. If you can't stop a yawn, try to suppress it by opening your mouth as little as possible.

TIPS FOR BOTH PROBLEMS

Grinding your teeth can cause jaw pain, too, so sometimes, solving one problem will in fact solve two.

Of food and drink

• **Avoid chewing gum**. Not only do your jaws get into the habit of chewing, but every time you chew, you tense your jaw muscles and give your temporo-mandibular joints an exhausting workout.

• Try to **steer clear of extremely crunchy and chewy foods**, such as apples, carrots, pork spare ribs, crusty rolls or dried crisp rolls. You want to spare your jaws from overwork, particularly when the aching and clicking are severe. What you want are soups, pastas and other easy-to-eat foods.

- Don't take big bites. Cut your food into **smaller pieces**, so you don't have to overwork your jaw.
- **Avoid caffeinated drinks**. Because caffeine is a stimulant, drinking coffee, tea or caffeinated soft drinks makes you far more likely to grind your teeth. Caffeine and TMJ problems don't go well together, either, as caffeine can increase muscle tension. Switch to decaffeinated drinks.
- **Don't bite your fingernails or chew a pencil.** When you work your jaws during the day, the pattern is likely to continue in your sleep. Instead, find a non-jaw-related way to get rid of your nervous energy – such as fiddling with worry beads or twisting a paperclip.

Be guarded

- A dental **mouthguard** – always worn by boxers and rugby players – works for teeth grinders, as well. Many types of protective mouthguards are available at sports shops, but dentists say that these don't fit snugly enough so tend to fall out when you're asleep. Your best bet is to have your dentist produce a made-to-measure mouthguard for you (though you will have to pay for it). Wear it to bed at night: the rubbery material will absorb pressure and save your teeth from damage.

Harness mineral power

- Take **calcium** and **magnesium** – in a two-to-one ratio – every day. These minerals help your jaw muscles to relax, particularly at night. Take 500mg calcium along with 250mg magnesium a day. If you can get the minerals in powdered form then do so: calcium/magnesium tablets are also available, but they don't dissolve as easily. When you use the powdered form, dissolve the supplements in an acidic liquid like orange or grapefruit juice.

Give your jaw a break

- During the day, make a conscious effort to **keep your jaw relaxed and your teeth apart**. Rest your tongue between your top and bottom teeth – if you start to bite down, you'll soon notice. Doctors have observed that people who break a daytime teeth-grinding habit are less likely to do it in their sleep.

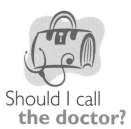

Should I call the doctor?

If you have jaw pain after two weeks of self-help remedies, see your doctor. And you need prompt medical attention if it's too painful to open your mouth or brush your teeth. For severe TMJ pain doctors may prescribe muscle-relaxing drugs or, if you have inflammation, inject corticosteroids into the joints. Your dentist can make a customized mouthguard to wear at night to reduce clenching or grinding if that's contributing to TMJ pain.

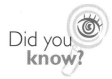

Did you know?

When you grind your teeth, you may be putting 550kg (1200lb) of pressure on the crowns and roots – that's as much as the weight of a horse. That recurring pressure is what can break or loosen your teeth.

Kidney stones

It's been said that the pain of passing a kidney stone is comparable to that of giving birth. Whether that's true or not, you'll probably want to stay home and take over-the-counter painkillers to take the edge off this experience. You can also put a hot-water bottle over the painful area to provide some measure of relief. After that, it's a waiting game. The stones might pass in a few hours, but sometimes it takes days. Fortunately, you can take measures to speed up the process a little.

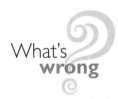

What's wrong

The pain in your back and side is so excruciating that you feel as though you might throw up. The cause is a nasty nugget formed from crystals that separate from the urine and build up on the inner surfaces of the kidney. Now that tiny stone wants to exit via the urethra, the spaghetti-thin tube that empties the bladder. Most kidney stones are made of calcium compounds. Heredity, chronic dehydration, repeated urinary tract infections and a sedentary lifestyle are all thought to contribute to kidney stone formation.

Flush it out

- To flush the stone into the bladder, drink at least **three litres of water** a day. If you're gulping enough water to do the job, your urine should run clear, with not a trace of yellow.
- During an attack, drink as much **dandelion tea** as you can. A strong diuretic, dandelion stimulates blood circulation through the kidneys, increasing urine output and helping to flush out the stone. To make the tea, add 2 teaspoons dried herb to 1 cup boiling water. Steep for 15 minutes, then drink.
- Consider drinking 2 or 3 cups a day of **buchu tea**. Like dandelion, this herb has diuretic properties which may help to flush out and prevent kidney stones. Place a sachet (2g) of buchu into a cup of boiling water and drink 1 cup three times a day before meals.

Stepping stone

- When you have a kidney stone, the slightest move is likely to be painful. But if you can bear to **take a walk**, try to do so. Walking may jar the stone loose. Despite the discomfort, you might pass the stone more quickly if you just keep moving.

The power of prevention

- Many experts believe that the single most important thing you can do to prevent kidney stones is the same thing you do to make them pass more quickly – that is, drink enough fluids. Anyone who is prone to kidney stones should drink at least **8 to 10 cups of water a day**, every day. The more you drink, the more you dilute the substances that form stones.

- Stick to a **low-salt diet** to reduce the calcium in your urine, which may reduce your risk of forming new stones. A good start is to limit your consumption of fast foods, tinned soups and other processed foods. **Read labels** carefully. The target is less than 6g salt (2,400mg sodium) a day.
- Drink two 250ml glasses of **cranberry juice** each day. Research suggests that it may help to reduce the amount of calcium in the urine. In one study of people with calcium stones, cranberry juice reduced the amount of calcium in the urine by 50 per cent.
- If you don't like cranberry juice, drink **orange juice** or real **lemonade** – 200ml (⅓ pint) at each meal. The citric acid these juices contain will raise the citrate level in your urine, helping to keep new calcium stones from forming.
- **Magnesium** has been shown to prevent all types of kidney stones. Eat more foods rich in this mineral, such as dark-green leafy vegetables, wheatgerm and seafood. You can also take 300mg a day in supplement form.
- Boost your intake of fruits and vegetables – especially bananas, oranges and orange juice, which are rich in **potassium**. In studies, people who ate a lot of fresh produce slashed their risk of kidney stones by half. If you suffer from stones regularly, ask your doctor whether potassium supplements might help you to ward off future attacks.
- **Cut back on coffee**. Caffeine increases calcium in the urine, which increases the risk of stone formation.
- If you know your stones are made of calcium oxalate (a urine test can tell you), **cut back on foods rich in oxalates**. These foods include rhubarb, spinach, chocolate, wheat bran, nuts (especially peanuts), strawberries and raspberries. Also **avoid drinking tea**, which is high in oxalates.

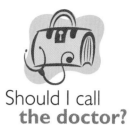

Should I call the doctor?

Most stones pass without a doctor's help, but the first time you get one, it's inevitable that you'll call the doctor. With pain like this, you definitely want to report your symptoms. They include nausea and vomiting, bloody or cloudy urine, needing to urinate but not being able to, a burning sensation upon urination or fever and chills (which may indicate infection). Even if you've had kidney stones before, call your doctor if the pain becomes excruciating. If your case is severe you may need prescription-only painkillers and hospital treatment.

Use a net to catch that stone

As distasteful as it may sound, medical experts recommend that during an acute attack, people with kidney stones should urinate through a piece of gauze, through cheesecloth or a fine-mesh strainer. The reason for this is to catch a stone, should they pass one, and take it to their doctor. The doctor can then have the stone's composition analysed, and based on that analysis, he or she will be able to give specific dietary advice on changes that will help to prevent a recurrence.

• If you have had uric-acid stones in the past, you need to keep your urine as alkaline as possible to prevent a recurrence. **Avoid foods that raise acid levels**, including anchovies, sardines, offal and brewer's yeast. Also, don't eat more than 100g meat or more than one serving of porridge, tuna, ham, lima beans or spinach in one day.

• **Calcium** in the diet may help to prevent calcium oxalate stones, probably because calcium combines with oxalate in the intestine and so prevents the body's absorption of pure oxalate. Foods rich in calcium include milk, cheese, yoghurt, dark green leafy vegetables, nuts and seeds. Taking calcium supplements during or just after meals may have a similar effect, but taking them between meals can increase the risk of stones.

Laryngitis

If you have laryngitis, the best way to get your voice back is to spend a week at the library (or in a Trappist monastery). In other words – be silent. This means not even whispering. (It may seem strange, but a whisper strains the vocal cords as much as a shout.) Resting your vocal cords will help to stop them from developing more serious problems, such as bleeding or the formation of nodules, polyps or cysts. And as you give your voice a rest, try one or more of these soothing remedies.

Don't clear your throat

• Whatever you do, **resist the urge to cough** or clear your throat. Either can damage your vocal cords. Try to suppress the feeling by sipping water or simply swallowing.

Coat your throat

• Drink at least 6 to 8 glasses of warm or lukewarm (not hot) **water** a day. Fluid keeps your larynx moist, which is critical for curing laryngitis.

• Other warm liquids, such as **chicken stock**, can also help ease the discomfort.

• Herbalists recommend drinking soothing laryngitis with teas made from **white horehound** and **Aaron's rod**. Horehound, a hairy-leaved member of the mint family, has long been used in proprietary cough sweets. Aaron's rod (or mullein) contains gelatinous mucilage, which soothes irritated tissues. To make either of these teas, put 1 or 2 teaspoons of the dried herb into 1 cup boiling water, steep for 10 minutes, strain and drink. Drink 1 to 3 cups a day. Both herbs are generally available from health-food shops.

• An old folk remedy for laryngitis is to drink a mixture of 2 teaspoons **onion juice** followed by a 'chaser' of 1 teaspoon **honey**. Take every 3 hours. If you don't have a juicer you can obtain onion juice by squeezing half an onion between two plates and collecting the juice that runs out.

• Try mixing up a tablespoon of **honey**, some **lemon juice** and a pinch of **cayenne pepper** and sip the mixture. Repeat as often as necessary.

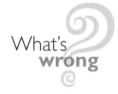

What's wrong

Your throat is sore and you can't make a sound. You've got laryngitis, an inflammation of the larynx (voice box), the part of the windpipe that houses your vocal cords. Normally, the vocal cords open and shut when you speak. When the vocal cords swell, they vibrate differently, which causes hoarseness. Along with overusing your voice, laryngitis can be caused by colds and other viral infections, smoking, allergies or a sinus infection, exposure to irritants like dust or fumes, and some medical conditions such as bronchitis and heartburn.

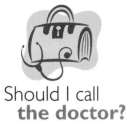

Should I call the doctor?

Steam your voice box

● **Inhale the steam** from a bowl of hot water for 5 minutes, two to four times a day. To help trap the steam, drape a towel over your head, forming a tent around the bowl, and breathe in deeply. The steam will help to restore the lost moisture in your throat and accelerate healing. Be sure to set the bowl on a sturdy table, and don't lean too close to the surface of the hot water or you risk a scald.

● For a more powerful healing inhalation, add 4 to 6 drops of antiseptic and anti-inflammatory essential oils, such as **lavender, sandalwood** or **camomile,** to the hot water.

● Make a **hot compress** using Aaron's rod, sage, thyme or hyssop tea. Apply the compress to your throat, then wrap a dry towel around your neck to keep the heat in.

The power of prevention

● **Breathe through your nose.** Your nasal passages are natural humidifiers. Mouth-breathing, on the other hand, exposes the voice box to dry, cold air.

● Use a **humidifier** in your bedroom, or stand a bowl of water on the radiator. Your vocal cords are lined with mucosa that needs to be kept moist in order to repel irritants.

● When you travel by air, chew **gum** or suck **lozenges.** The cabin air is excessively dry and your vocal cords suffer. If you keep your mouth closed and increase saliva production, you help to prevent dehydration.

● Another trick when flying is to hold a **wet cloth or flannel over your nose** and mouth periodically to moisten the air passing through your airways.

● Check with your doctor to see if any medication you take might be causing your hoarseness. Certain **drugs,** including **blood pressure** and **thyroid medications** and **antihistamines,** can be very drying to your throat.

● **If you smoke, quit.** It's a major cause of throat dryness. And avoid smoky bars, clubs and restaurants

Memory problems

Do you remember the title of the last book you read? Do you scratch your head and wonder whether you've taken your pills this morning? Are names sometimes just beyond your brain's reach? While forgetfulness isn't necessarily a sign that something's wrong, it can be frustrating. Memory boosters and simple do-it-yourself remedies can help to sharpen your memory now and keep it honed for years to come.

Catch the scent

- Buy a small bottle of either **rosemary** or **basil** essential oil from a health-food shop. Tests of brain waves show that inhaling either of these scents increases the brain's production of beta waves, which indicate heightened awareness. All you need to do is put a trace of the oil in your hair, wrists or clothing – anywhere you can get a whiff. Or put some of the oil in a diffuser and let it fill the air.

Count on coffee

- If you drink **caffeinated drinks**, you'll get a short-term boost in your ability to concentrate. And there may be long-term benefits as well. At the Faculty of Medicine in Lisbon, Portugal, researchers found that elderly people who drank 3 or 4 cups of coffee a day were less likely to experience memory loss than people who drank a cup a day or less.

Give it oxygen

- Take 120mg of **ginkgo biloba** a day. The herb appears to improve bloodflow to the brain, which helps brain cells to get the oxygen they need to perform at their peak. In Germany, where the government's Commission E reports regularly on the effectiveness of herbal medicines, a standardized extract of ginkgo is frequently prescribed to prevent memory loss as well as stroke. If you're perfectly healthy, you probably won't see any beneficial effect from ginkgo. But if you have diminished bloodflow to the brain, it may help.
- Another way to increase the flow of blood to the brain is to **get moving**. There's even some evidence that exercise may

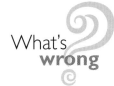

What's **wrong**

Patchy forgetfulness, when you can't remember where you put your keys or glasses, or you forget names, can be disconcerting. Ageing is the main culprit. As we get older, there are changes in the way the brain stores information, making it harder to recall facts. Physical problems, including thyroid disorders, can affect memory, as can medications, including those for high blood pressure and anxiety. Alzheimer's disease also causes memory problems, but the symptoms are much more severe than the more common, normal memory lapses.

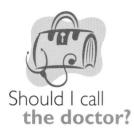

Should I call the doctor?

It is almost impossible for anyone to determine the seriousness of their memory problems. Make an appointment with your doctor if you feel that your memory has become significantly worse over the last six months. See a doctor as soon as you can if you have trouble remembering how to do things you've done many times before or can't remember how to get to a familiar place. You should also tell your doctor if you have trouble accomplishing activities that involve step-by-step instructions, such as following a recipe.

increase the number of nerve cells in the brain. Any type of regular exercise, but especially aerobic exercise like walking and cycling, will do. Exercise also helps to prevent illnesses like diabetes, stroke and high blood pressure, all of which can contribute to memory lapses.

Keep your blood sugar steady

- New research has uncovered a link between mild glucose intolerance and age-related memory loss. Food converted by the digestive system to glucose (blood sugar) is the main fuel that powers the organs, including the brain. But many people, especially those past their youth, have poor glucose tolerance, meaning they have trouble processing glucose out of the bloodstream and into cells. According to the new research, even mild, non-diabetic glucose intolerance appears to reduce short-term memory in middle age and beyond. What can be done? Eat **regular reasonably-sized meals**, emphasizing fibre-rich **whole grains** and **vegetables** over 'white' carbohydrates such as white pasta, white bread, potatoes and white rice.
- Focus on good fats – those found in **vegetable oils, nuts, seeds, avocados** and **fish**. They help to keep your blood sugar levels steady without clogging up your arteries.
- Lace up your walking shoes. **Regular exercise** is another way to prevent blood sugar problems.

Smarten up your diet

- The brain is 85 per cent **water**. So if you don't drink at least 8 large glasses a day, it's time to get into the habit. Dehydration leads to fatigue, which can take its toll on memory.
- Make sure that you get enough of the **B vitamins** in your diet. These include vitamins B_6, B_{12}, niacin and thiamin. These nutrients help to make and repair brain tissue, and some of them help your body to turn food into mental energy. Bananas, chickpeas and turkey are rich in vitamin B_6; whole grains and meat are good sources of all the Bs. Nuts and seeds, wheat germ and fortified breakfast cereals are other good sources.
- While you're eating more of the good stuff, **cut back on foods high in saturated fat**. You probably already know that it clogs the arteries that feed the heart. But high-fat foods also clog arteries that feed the brain; this in turn reduces the brain's

supply of oxygen. Just as harmful as saturated fats are the **trans fatty acids** found in soft margarine and many packaged baked goods, such as biscuits, cakes and other snack foods.

- Eat **fish** two or three times a week. Oily fish such as salmon, mackerel, herring and fresh (not tinned) tuna contain omega-3 fatty acids. You may know that these fats are good for your heart because they help to 'thin' the blood and prevent clogged arteries; they're good for your brain for the same reasons.

Buy extra insurance

- Take a **multivitamin** every day. Make certain it has 100 per cent of the adult daily requirement for folic acid and B_{12}, as it can be hard to get enough of these vitamins in your diet. Even moderate shortfalls may contribute to mental decline.

Sound out the problem

- **Listen to music** often, and try various types. Researchers have found that listening to music can improve your ability to concentrate and help you to remember what you've learnt. Some types of music actually cause brain neurons to fire more quickly. The faster the beat, the more the brain responds.

Challenge your mind

- If you're really keen to sharpen your memory, take up a **musical instrument**. Whether you want to play the drums or the piano, learning to play will develop your motor skills while it fine-tunes your brain's ability to analyse and focus.
- Go out of your way to stay mentally active. A study conducted on nuns, and known, not surprisingly, as the Nun Study, found that those with the most education and language abilities were the least likely to develop Alzheimer's. But what really counts is not the amount of book learning you did at school or university, it's how much you actively use your mind. **Doing crossword puzzles, learning a second language**, or **playing Scrabble** can exercise your brain.

Put stress in its place

- Find ways to **reduce stress**. Tense people have high levels of stress hormones in their bodies. Over time, these hormones can affect the hippocampus, the part of the brain that controls

Mental gymnastics

Try these exercises to challenge your brain and help you perfect the art of recall:

MEMORY BOOSTER 1

If you want to grow some new brain circuitry, use the 'wrong' hand to do an everyday task several times a day. For example, if you normally brush your teeth with your right hand, use your left instead. If you always zip up your jeans with your left hand, use your right. The brain 'knows' when you're using the wrong hand, because of the sensory and motor information it receives from that hand. It's that confusion that stimulates new brain circuits, as the brain struggles to master a new task. (Stick to simple tasks, though. You don't want to try this when you're using a power drill.)

MEMORY BOOSTER 2

If you're trying to remember a fact, think of a mnemonic – a phrase, formula or rhyme that will help your recall. Many people, for instance, remember the colours of the rainbow – red, orange, yellow, green, blue, indigo and violet – by recalling the phrase '**R**ichard **of Y**ork **g**ave **b**attle **i**n **v**ain'. You can use the same trick to memorize lists. If you need to visit the library, post office and chemist, make up a phrase like 'Lois puts on a coat'. Or you may have a shopping list that includes jam, apples, paper towels, eggs, milk and cheese. How about 'Jane and polly eat mouldy cheese'? Or you could write a list…

MEMORY BOOSTER 3

Another way to remember which errands you have to run is to make up a short story – the more fantastic, the better – about them. Suppose your list includes bank, library, butcher and a stop at your friend Bob's to return a book he lent you. The story might go like this: Beefy Bob the butcher robbed the bank at gunpoint and then hid in the library.

memory. You don't have to chant or meditate – just do something that's simple and fun, from swinging in a hammock to finger painting with your children or grandchildren.

- Consider taking **Siberian ginseng**, which helps to protect the body from the effects of stress and is said to heighten mental alertness. Take 10–20 drops tincture (1:3 in 25 per cent alcohol) in water three times a day after meals; or take up to six 50mg capsules a day with water. Don't use for more than a month at a time: give your body a break for two months before restarting.

Favourite food of elephants

- **Gotu kola**, a herb elephants love, has been used to increase mental acumen for thousands of years. There is some research to support the use of the herb to boost memory. Take two 300mg capsules twice a day with food.

Menopause

Some women sail through the menopause with few symptoms. For the rest of us, there are many options to help us to cope with annoying afflictions such as mood swings, hot flushes and night sweats. Hormone replacement therapy is one answer, but natural therapies can also be very helpful. Remember that menopause is not a disease and it won't last for ever. And try some of these approaches for relief in the meantime.

Say 'yes' to soya

- Eat 200mg **tofu** every day. Tofu is high in phytoestrogens – compounds with mild oestrogen-like qualities that have been found to ease menopausal symptoms. Certain kinds of phyto-estrogens, called isoflavones, found in soya products can help to ease hot flushes and vaginal dryness. The recommended amount is 60mg a day of isoflavones, which is what you'll get by eating 200mg of tofu.
- One 50mg supplement of **isoflavones**, taken daily, can meet most of your needs if you can't face eating tofu every day. Look for brands that contain genistein, daidzein or red clover.
- **Flax seeds** are another source of phytoestrogens. Grind some in a spice mill or coffee grinder and add 1 to 2 table-spoons to cereal or yoghurt.

Ease night sweats

- To tame night sweats, take 3 to 15 drops **sage tincture** three times a day in half a cup of water or tea. The genus name of this herb, *Salvia*, comes from the Latin *salvere* (to heal) and the extract of sage leaves has been used to treat more than 60 different health complaints. The herb has astringent qualities that can help to dry up abnormal sweating within a day or so.
- Some women find that taking **vitamin E** can help to relieve hot flushes and night sweats as well as mood swings and vaginal dryness. The suggested dose is 250mg twice a day – within the 540mg a day limit considered safe in the UK. However, you should talk to your doctor before you start taking vitamin E regularly. This is especially important if you have diabetes, bruise easily or have high blood pressure.

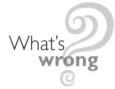

What's **wrong**

A woman has officially passed the menopause when she hasn't menstruated for one year. But in the years preceding menopause, called the perimenopause, her ovaries are producing less of the female sex hormones oestrogen and progesterone, while ovulation (the monthly release of an egg) also becomes less frequent. This hormonal fluctuation can result in a variety of uncomfortable symptoms, including hot flushes and night sweats, vaginal dryness, mood swings, sleep problems and unusually light or heavy periods.

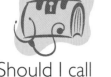

Should I call the doctor?

• **Black cohosh** is a very popular remedy for hot flushes and night sweats. It is taken in tincture form two to four times a day, with half a glass of juice or water added to make it more palatable. It can have other benefits as well, such as relieving vaginal dryness, nervousness and depression. Recent research has, however, suggested a strong link between taking black cohosh and liver problems.

• Any herbal treatment for hot flushes is potentially oestrogenic and if you prefer to avoid taking anything like that, a simple measure such as **turning down the central heating** may have the effect you are seeking.

• To help to stay cool, wear lightweight clothing made of **natural fibres**. And carry a small, battery-powered **fan** with you to cool the hot flushes.

• Some women find that taking a **tepid bath** in the morning for 20 minutes prevents hot flushes for the whole day.

Exert yourself

• Increase the amount of **aerobic exercise** you get to at least 20 minutes a day. Besides helping you to lose weight, exercise has other positive effects for women going through the menopause. Studies show that daily vigorous physical activity decreases hot flushes and night sweats, helps to improve mood and sleep and improves the balance of hormone levels. Weight-bearing activities such as walking, running and resistance training also help to keep your bones sturdy.

Stay chaste

• Women have used **chasteberry** (*Vitex agnus castus*) for around 2,000 years. Made from the berries of the chaste tree, the remedy helps to restore progesterone levels, which decrease

A liver saver

If you take synthetic hormones (HRT), you may have symptoms related to excess hormone levels – such as breast tenderness, bloating or headaches. But some of these symptoms can be alleviated with milk thistle, a herb that helps the liver to clear away some by-products from the synthetic hormones. Milk thistle also helps to repair and regenerate liver cells. Take 200mg three times a day between meals. After six to eight weeks cut down the amount to 280mg a day in divided doses.

significantly during menopause. Chasteberry may be particularly useful for combating very heavy bleeding, which some women experience during the perimenopause. It may also help with other symptoms, including hot flushes and depression. Take two 250mg capsules morning and evening with water; or take 30 drops of tincture (1:3 in 25% alcohol) in a little cold water. Be patient: you may not notice any effects for three months or so.

Meal plans

- If you've been having hot flushes, **keep off alcohol, coffee, spicy foods** and **hot drinks**. Many of these foods are triggers.
- To help prevent accelerating bone loss – osteoporosis – make sure you get enough **protein**. It doesn't take much chicken, fish or meat to supply your daily requirement of protein. As long as you have a serving that's about equal to the size of the palm of your hand, you're getting enough.
- Take a daily supplement containing 600mg **calcium**, 300mg **magnesium** and 10mcg **vitamin D**. Low-fat dairy products are good sources of calcium: a cup of skimmed milk, for instance, provides 300mg calcium.

Look to lubricants

- Vaginal dryness, the result of waning oestrogen levels, is enough to put anyone off sex. It hurts. Try a **water-soluble lubricant**, such as K-Y Jelly. Avoid oil-based lubricants such as petroleum jelly (Vaseline). Studies suggest that oil-based moisturizers don't work as well and can actually increase irritation if used long-term.

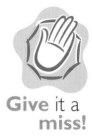

Give it a miss!

Some women turn to progesterone creams or suppositories to ease menopause symptoms. But doctors and researchers are concerned that overuse of progesterone might increase the risk of breast cancer. Talk to your doctor before using the cream.

Menstrual problems

Many women experience mild discomfort just before and on the first day or two of their menstrual periods – usually mild cramps and perhaps a headache. But for others, premenstrual symptoms are severe enough to disrupt their daily lives. These can include mood swings, irritability, depression and anxiety, along with bloating, breast pain and weight gain. You can get quick relief from cramps and headaches by taking ibuprofen or paracetamol. But there are also things you can do to control PMS symptoms and – hopefully – prevent or at least lessen next month's discomfort.

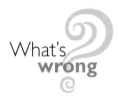

What's **wrong**

Cramps, bloating, backache, nausea, headache and fatigue – any or all of these menstrual problems can result from hormonal fluctuations in a woman's monthly cycle. Some of them are related to prostaglandins, hormone-like substances that cause the muscles in the uterus to tighten, leading to cramping. During the week to 10 days before your period, there's also a drop in production of the hormone progesterone, which causes your body to retain salt and water. And an imbalance between progesterone and the hormone oestrogen contributes to emotional symptoms such as depression, anxiety and irritability.

Take anti-cramp action

• When you feel cramps coming on, go for a walk or run. Or go swimming. Or get on an exercise bike. Any kind of **exercise** helps to inhibit prostaglandin production and boosts the release of painkilling endorphins. As a bonus, exercise can also help to relieve bloating.

• Soak in a **hot bath**. The warmth helps to relax knotted-up muscles in the uterus. Or lie down with a hot-water bottle or heating pad on your abdomen.

• Try a homeopathic remedy. For severe cramps experts recommend **mag phos** (phosphate of magnesia). Take five pellets of 6C or 12C every hour for five doses. If the cramps don't improve, take the same dosage of **pulsatilla** or **nux vomica**. Pulsatilla is advised when you find yourself not only cramping, but crying as well while nux vomica is usually recommended for cramps accompanied by constipation and extreme irritability.

Tame cramps with tea

• During the day, drink 3 cups of warm **red raspberry-leaf tea**. (Look for raspberry-leaf tea bags at the supermarket or a health-food shop.) The leaves contain fragrine, a substance that tones the uterus and helps to ease cramping. It can also lighten excessive bleeding.

• As its name implies, **cramp bark** (*Viburnum opulus*) can take the edge off cramps. Buy the dried bark (usually available at health-shops) and make a tea using 1 teaspoon bark in 1 cup water, or buy the tincture and follow the dosage directions on the label.

- Good old **camomile tea** has antispasmodic properties to unclench your uterus. Use 2 to 4 teaspoons of herb per cup of hot water, or buy camomile tea bags. Peppermint is another antispasmodic herb.

- **Ginger** is another tried and trusted cramp remedy. It is thought to work by inhibiting the production of prostaglandins. To make ginger tea, grate 1 teaspoon fresh root ginger, add a cup boiling water, steep for 10 minutes, then strain.

Beat bloating

- To deal with bloating, **reduce the salt** in your diet and take **vitamin B$_6$** during your period. During the week before your period, add as little salt to your food as possible and cut back on high-sodium foods, such as processed meats, tinned soups and salty snacks. Meanwhile, take up to 50mg of vitamin B$_6$ every day. This vitamin appears to have a mild diuretic effect. Note that the Safe Upper Limit for B$_6$ is 10mg a day, though 25-50mg daily is often recommended for PMS. If you get any symptoms of tingling in your fingers or toes, stop taking B$_6$.

- **Eat diuretic foods**. Certain foods work well as natural diuretics – try asparagus, dandelion leaf (eat in salads), celery, garlic, watercress and parsley.

Manage the flow

- Every day take 1000mg **vitamin C** and 1000mg **bioflavonoids** in divided doses – 500mg of each in the morning, then another 500mg in the evening. Both supplements help to strengthen the walls of the blood vessels to reduce excessive bleeding. Bioflavonoids are found in grape skins, blackberries, blueberries and citrus fruits, especially in the pulp and white rind.

- **Chasteberry** also helps to regulate the menstrual cycle by balancing levels of sex hormones. (In men it can lower libido, so in days of old it was fed to priests, hence the name chasteberry.) Try it to lighten a heavy flow. Take two 250mg capsules morning and evening with water; or take 30 drops of tincture (1:3 in 25% alcohol) in a little cold water.

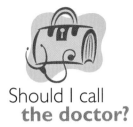

Should I call the doctor?

Contact your doctor if your cycles are shorter than 21 days, if you go more than 35 days between menstrual periods, or if you have any spotting or bleeding between periods. You also want to see your doctor if you bleed heavily for more than a week, quickly soaking through your tampons or pads, or if you pass large clots of blood. (Small clots, no larger than the size of a 50p piece, are normal.) And the doctor might be able to help if you experience severe cramps that over-the-counter painkillers don't relieve.

The power of prevention

- Every day take 1000mg of **calcium citrate** in divided doses with food. Calcium is a natural tonic and muscle relaxant. It helps to reduce the ferocity of menstrual cramping. (Avoid calcium supplements from dolomite oyster shell or bonemeal: they may contain high levels of lead.)

- Anyone taking calcium should also take **magnesium** in a ratio of 1:2. So if you take 1000mg calcium a day, take 500mg magnesium as well. Magnesium helps to prevent menstrual cramps, but the citrate and oxide forms also have a laxative effect. Use magnesium gluconate if you don't need to worry about regularity.

- Essential fatty acids slow down the production of prostaglandins, which contribute to cramps. Get yours by taking 1000mg **evening primrose oil** three times a day or 1 tablespoon of **flax seed oil** a day (use it in salad dressings in place of other oils).

- During the last two weeks of your cycle, take 40mg **black cohosh** extract (often prescribed for menopause symptoms) three or four times a day. This herb is an antispasmodic, which means it relaxes the uterus and reduces cramping. Some researchers have expressed concern about taking this herb for more than six months, as it has been recently associated with liver toxicity (though this was not definitely attributable to black cohosh). If you are worried, talk to a medical herbalist.

(See also *Premenstrual syndrome (PMS)*, page 318)

Morning sickness

You may be joyfully embracing the notion that a new life is growing inside you, but your body seems to be doing anything but. Considering how queasy you're feeling, you have a perfect right to mutter a few unprintable words and snap at your partner now and then. You also have a right to some relief. When your stomach feels like it's riding a rollercoaster, try these strategies to calm, soothe and settle. Treat any herbal remedy with the same caution as you would medication in pregnancy – it's best to check with your doctor or midwife first.

Give your tummy a treat

• Nothing beats morning sickness like a cup of **ginger tea**. The same spicy herb is used to counter motion sickness. To make ginger tea, use a ginger teabag, available in health-food shops and supermarkets, or add ½ teaspoon grated root ginger to 1 cup of very hot water, leave to infuse for 5 minutes, strain and sip.

• Herbal teas made with **camomile, lemon balm** and **peppermint** are also known to reduce nausea. Use 1 to 2 teaspoons of the dried herb per cup of hot water. Avoid peppermint tea if you have heartburn, however.

• Brew yourself a cup of **raspberry-leaf tea**. The herb is used to help with morning sickness – and a lot of women drink it in gradually increasing doses in later pregnancy to ease labour because it acts as a uterine tonic. Use 1 to 2 teaspoons of the dried herb per cup of hot water. Drink no more than 1 cup a day in the first three months of pregnancy (and avoid raspberry leaf tablets). Some people advise that raspberry leaf shouldn't be taken in early pregnancy and should be avoided by women at risk of miscarriage or premature labour but there appears to be no scientific evidence of ill-effects, despite widespread worldwide use for centuries. However, to be on the safe side, consult your midwife or doctor.

• Drink flat, room-temperature **ginger ale** to settle your stomach. Although no one knows why (there's not enough ginger in shop-bought ginger ale to have an effect), it works for many nauseated mums-to-be. Don't drink ginger ale with

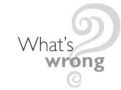

What's **wrong**

When a pregnant woman has daily bouts of nausea, it's no surprise. But that doesn't mean it can be explained. Doctors think morning sickness – which doesn't necessarily occur in the morning – may be the result of rising levels of oestrogen, mild dehydration (not enough water intake to keep your body wet enough on the inside), or the lower blood sugar characteristic of early pregnancy. Stress, travelling, some foods, antenatal vitamins and certain smells can aggravate the problem.

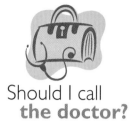

Should I call the doctor?

fizz, though. The bubbles promote the production of more stomach acid – just what you don't need.

- Chew on **anise** or **fennel seeds**, which are known to soothe upset stomachs.

Feel better with B$_6$

- In studies, women who took 25mg of **vitamin B$_6$** three times a day (a total of 75mg per day) for three days reduced nausea and vomiting associated with pregnancy. But you should be aware that the Safe Upper Limit for vitamin B$_6$ is 10mg a day, and in common with other vitamins, **if you're pregnant, don't take B$_6$ without talking to your doctor or midwife first**.

Wrist business

- Try wearing the **acupressure wristbands** designed for people who get seasick. Available in chemists, they apply constant pressure to acupressure points for nausea.
- If you can't find a wristband, **use your fingers to apply pressure**. Turn your arm over, forearm up. Locate the point two thumb widths from the crease at your wrist, dead centre between the ligaments. Press this point with your thumb while you count slowly to 10. Repeat three to five times, or until the nausea subsides.

Drown the nausea

- **Water** is the best medicine. Amazing as it seems, women who drink a glass of water every hour have a lot less morning sickness. Also, drink a glass of water every time you get up in the night to go to the loo. This helps to ensure you start your day feeling as good as you can. Check the water in the toilet

Is morning sickness really a good sign?

People have long believed that if you suffer from morning sickness during pregnancy, you're less likely to miscarry. But is it true? Yes. Morning sickness is associated with fewer miscarriages, as well as lower risks of premature labour, low birth weight and perinatal death. Morning sickness may also play a role in promoting healthy placental development. So while you may feel ghastly, you can think positive and feel encouraged. That sickness is a sign that your pregnancy is going well – and it *will* pass.

before you flush. If you are drinking enough water, your urine should be almost clear. If it's dark, sinks to the bottom or has an extra-strong smell, you need to drink more.

- If nothing wants to stay down, treat yourself to a **frozen-fruit ice lolly**. It helps to replace sugars lost through vomiting. And since an ice lolly is made with frozen water, it also helps to keep you hydrated.

Try a citrus cure

- Sniff a slice of **lemon**. Some pregnant women report that, for unknown reasons, it helps with morning sickness.
- You might also try drinking water with lemon or another **lemon-based drink**.
- Grate a little **grapefruit, orange** or **tangerine zest** (the coloured part of the rind) and add it to your tea. But be sure to rinse any wax off the fruit first.

Don't run on empty

- In the morning, you might be able to prevent nausea by eating before you even get out of bed. Keep some **cream crackers** by your bed and have a few as soon as you wake up.
- Eat a number of **small meals** throughout the day. Small amounts of food are much easier to tolerate than a large meal. In fact, you might want to have a snack every hour or two, keeping the servings small. A bunch of grapes, an apple, a few nuts or a slice or two of cheese are all good choices.
- **Take your antenatal vitamins with food** to help them stay down. Even a cracker or wheat thin can help.
- **Avoid fried, fatty foods**, which tend to cause and intensify the nausea. It's not known why – perhaps because fatty foods are digested more slowly.

Smell no evil

- Morning sickness is largely provoked by smell – women with anosmia (an inability to smell) hardly ever get it. If you're prone to morning sickness, try to stay in **well-ventilated rooms** that don't accumulate cooking smells or cigarette smoke. You may also find yourself asking the family to brush more – as bad breath can also cause nausea. This sensitivity usually passes by the 12th to 14th week . . . so you're not going to be finicky forever.

Motion sickness

Many of us have been unlucky enough to experience the misery of nausea or vomiting when travelling by air, road or sea. And although travel sickness can be prevented, it is very hard to cure once it sets in. So if you know you're going on a journey, take steps to prevent motion sickness before it begins. The discomfort of motion sickness is often worsened if you are anxious – so try practising yoga or other relaxation techniques to keep your mind and body in control.

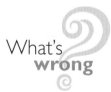

What's wrong

Motion sickness occurs as a result of a 'mismatch' occurring between sensory information from the eyes and ears (as well as other balance receptors). This is why motion sickness is worse when you're looking at a book: your eyes are telling you that the world is still while your inner ear and joint receptors know that it's moving. This can cause nausea and vomiting and, in severe cases, sweating and a headache. It is especially common in children, whose balance mechanism is more sensitive than that of adults. Focusing on the scenery should help because the eyes and ears are receiving similar information. Most people suffer less as they get older. The sickness usually evaporates quickly at the end of the journey.

Choose a sensible seat

- If you're an **adult** passenger travelling by car, **sit in the front seat** or, better still, drive. Motion sickness never seems to affect a car's driver. (However, children should always sit in the back. It's much safer.)
- If you are flying, ask the airport staff to allocate you a **seat over the wing** and **by a window** where movement is least. Explain your reason – the thought of a full sick bag may get you just the cooperation you need.
- On a boat, you want to **locate yourself amidships** where the effect of any swell is least.
- **On a train**, don't sit in backwards-facing seats.

Breathe cool air

- Anyone who's ever felt carsick knows the feeling of relief that comes from opening a window. Check with the other passengers, then **let the fresh air in**. If you're on a boat, go up on deck – whatever the weather to escape from the stuffy interior. And on a plane, use your personal overhead vent. The air may not be that fresh but at least it's cool.

Assist your beleaguered inner ear

- **Look straight ahead** at the road if you're in a car, or at the horizon if you're at sea.
- Keep your **head still** to limit visual stimulation.
- **Don't read** or attempt any activity that involves focusing on nearby objects. Tell the driver that asking you to map-read may not be a great idea.

Don't talk about it

- If your child is prone to motion sickness, don't increase his or her anxiety by talking about it before or during the journey. If you do the child will probably reward you by throwing up.
- Don't read or attempt any activity that involves focusing on nearby objects.

Don't travel on a full stomach

- **Avoid large meals** before travelling: a full tummy makes the condition worse.
- In particular, stay away from **fried, fatty foods**. These make nausea worse, probably because your digestion has to work harder to deal with them.

Avoid unpleasant smells

- The nausea of motion sickness is made worse by **certain smells**. If you're on a ferry or about to fly, stay away from people who are smoking (smoking is banned on most airlines, so the problem won't arise once you've boarded). And if you are about to experience a rough crossing, find yourself a seat well away from any food outlets – and their related cooking smells – or, better still, on deck.

Get some spicy relief

- Two hours before you travel and every four hours after that, **take ginger**. It takes effect almost instantly and has none of the side effects of conventional drugs, such as drowsiness or blurred vision. Take 100mg to 200mg of standardized extract in capsule form; or chew fresh ginger; or drink ginger tea or a few drops of ginger tincture in warm water. You can even eat delicious crystallized root ginger or nibble on gingernuts or other ginger biscuits.

Travel supplements

- A good general tonic for calming the nerves and thus easing motion sickness is **magnesium**. Take 500mg, with food, one hour before travelling.
- **Vitamin B$_6$** can help to relieve nausea. The recommended dose is 100mg an hour before travelling and another 100mg two hours later.

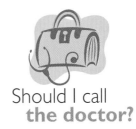

Should I call the doctor?

Motion sickness is unpleasant but it is not a disease. It may, however, mask another condition. If your 'motion sickness' is accompanied by a fever or severe headache or you feel faint or dizzy, you should talk to a doctor. You also need medical attention if symptoms don't lessen within 24 hours. Get help right away if you have severe abdominal or chest pain.

Homeopathic remedies

● Take one dose of an appropriate remedy just before you set off and then as necessary throughout your journey. All symptoms of motion sickness are eased with **cocculus**; or choose **tabacum** if the slightest movement brings on nausea or vomiting – especially if you are pale or sweaty.

Wrist bands can really help

● Try wearing **acupressure wristbands** specially designed for people who get carsick, seasick or airsick. Available in pharmacies, they apply constant pressure to acupressure points for nausea.

● If you can't find a wristband, **use your fingers to apply pressure**. Turn your arm over, forearm up. Locate the pressure point about two thumb widths above the crease at the front of your wrist, dead centre between the tendons. Press this point with your thumb while you count slowly to 10. Repeat three to five times, or until the nausea subsides.

Visit the pharmacy

● If all else has failed on previous journeys and you want to feel confident that you're not going to succumb, then buy an **over-the-counter drug** such as Kwells or Sea Legs. These medicines must be taken before you travel or they won't work. Read label directions to see how many hours in advance the tablets should be taken.

● There are few nastier experiences than cleaning sick off the back seat, but there are several good **travel sickness remedies for children**. The most effective drug for motion sickness prevention is hyoscine, the active ingredient in JoyRides (for over 3s) and Junior Kwells (for over 4s). A sedating anti-histamine is sometimes useful: try Phenergan elixir (for children over 2), which even tastes okay, according to a very small sample (our children). Very young children, under 2, tend not to suffer from motion sickness. If yours does, ask your doctor for advice.

Mouth ulcers

Those little sores in your mouth cause more pain than anything so small deserves to. You can be sure that in a week or two, your mouth ulcer will have healed completely and you will be able to eat an orange, crunch salt-and-vinegar crisps, drink a cup of coffee or smooch your spouse without regretting it. Meanwhile, here are some ways to numb the pain and get rid of your mouth ulcers more quickly.

Seal the sore

- Over-the-counter products such as **Orabase** form a long-lasting protective coating over the sore to speed up healing and provide fast pain relief. Dry the sore with a cotton bud before applying the paste.
- A form of liquorice known as **deglycyrrhizinated liquorice** or **DGL** also coats ulcers. It's available as chewable wafers from some health-food shops (you may need to order them): chew one or two wafers two or three times a day.
- The sap of **aloe vera** – the ubiquitous 'first aid plant' – can bring welcome relief. Squeeze a bit of gel from an aloe vera leaf. Dry the ulcer with a cotton bud, then dab on the gel. Repeat as often as you like.
- Cut open a **vitamin E** capsule and squeeze some of the oil on to the sore several times a day.

Put it in neutral

- Munch a chewable **Pepto-Bismol** or **Tums** tablet or put it on the ulcer and allow it to dissolve. The niggling pain of mouth ulcers is caused by acids and digestive enzymes eating into the tissue in the sore. The antacid tablets will neutralize the acids and may also speed up healing. Do not exceed the recommended dose.
- Use a small amount of **milk of magnesia** as a mouth wash, or apply it to the ulcer three to four times a day.
- Apply a damp **tea bag** to the sore for 5 minutes. Tea is alkaline, so it can neutralize the acids that make mouth ulcers painful. It also contains astringent compounds, which may help to relieve the pain.

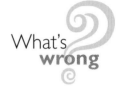

What's **wrong**

A mysterious condition known medically as *aphthous stomatitis*, ulcers often appear in crops inside the lips or cheeks, around the gums or on the tongue. They are white or yellowish, with a halo of red, ranging from the size of a pinhead to much larger sores. Experts aren't sure what causes them, but an immune-system malfunction is thought to play a role. A stressful episode or a mouth injury often precedes a break-out. Recurrent sores can also be brought on by eating certain foods.

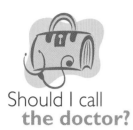

Should I call the doctor?

Get that numb feeling

- Dab on a **topical anaesthetic** such as **Anbesol** liquid or **Rinstead** gel. These don't stick, so you need to reapply them several times a day.
- Try a babies' **teething gel**: these also have a mild numbing effect – as babies know.
- Let a **pain-relieving lozenge**, such as **Chloraseptic**, dissolve in your mouth and numb the soreness.

Battle bacteria

- Mix a tablespoon of 20 vols **hydrogen peroxide** into half a glass of water. Add 1 teaspoon of **bicarbonate of soda** and 1 teaspoon of **salt** and stir until they dissolve. Swish the solution around in your mouth and spit it out. Hydrogen peroxide is a strong disinfectant – useful because an ulcer is an open wound and therefore vulnerable to infection, which will make the pain worse. And bicarbonate of soda is alkaline and gives further relief by neutralizing acids.
- To speed up healing, apply a liquid form (tincture) of the herb **goldenseal** to the sore three times a day, at least an hour before eating. Goldenseal has mild antibacterial properties.
- Put a single drop of antiseptic **tea tree oil** on the sore.
- Make a tea from **calendula**. Better known as the garden marigold, it has been used for centuries for treating minor cuts, cracked or itching skin and insect bites. Pour a cup of boiling water over 1 to 2 teaspoons of dried petals. Let it steep for 10 minutes, strain and leave to cool until lukewarm. Gargle and rinse your sore mouth with this tea as often as you like.

Take extra measures

- Many experts think **lysine**, an amino acid, may be needed to remedy a deficiency associated with ulcers. Take 1000mg of lysine three times a day on an empty stomach.
- **Echinacea** is a herb thought to boost the immune system. Take 200mg two or three times a day as soon as you first notice the onset of an ulcer. (*Alert* Do not take echinacea if you have an autoimmune disease such as lupus, or a progressive disease such as multiple sclerosis or tuberculosis.)
- **Vitamin C** with **flavonoids** will help to heal the mouth's mucous membranes. Citrus fruits supply dietary vitamin C, but

these can trigger mouth ulcers in some people. Instead, take 250mg each of vitamin C and flavonoids (which enhance vitamin C's effectiveness) three times a day.

- **Zinc** may help mouth injuries like ulcers to heal faster. At the first sign of a sore, take up to 25mg of zinc a day, in the form of lozenges, until it clears up. (*Alert* Do not exceed this dose as too much zinc is toxic.)

The power of prevention

- **Avoid ulcer-triggering foods**. Potential troublemakers include whole wheat, rye, barley, shellfish, pineapple or citrus fruits, figs, chocolate, tomatoes, green peppers and strawberries. To find out which, if any, cause your ulcers, cut all these foods out of your diet. Then slowly reintroduce them, one at a time, and see if any make the problem recur.
- Eat **live yoghurt** that contains *Lactobacillus acidophilus*. This friendly bacteria might help to fight off the baddies in your mouth. Eat 3 or 4 tablespoons a day for prevention.
- Check the label of your favourite toothpaste for an ingredient called sodium lauryl sulphate, or SLS. This foaming agent, found in almost every brand of toothpaste, can trigger ulcers in some people. And it really isn't necessary for teeth cleaning. If you get frequent ulcers, ask in your health-food shop for **toothpastes that don't contain SLS**.
- Tiny cuts and grazes inside your mouth can cause ulcers. **Take care when eating sharp edged foods** like crisps and baguettes. When you brush your teeth, **use a soft-bristled brush** so as not to scratch your gums.
- See your dentist if you have any kind of tooth problem that could be irritating the inside of your mouth. **Ill-fitting dentures**, in particular, can cause trouble.
- People plagued with frequent ulcers may be deficient in B vitamins. Try taking a **daily B-vitamin complex**. (*Alert* If you notice tingling in your fingers or toes, stop taking vitamin B). To get more B vitamins into your diet, incorporate beans, wheatgerm and fortified breakfast cereals.
- Stress can trigger ulcers because it causes the body's immune system to overreact to bacteria normally present in the mouth. If you suffer from stress, try a relaxation technique such as **yoga** or work it off through **aerobic exercise**.

Muscle cramps

Something as simple as heat or massage can quickly take care of muscle cramps. Once the agony is over, it's important to mount an anti-cramp campaign. Your body is probably yearning for potassium, magnesium and calcium – the trio of minerals that helps to regulate activity in your nerves and muscles. (You have plenty of potassium if you eat fruit and veg, but you may lack potassium if you're on a high-protein diet.) You'll also need to drink plenty of water and exercise regularly.

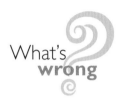

What's wrong

Sometimes you get cramp during a workout. But it can also happen when some part of your body has remained frozen in one position for hours – say, gripping a pen or a paintbrush. In either case, the cramps are caused by overuse of a muscle, dehydration, stress or fatigue. But if your calves cramp painfully when you're trying to sleep, or a muscle often locks up for no apparent reason, the root cause is a faulty chemical signal from the nervous system that 'tells' the muscle to contract. Often the problem is linked to an imbalance of potassium and sodium.

Put the heat on
• Place an electric **heating pad** or a **hot flannel** on the misbehaving muscle to relax the cramp and increase bloodflow to the affected tissue. Set the pad on low, apply for 20 minutes, then remove it for at least 20 minutes before reapplying.
• Take a long, warm shower or soak in the bath. For added relief, pour in half a cup of **Epsom salts**. The magnesium in Epsom salts promotes muscle relaxation.

Press out pain
• Find the central point of the cramp. Press this spot with your thumb, the heel of your hand or a loosely clenched fist. Hold the pressure for 10 seconds, ease off for 10 seconds, then press again. You should feel some discomfort but not excruciating pain. After several repetitions, the pain should start to diminish.

Rub it in
• Mix 1 part **oil of wintergreen** (available from chemists or essential oils suppliers) with 4 parts **vegetable oil** and massage it into the cramp. Wintergreen contains methyl salicylate (related to aspirin), which relieves pain and stimulates bloodflow. You can use this mixture several times a day, but not with a heating pad – you could burn your skin. (*Alert* Note that wintergreen is highly toxic by mouth.)

Banish night-time leg cramps
• Before bed, drink a glass of **tonic water**, which contains quinine, a popular remedy for leg cramps. Research has

supported the use of quinine for nocturnal leg cramps, but **don't take quinine tablets**; they can have serious side effects, such as ringing in the ears and disturbed vision.

- To prevent night-time calf cramps, **try not to sleep with your toes pointed**. And don't tuck in your sheets too tightly – this tends to bend your toes downwards, causing cramp.

- Take 250mg **vitamin E** a day to prevent nocturnal leg cramps. Studies suggest that taking vitamin E improves bloodflow through the arteries.

Mind your minerals

- Low levels of minerals known as electrolytes – which include potassium, sodium, calcium and magnesium – can contribute to cramps. You probably don't need any more sodium (salt) in your diet, but you may need more of the others. Good food sources of **magnesium** are wholegrain breads and cereals, nuts and beans. You can get **potassium** from most fruits and vegetables, especially bananas, oranges and cantaloupe melons. And dairy foods supply **calcium**.

- If you change your diet and you still get cramps, take 500mg of **calcium** and 500mg of **magnesium** twice a day, adding up to 1000mg of each supplement. Some people who get leg cramps due to a magnesium deficiency obtain rapid relief from supplements. Don't take magnesium without calcium; the two minerals work as a pair.

- If you take **diuretics** for high blood pressure, your increased need to urinate may be robbing you of potassium. The result is a condition called hypokalemia, which can cause fatigue, muscle weakness and muscle cramps. Ask your doctor if you can switch to a blood-pressure medication that isn't a diuretic.

Drink your fill

- Cramps are often caused by dehydration, so if you get cramp frequently, **drink more water**.

- If you tend to get cramps during exercise, drink at least 2 cups of water 2 hours before each workout. Then stop and drink 100ml to 250ml every 10 to 20 minutes during your exercise sessions. If you sweat a lot, consider a **sports drink**, such as Lucozade Sport, that replaces lost sodium and other electrolytes.

Should I call the doctor?

Muscle cramps are usually temporary and don't cause permanent damage. But contact your doctor if the cramp or spasm lasts for more than a day, or if it continues to bother you despite trying these home remedies. And call immediately if the spasm occurs in the lower back or neck, accompanied by pain that radiates down your leg or into your arm. Finally, if abdominal cramps occur in the lower right hand part of your belly, it could signal appendicitis.

DO-IT-YOURSELF HEALING
CRAMP-QUELLING STRETCHES

Next time you get a cramp, stretch it out with one of these moves. Hold each stretch for 10 to 20 seconds and repeat 3 times.

NOCTURNAL CRAMPS

If calf or foot cramps wake you up at night, do this stretch three times a day, especially before bedtime. Stand about 75cm (2ft 6in) from a wall. Place your palms on the wall near eye level. Keeping your heels on the floor, gradually move your hands up the wall until you're reaching as high as you can. Hold, then return to the first position.

CALF CRAMP

Stand with your legs apart, feet facing forward. Shift your weight to the front leg, keeping the back leg straight.

FRONT-THIGH CRAMP

Holding on to a chair, bend the cramped leg and grab the foot, bringing the heel as close to your buttock as you comfortably can. Keep the knee pointing down.

HAMSTRING CRAMP

Place the heel of the leg with the cramp on a low stool or step. Slowly lean forward from the waist until you feel a stretch at the back of your leg.

Nail problems

Some people really look after their nails, while others couldn't care less. Whether or not you're the manicure type, though, you'll want to seek some help when brittleness, discoloration, ridges or fungal infection turn fingernails or toenails into eyesores. Here are some ways to get them back in shape fast with better nutrition, selected supplements and fungus-fighters.

Foil fungus

- To fight stubborn nail fungus, try **tea tree oil**. A powerful antiseptic, it can help to make nail fungus disappear. In fact, in one study it proved to be as effective as a prescription antifungal medicine. Once or twice a day, apply a drop or two to the discoloured nail. A good time to do it is after you bath or shower, when your skin is softest.
- Alternatively, you can use an **antifungal powder** that absorbs moisture and prevents fungus. Some good ones are Canesten-AF powder or Daktarin powder (often recommended for athlete's foot). You can sprinkle a medicated antifungal powder into your socks too.
- If your feet are sweaty when you get home, change into a **fresh pair of socks** straight away. And if you have an office job, take along a pair of clean socks – especially on hot summer days – so you can change before you start work.
- **Don't clip your cuticles.** When you do this, you remove your nail's protective barrier. Fungi and bacteria find it easier to get a grip around the base of the nail after the cuticle has been removed.

Say no to weak nails

- Take 300mcg of **biotin**, a B vitamin (also known as vitamin H), three times a day with food. Long ago, vets learned that this vitamin could strengthen horses' hooves – and hooves are made primarily from keratin, the same material that makes up human nails. If your nails are weak or brittle, biotin might be all you need to strengthen and thicken them. However, it doesn't work instantly. You'll need to take this treatment for six months

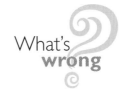

What's **wrong**

Apart from ingrowing toenails (see page 246), nail fungus is probably the most disagreeable nail problem. When you get this affliction – usually on a big toenail – the nail becomes thick, discoloured and crumbly. Other nail problems include brittle nails, which can be the result of age or too much or too little moisture, or nutritional deficiencies. And certain skin diseases can affect the nails, including psoriasis (it can cause a thickening and pitting of the nails) and the patchy hair loss known as alopecia areata (it can cause ridged, pitted, rough nails).

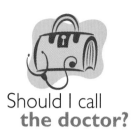

Should I call the doctor?

Unless you suspect you have an underlying nutritional deficiency, brittle nails are a cosmetic issue rather than a health problem. As for nail fungus, it's tenacious and it can take months – or years – to clear up on its own, so ask a doctor if you might benefit from prescription medication.

or more before you will see a noticeable difference. Food sources of biotin include barley, nuts, rice and soya.

- Drink a cup of **horsetail** or **nettle tea** once a day. These herbs are high in silica and other minerals that nails need to grow. Both herbs are sold as tea bags in health-food shops.

Eat for beautiful nails

- If your nails are brittle or flaking, try getting more essential fatty acids. These are found in foods such as **oily fish** (mackerel, sardines and salmon) and **flax seeds** or **flax seed oil**. If you don't eat much fish, take 1 tablespoon flax seed oil a day (use it in place of other oil in salad dressing) or sprinkle ground flax seeds on your cereal or other foods.
- **Evening primrose oil** is another source of essential fatty acid. Take 1000mg three times a day with meals.
- If your nails have white spots, you may be deficient in **zinc**. Increase your dietary intake of zinc by eating beef, pork, liver, poultry (especially the dark meat), eggs and seafood. It's also found in cheese, beans, nuts and wheatgerm.

Moisturize and protect

- If they are dry and brittle, rub **petroleum jelly** or a thick cream into your nails to hold moisture under and around them. If you do this at bedtime, slip a pair of thin cotton gloves on your hands before you go to sleep.
- Wear **rubber gloves** every time you wash up or do other wet household chores.
- Avoid nail varnish removers that contain acetone or formaldehyde. They're terribly drying to nails. Use **acetate-based** removers instead.

False nails breed fungus

For women who have problems with weak, soft, brittle nails, false nails must seem like a godsend. But if you want to avoid nail fungus, forgo the fakes, no matter how much you long for elegant nails. False nails are glued on top of your real ones, and the gap between creates a breeding ground for fungus. Even worse, this is an area where you can develop a painful bacterial infection. False nails are the most common cause of nail fungus infection in women.

Nappy rash

The sight of a baby's raw, red bottom can fill a parent with unrelenting guilt, especially if the baby is crying because of the discomfort. The best treatment for nappy rash is to leave the baby's nappy off. This is easy in the garden or on a washable kitchen floor. Otherwise, change the nappy as often as you can. What else can you do? Try a new cleansing technique and use the right ointment to provide protection.

Clean with care

- When you remove stools from a baby's bottom, do it as gently as possible. Fill a spray bottle with **warm water** and a few drops of **baby oil**, spray on the mixture, and then gently wipe the area with a clean cloth.
- If you use baby wipes, look for a brand labelled 'sensitive' that **does not contain alcohol** or **fragrances**.
- If wiping seems too painful, rinse the baby's bottom in a basin of lukewarm water or baby bath, and pat dry with a soft muslin cloth. **Do not use soap**, which is irritating.

Bring out the hair dryer

- If your baby's bottom is too sore to towel-dry after a bath or a change, use your **hair dryer,** set on the coolest setting. (Keep checking to ensure it's not too hot.) Hold it at least 20cm (8in) from your baby's skin, and keep it moving back and forth.

Give your baby some air

- When the nappy is off and your baby is all cleaned up, give him or her an **air bath** for 10 to 15 minutes, leaving the nappy area exposed to air. As long as the infant's happy, he or she can remain chest down, on a towel placed on top of a waterproof sheet. The longer he or she remains nappy-free, the better.

Opt for the right ointment

- Use an ointment made with **zinc oxide**, which has weak antiseptic properties and provides a barrier between your baby's skin and the moisture that irritates it. Sudocrem or Mothercare's own brand both contain this ingredient.

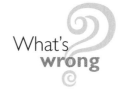

What's wrong

Every parent knows that the red, bumpy, painful-looking rash on a baby's most tender parts is caused by a wet or dirty nappy. Much of what is usually called nappy rash is actually a burn from ammonia, which is produced when urine comes in contact with bacteria from faeces. The stools alone are also an irritant.

Could it be a yeast infection?

If your baby's rash is a beefy red with round pink spots inside the reddened area, it may not be nappy rash at all – it may be a yeast infection (known as thrush or candida). Damp nappies are a breeding ground for yeast. Yeast infections aren't serious and are easily treated. Your baby may also have thrush in the mouth, and if you are breastfeeding, you may have sore nipples. See your doctor who can treat you both with an appropriate anti-fungal medication.

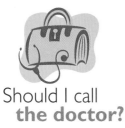

Should I call the doctor?

The chances are your baby's nappy rash will clear up quickly using one or more of the measures recommended here. If it doesn't clear completely in three or four days, see your GP. The doctor will want to know if the rash has spread to other areas, if the creases between your baby's legs are red and raw, or if blisters have developed. A pimple or blister in the nappy area could be a staphylococcus infection that will require antibiotic treatment. If your baby has a rash that is ulcerated and bleeding, and creams aren't working, you should consult your doctor as soon as possible.

• For a rash that is deep red, has an irregular border and tiny dots around the edges, see your doctor who will probably prescribe an **antifungal cream,** such as Canestan, perhaps with a mild steroid to reduce inflammation. You will need to apply the cream to the genital area, the buttocks, groin and any creases that look inflamed. Then, on top of that, apply a **barrier cream**, such as **Sudocrem**, that protects the baby's skin from irritating substances. (Don't use petroleum jelly as a barrier cream. It prevents the nappy from absorbing urine.)

• For an all-purpose cream that clears up diaper rash caused by yeast and ammonia, mix together equal parts of **Nivea cream, Canesten cream, cornflour** and **Sudocrem**. Apply this mixture with each nappy change.

Sit your baby in the bath

• A **bath** may also ease your baby's discomfort. Several times a day, fill the tub with a few inches of warm water and let your child sit and play with toys for five or ten minutes, making sure you stay right there, too, of course. For babies who cannot sit, get in the bath as well – mums and dads make the best made-to-measure baby bath support.

• Don't add bubble bath or anything else to bathwater. They may contain substances that will further irritate a sore bottom.

The power of prevention

• If you use disposable nappies, buy the **ultra-absorbent** types. They draw more urine towards the gel-filled heart of the nappy – away from the skin. You should still change the nappy just as often – as soon as you become aware of a dirty nappy, and as many as **ten times a day** while the rash is severe.

- If you use terry or fabric nappies and launder them yourself, add 4 tablespoons of **white vinegar** to the final rinse. The acid in the vinegar will discourage the growth of bacteria and bring the pH of the nappy closer to the neutral pH of your baby's skin.

- Unless you absolutely have to, **don't cover cloth nappies with plastic pants**. The plastic holds in moisture, which encourages the onset of nappy rash.

- Whether you use disposable or cloth nappies, **put them on more loosely** than you see on the TV ads. Super-snug nappies prevent the circulation of air and contribute to skin irritation.

- Mums and grandparents love the evocative 'baby' smell of baby powder. But some baby powders contain additives that can actually cause a rash, rather than prevent it. And the powder contains fine granules that babies should not inhale, as it can trigger breathing problems. If you want to use a powder, use **cornflour** (which has no irritating additives). Mix it with a gentle cream like Nivea and apply it to the baby's bottom.

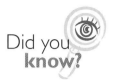

Did you **know?**

Babies who are breastfed have half the risk of bottle-fed infants of developing nappy rash. Doctors speculate that the urine and faeces of a breastfed baby contain fewer irritants. If you breastfeed and your baby develops nappy rash, check your diet for potential irritants, such as spicy foods, acidic juices or fruit, alcohol or caffeine.

Nausea

When nausea tells you that something inside your stomach wants to get out, doctors agree that you shouldn't try to make yourself vomit. But if it's going to happen naturally, then go ahead and let it. If you have a milder case of queasiness, try these tummy tamers to help your stomach feel as though it's back on dry land instead of tossing on stormy seas.

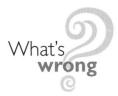

What's wrong

Nausea occurs when the nausea and vomiting centre in the brain stem is activated. It can be caused by motion sickness (see page 282), morning sickness that accompanies pregnancy (see page 279) and gastric flu. Sometimes it's a natural reaction to something you've eaten – something bad the body wants to get rid of. Concussion, a heart attack, some types of cancer and chemotherapy can also trigger nausea. So can certain prescription drugs and over-the-counter medications.

Teas for the queasy

• One of the oldest and perhaps the best remedies is ginger, proven to allay both nausea and motion sickness. Try a warm cup of **ginger tea**. You can buy ginger teabags or, to make a stronger tea yourself, peel the skin from a piece of the fresh root, then chop or grate the yellowish part of the root until you have a full teaspoon. Put the gratings in a mug, add a cup of boiling water, cover with a saucer and let it steep for 10 minutes. You can drink the tea when it's still hot or after it has cooled down a bit. Alternatively, try eating a few ginger-nuts or a piece of crystallized ginger.

• Second to ginger is **peppermint**, which has a calming effect on the lining of the stomach. There are many brands of peppermint tea, sold in teabags or loose-tea form, and you can drink a cup whenever you feel nauseous.

Sip something sweet

• Concentrated sugar is likely to calm a shaky stomach. One recommendation is **cola syrup** (a concentrate used as a base for homemade fizzy cola drinks), which can be found in some pharmacies. Or try a spoonful of golden syrup or honey.

• Make a homemade **anti-nausea syrup**. Put half a cup of white sugar with a quarter of a cup of water into a saucepan, turn the heat to medium and stir steadily until you have a clear syrup. After the syrup cools to room temperature, take 1 to 2 tablespoons as needed.

• Open a bottle of **cola** and stir it until it goes flat. Drink it at room temperature. Some people swear by flat **7-Up** or **ginger ale**, also at room temperature.

Replace your fluids

If nausea leads to vomiting, you may lose a lot of salts and fluids. To recover – and avoid dehydration – you need to replace what you've lost. One way is to make a rehydration drink by dissolving 8 level teaspoons of sugar and 1 teaspoon of salt in 1 litre of water.

Take small sips to begin with, then more as your stomach settles down. Alternatively, an energy drink such as Lucozade Sport will do the trick. (However, don't drink ordinary Lucozade, as this doesn't contain the right electrolytes.)

Be still

● When you're nauseated, **lie still**. Moving around disturbs the balance mechanism in your middle ear, which can worsen nausea and lead to vomiting. While you're lying down, place a cool flannel on your forehead and focus on your breathing so you don't think as much about your stomach.

Press the anti-nausea point

● Try this **acupressure** trick: place your right thumb on the inside of your left forearm, about two thumb-widths from the crease of your wrist. Press firmly for about a minute, then move your thumb a little closer to your wrist and press for another minute. Repeat on the other forearm.

Calm with carbohydrates

● If you're hungry (despite the nausea) and you think you can handle it, eat some **toast** or a few **crackers**, foods that are high in carbohydrates. As your stomach starts to calm down, add a bit of light protein – poached chicken breast, for instance. But don't eat foods that contain fat until you're feeling a lot better.

See also *Morning sickness*, page 279 and *Motion sickness*, page 282.

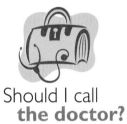

Should I call the doctor?

If you've been feeling queasy for several days, tell your doctor. And be sure to call the doctor if you start to vomit profusely, if the vomit is bloody, if you've been unable to keep food or liquids down for 24 hours or if you've had a bad fall or a severe blow to the head. Heart attacks are sometimes accompanied by nausea, so dial 999 immediately if your nausea is accompanied by severe, sudden chest pain.

PUTTING ON THE PRESSURE

Who would believe that you could stop a toothache simply by pinching the web of skin between your thumb and index finger? Or fall asleep faster simply by pressing your index fingers against the centre of your forehead, between your eyebrows? Well practitioners of acupressure have used these techniques for 5,000 years. Think of this therapy as a DIY, needle-free version of acupuncture.

Acupressure requires nothing more than applying some pressure with your fingertips. When you press on specific points on your body, you rebalance or unblock qi (pronounced 'chee'), a subtle form of energy that flows along pathways that crisscross the body like so many roads. At least that's the explanation given by practitioners of traditional Chinese medicine.

Western-trained doctors still aren't sure exactly how acupressure works, though recent studies suggest that these energy pathways do indeed exist and that finger pressure can cause the body to release natural painkillers known as endorphins. These compounds ease muscle tension and promote better blood circulation while triggering a wonderful sense of well-being.

Acupressure is no substitute for proper medical care, nor does it guarantee instant relief. But here are a few examples of what it might be able to do for you.

Fight nausea

When your stomach is churning, you want relief – fast. Unfortunately, anti-nausea drugs don't always work, and they can make you very drowsy. So next time you feel the first telltale twinge of queasiness, try pressing firmly on the inside of your wrist, between the two large tendons, about two thumb-widths above the crease at the front of your wrist. Keep pressing until you feel better.

If you're planning a long trip by car or boat, you might want to pick up a set of the acupressure wristbands that are sold in many pharmacies and boat yards. These elastic bands have a small bead that automatically presses against the anti-nausea pressure point in the wrists.

Acupressure is so effective at relieving nausea that some surgeons now use it to relieve nausea caused by anaesthesia. In a recent study of 80 women who had under-gone surgery, 40 received acupressure, while the other 40 received a sham treatment (finger pressure on a non-acupressure point). Only 16 of the women in the acupressure group continued to feel nauseous, compared with 28 in the placebo group.

Ease back pain

What did you do or take for relief the last time you put your back out? If you're like most people, you swallowed a few painkillers and crawled into bed. But painkillers can have side-effects, and doctors now know that bed rest is just about the worst thing you can do for a bad back.

Many people have found that acupressure can ease the pain. All you need to do is press against the creases in the skin behind each knee while lying on your back with your knees bent and your feet flat on the floor. Next, lift your feet, and gently rock your legs back and forth for a minute or two.

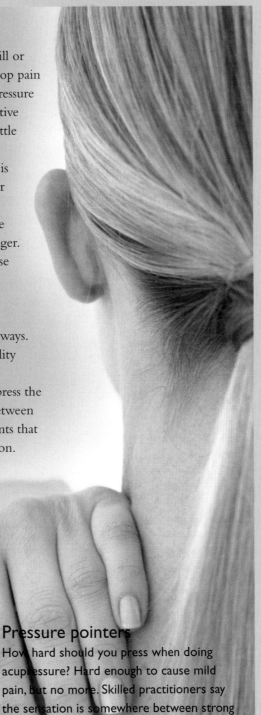

Soothe repetitive strain injuries

If you spend a lot of time writing, working at a till or on a keyboard, there's a good chance you'll develop pain and tingling in the wrists, hands or elbows. Acupressure is no panacea for this condition (known as repetitive strain injury or RSI). But it can ease the pain a little and is even more effective for preventing RSI.

• **Elbow pain:** Bend your arm so that your palm is facing your chest, then press against the elbow for a minute or two.

• **Hand pain:** Press against the web of skin on the back of the hand between the thumb and forefinger.

• **Wrist pain:** Press against the centre of the crease on the back of the wrist.

Conquer cold symptoms

Acupressure helps to fight colds in two different ways. It stimulates the immune system, boosting its ability to combat viruses and helps to ease congestion.

Reach over each shoulder (one at a time) to press the tender spots in the upper back. Aim for a spot between the spine and the tip of the shoulder blade – points that help to stimulate our natural resistance to infection.

To ease nasal congestion, press the inner corner of each eye (just next to the bridge of the nose) and then against the points at which the nostrils meet the upper lip. This four-point acupressure technique also helps to relieve itching, burning eyes.

Ease headaches

When a headache strikes, people tend to rub the area around the eyes. No wonder. It is one of the main acupressure points for easing tension headaches and migraines.

For maximum relief, press a spot about 1cm (½cm) above each eyebrow, directly above the pupils. Don't press too hard or your head-ache might get worse. Next, apply pressure under the cheekbone, directly below the pupils. Press upwards into the notch on the bottom of the cheekbone.

Pressure pointers

How hard should you press when doing acupressure? Hard enough to cause mild pain, but no more. Skilled practitioners say the sensation is somewhere between strong pressure and outright pain.

If you bruise easily, have a history of orthopaedic injuries, are taking blood-thinning drugs, have osteoporosis or are pregnant, check with your doctor before trying acupressure.

Neck and shoulder pain

Most of us have slept in a funny position or sat too long in front of a computer, or been too busy knitting or woodworking – only to suffer from painful neck or shoulder stiffness as a result. Or maybe you've chatted for ages on the phone with the handset cradled between your ear and shoulder – and paid the price. Anti-inflammatory drugs like aspirin or ibuprofen can help and there are other ways to relieve the tension.

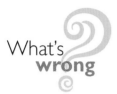

What's wrong

Neck pain usually results from nothing more aggressive than staying in the same position too long. Shoulder pain is often caused by tendinitis – an inflammation of the cord that connects muscle to bone. But it could also be bursitis, resulting from inflammation of the sac, or bursa, that encases the shoulder joint (see *Bursitis and tendinitis*, page 97). Often, shoulder pain is 'referred pain' – it originates elsewhere in the body. Referred pain in the shoulder can come from abdominal organs such as the stomach or gall bladder (due to impulses travelling up the phrenic nerve if the diaphragm is irritated) or from the lung. Injury, arthritis and Lyme disease are other causes of neck and shoulder pain.

Heal with heat

● Heat helps to relieve pain, relaxes the muscles, reduces joint stiffness and speeds up healing. You can use a **heating pad** set on low, a **hot-water bottle**, an **infra-red lamp** or a **heat pack**. Or simply take a hot bath or shower.

● Moist heat eases a stiff, sore neck caused by muscular tension. Make a **neck compress** by soaking a towel in hot (not boiling) water. Fold the towel and wring it out well. Unfold and place it over the back of your neck and shoulders. Cover the wet towel with a dry one and leave both in place for 10 minutes.

● For easy, fast relief, simply set a **hair dryer** on warm and blow the air onto your neck.

Apply some pressure

● Try this simple trick: with your thumb or fingertips, apply **steady pressure** on the painful spot on your neck for 3 minutes. This should lessen your pain significantly.

● A gentle **massage** can work wonders on neck and shoulder pain. Place the fingers of your left hand on the right side of your neck just below your ear, and stroke the muscles in a downward motion towards your collarbone. Do this three times and repeat on the other side. Using a massage oil or lotion to which you have added a few drops of **lavender** or **geranium oil** will enhance the soothing effects.

Rub on a liniment

● Apply a cream known as a counter-irritant. These products irritate nerve endings, diverting the brain's attention from the pain. Over-the-counter brands include the delightfully named Fiery Jack, Algipan and Ralgex.

The power of prevention

• If you usually sleep on your front, you can do your neck a favour by **changing your night-time posture**. Sleep on your back instead. And try using a special **neck-supporting pillow**, available at department stores, some pharmacies and online from medical supply outlets. You should also consider investing in a new mattress if yours is old and sagging.

• Make sure you sit in chairs that give you **good back and head support** (buy a lumbar support roll if you need one, or use a rolled-up towel or small pillow behind your lower back), and be sure not to hunch forward.

• Whether you're standing or sitting, keep your ear, shoulder and hips in a **straight line**.

• Do you wedge your phone in the crook of your neck? To avoid neck strain, **hold the handset**, or if you're on the phone a lot, buy a **headset** or **speaker phone**.

• If you're a woman with large breasts, wearing a **sports bra** can help to relieve neck and shoulder pain. The bra offers more support, and because it has wider straps than a standard bra, it distributes the weight more evenly across your shoulders.

• Don't overload a shoulder bag. The bag not only puts weight on the shoulder, it also throws your posture out of alignment. The best alternatives are a **rucksack** – but use both shoulder straps or buy the sort with a strap that crosses your chest – or a **beltbag**. For dressy occasions, carry a strapless evening bag.

• If you spend hours at a computer, make sure the **screen is angled and raised** so that you don't have to bend your neck or tilt your head to see it.

• **Avoid wearing high-heeled shoes**. They can contribute indirectly to neck pain by tilting your spine out of alignment, making your neck jut forwards.

• **Wear a scarf** whenever the weather is cold and damp. Wintry conditions can aggravate neck stiffness and pain.

• Don't sit or sleep **in a draft**. Wear a scarf in bed if you find yourself sleeping in a cold room.

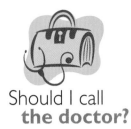

Should I call the doctor?

If home remedies don't work and the pain lasts for more than three days, see your doctor. You also need attention if you have the kind of pain that prevents you from lifting your arm above your head or if you can't move your shoulder. Get in touch with your doctor at once if shoulder or neck pain begins just after a fall or accident. And seek **urgent** medical attention if the neck is not only painful but also stiff, and there is a headache, raised temperature, dislike of light and a non-fading rash. These are symptoms of meningitis.

DO-IT-YOURSELF HEALING
NECK AND SHOULDER PAIN

SHOULDER STRETCHES

The best way to shrug off shoulder pain is to keep your shoulder muscles strong and flexible. The following exercises can be done in one session.

To help resolve shoulder pain, hold a small soup can in one hand. Bend over, letting the weight-bearing arm hang straight. Keeping your shoulder relaxed, slowly trace a figure-of-eight with the soup hand. Repeat 10 to 20 times. Stop if you feel numbness, pain or tingling.

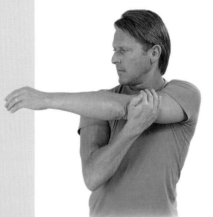
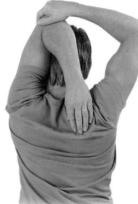
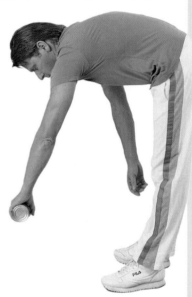

Cross your left arm in front of your body. Use your right hand to press on the outside of the biceps and push the arm towards your collarbone. Press for 15 seconds, then release for 15 seconds and press again. Repeat five times, then switch sides.

Raise your left arm and bend it behind your head so your left hand touches the right shoulder blade. Then place your right hand on your left elbow and pull that elbow towards the right. Hold for 15 seconds, release for 15 seconds, and repeat five times. Switch sides.

EASY-DOES-IT NECK RELIEF

To relieve a sore neck, try these two stretches. Stretch slowly and smoothly, without any jerky motions that could tear a muscle or ligament.

Relax your neck muscles and let your head tilt to the left as far as it will go without straining your neck or lifting the shoulder. Hold for 10 seconds. Return your head to an upright position. Then tilt your head to the right, hold it, and return to the upright position. Repeat four times.

Keeping your shoulders relaxed, slowly drop your head forwards. Hold for 10 seconds. Repeat four times.

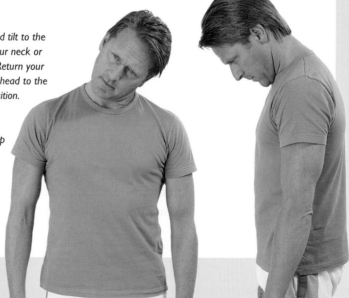

Nosebleed

They tend to occur at the most inconvenient moments, and the sudden gushing of blood from your nose can be both embarrassing and frightening, especially as a small amount can seem like gallons when it's soaking through tissue after tissue. Don't panic. Usually you can halt a nosebleed in a matter of minutes. Here are some effective ways to do it.

Pinch and pack

• The simplest remedy for a bloody nose is the time-honoured **pinch cure**. Sit up straight with your head tilted slightly forwards (to keep the blood from running down your throat). First, gently blow out any clots that could prevent a vessel from sealing. Then pinch the soft part of your nose and press firmly towards your face. Hold that position for at least 10 minutes. If the bleeding doesn't stop, pinch again for another 10 minutes. This usually works.

• If you're still bleeding you can try **packing the nose** itself with a piece of rolled gauze, and pinching for a further 15 to 20 minutes. Then, if the bleeding has stopped, leave the gauze in place for 2 hours. If it is still bleeding, seek medical attention – it may need professional packing or cauterizing.

• A little **lemon juice or lavender oil** dabbed onto the bleeding area (if you can identify where it is – usually on the septum at the front) can help.

• Apply an **ice pack** or a cold compress soaked in **witch hazel** to the outside of the nose alongside the bleeding nostril. The cold narrows the blood vessels in the nose to slow the flow.

Of buttons and brown paper?

• One old fashioned remedy suggests tearing a small square of **brown paper** (from a paper bag), sprinkling it with **salt** and then sticking it between your gums and upper lip in the area right under your nose. Another calls for placing a **coin** or a small, flat **button** under your upper lip, again beneath the affected nostril. However, there's no scientific evidence that these remedies work.

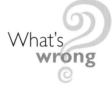

What's wrong

Most nosebleeds occur for no apparent reason in people prone to them. They can also be caused by bruising or picking the nose, and in small children are often the result of a foreign body – such as a bead – being pushed into a nostril. Regardless of the cause, a nosebleed occurs when blood vessels rupture inside a nostril. That can happen when the sensitive inner lining of the nose becomes irritated by dry indoor heat or air conditioning. People with hardening of the arteries are vulnerable to nose-bleeds, as are those who take certain medications, including anti-inflammatory drugs such as aspirin or ibuprofen or blood thinners such as warfarin.

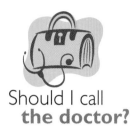

Should I call the doctor?

The power of prevention

• If you want to avoid nosebleeds, you need to keep your mucous membranes moist by drinking **8 large glasses of water a day.** You are properly hydrated if your urine is pale, not dark.

• In winter, counter the drying effects of central heating by adding moisture to the air: run a **humidifier** or dry damp laundry on the radiators.

• Wipe the insides of your nostrils with **petroleum jelly**, or moisturize your nostrils liberally with a **saline nasal spray;** you can make your own by stirring a teaspoon of salt into about 500ml (1 pint) boiled water. Either method will help to keep nostrils moist. This approach is helpful if you're about to fly, if you've just recovered from a cold or sinus infection or if you live in a very dry climate.

• **Watch your aspirin intake.** Aspirin can interfere with blood clotting, and that's not a good thing if you get frequent nosebleeds. Don't stop taking daily aspirin if it has been prescribed by your doctor for blood thinning. Talk to your doctor.

• If you have **nasal allergies**, treat them promptly. Between the constant irritation caused by allergens and the damage done by blowing your nose, nasal membranes take a real hammering when you have an allergic reaction.

• If you often have trouble with nosebleeds, include plenty of **vitamin C-rich foods** in your diet. Go for oranges, grapefruit, kiwi fruit and lots of greens. You could supplement, too. Take up to 1000mg vitamin C every day. Vitamin C helps to strengthen capillary walls and is also a vital component of collagen, a substance that gives your nostrils a moist, protective lining. Along with vitamin C, take 500mg a day of a **bioflavonoid supplement** such as grapeseed extract, pinebark extract, pycnogenol or proanthocyanins. Flavonoids are known to heal capillaries.

Oily skin

Look on the bright side: oily skin tends to age better and develop fewer wrinkles than dry or normal skin. But it does require more attention, as you need to keep cleansing those overproductive pores. The key is a firm but gentle hand. You want to wash away dead skin cells, dirt and excess oil without scrubbing so hard that you cause irritation. Ironically, if you overdo the scrubbing, your skin produces even more oil.

Keep your skin clean

- Wash your face with **warm water**. It dissolves oil more effectively than cool water.
- Choose the **right cleanser**. Whether you prefer soap bars or liquid cleansers, avoid creamy products such as Dove, that have added moisturizers. Bar soaps like Neutrogena or Simple Soap are perfectly effective, although you can also use cleansers formulated specifically for oily skin (they're likely to be more expensive).
- If you have periodic **acne outbreaks**, choose a soap formulated for spots, such as Boots ACT wash bar. These discourage the growth of acne-causing bacteria.
- Use a liquid face wash that contains **alpha-hydroxy acids (AHAs)**, such as citric acid, lactic acid or glycolic acid. The AHAs work in several different ways; they help to wash away dead skin cells, they reduce the oil in your pores and they also combat infection.

Make your own toner

- After you've washed your face, soak a cotton pad in **witch hazel** and dab it all around. Use it twice a day for two to three weeks. After the third week, apply it once a day. Witch hazel contains tannins, which have an astringent effect, making the pores tighten up as they dry.
- The herbs **yarrow, sage** and **peppermint** have astringent properties. To make a homemade skin toner that will improve the look and feel of oily skin, put a tablespoon of one of these herbs in a cup, then fill to the top with boiling water. Leave to steep for 30 minutes. Strain the liquid and let it cool before

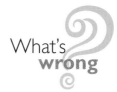

What's wrong

If you have oily skin, your sebaceous glands are pumping out an overabundance of sebum, the waxy substance that protects your skin. When there's too much, skin looks oily, and that excess sebum may contribute to acne. Heredity plays a part – for instance, people with dark hair tend to make more oil than fair-haired people. But there are other contributing factors, including stress and changes in hormone activity. Pregnant women and those taking oral contraceptives are more likely to have problems with oily skin.

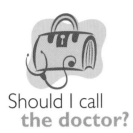

Should I call the doctor?

you dab it on your face. Whatever is left over can be stored. It will stay fresh for three days at room temperature, or five days if you keep it in the refrigerator.

- **Hyssop**, a member of the mint family, also makes an excellent herbal toner. In folk medicine, it has long been considered good for the complexion. Add 1 tablespoon hyssop to about 250ml (½ pint) water. Simmer gently for 10 minutes and strain. Let the mixture cool. After cleansing your skin, apply the toner with a cotton wool ball.
- A combination of **lavender water** and **neroli essential oil** (derived from orange blossoms) acts as a beautifully scented skin cleanser and toner. Pour some lavender water into a hand sprayer and add a drop of neroli oil. Spray the mixture onto your skin several times a day.

Give your face a massage

- A fine-grain powder can help to absorb oil and get rid of dead skin cells that clog pores. Grind and sift 2 teaspoons of **dry oats**, then moisten with some **witch hazel** to form a paste. Using your fingertips, massage this paste gently into your skin, then rinse it away with warm water.
- Several times a week, massage your face with **buttermilk** after washing it. The active cultures in buttermilk contain acids that help to clean away dirt and tighten pores. Leave it on for a few minutes, then rinse.

Use a grease-busting face mask

- **Clay masks** or **mud packs** reduce greasiness and help to tone your skin and draw out impurities. The masks are available from most chemists. Or you can make your own using facial clay (available at some health-food shops and online) and **witch hazel**. Don't use pottery clay; it won't have the same effect. Add 1 tablespoon witch hazel to 1 teaspoon facial clay, and stir until smooth. If you like, add 2 drops cypress oil and 2 drops lemon oil for fragrance and to help to control overactive oil glands. Apply the mask – keeping it away from your eyes – sit back and relax. Leave the clay on for 10 minutes or until the clay is dry, then rinse it off.
- Egg-white masks are said to firm the skin and soak up oil. Mix 1 teaspoon of **honey** with an **egg white** and stir well.

Then add just enough flour to make a paste. Apply the mask to your face, avoiding the eye area. Let it dry for about ten minutes, then wash it off with warm water.

• Some Indonesian women use **mango** to make a face mask to dry and tone the skin. To make the mask, mash a mango until it turns into soft pulp, massage it into your skin, leave it on to dry for a few minutes, then rinse off. It is said to help unblock pores.

• **Lemon juice** is used in another grease-cutting mask, along with astringent herbs and **apple** as the base. Peel an apple and put it in a pan with enough water to cover; then simmer until it's soft. Mash the apple, then add 1 teaspoon lemon juice and 1 teaspoon of either dried **sage, lavender** or **peppermint**. Apply this mixture to your face, leave it on for 5 minutes, then rinse with warm water.

Take off the shine

• Throughout the day, powder your face with **loose face powder**, which will blot up excess oil. Don't use pressed powder – it contains oil and it may trigger blemishes or make existing acne worse.

• Look in the skin-care section of the pharmacy for **alcohol wipes** for oily skin. These often come in hand-bag (or pocket) sized tubs, or as individual foil-wrapped sachets. Keep some to hand to use whenever you need them. The alcohol cuts through the oil to temporarily de-shine your face.

The power of prevention

• Take a tablespoon of **flax seed oil** a day. While it may sound weird to add oil to your diet, there's a good reason for it. Flax seed oil is high in essential fatty acids, which have been shown to help improve many skin conditions, including oily skin. You'll find flax seed oil in health-food shops. Store it in the fridge as the oil deteriorates when exposed to light or heat.

Palpitations

About 36 million times a year the heart beats exactly when it's meant to – which is why it's so unnerving when it occasionally loses its rhythm. Fortunately, there are ways to stop palpitations almost as soon as they start. Better still, you can prevent them from happening in the first place by practising stress-reducing techniques, asking your doctor to check any medications you are taking and adding certain foods and supplements known to benefit the heart to your diet.

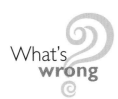

What's wrong

Steady electrical impulses make the heart beat with such regularity that you don't even notice it. But if the system develops a glitch, you may experience palpitations – a fluttering or pounding sensation in your chest – as your heart beats too fast or 'skips a beat'. Palpitations occasionally indicate a serious heart problem, but most cases are caused by fatigue, worry, illness or stress. Although they can make you feel anxious, they don't usually need medical treatment.

Calm a flutter

- As soon as you notice an irregular heartbeat, sit down and prop your feet up. Breathe slowly and deeply, letting your abdomen expand with each inhalation. If you focus on **slow, steady breathing**, your heartbeat will probably return to its normal rhythm straight away.
- If the fluttering continues, do the **Valsalva manoeuvre**. Pinch your nose, close your mouth and try to exhale. Because you can't – your nose and mouth are closed – you will strain as if having a bowel movement. The brief rise in blood pressure that occurs as a result should help to reset your heart. The Valsalva technique was named after an 18th-century Italian anatomist, Antonio Maria Valsalva.
- **Cough forcefully.** Like the Valsalva manoeuvre, coughing increases pressure inside your chest. Sometimes that's all you need to restore your heart to its regular rhythm. Or blow up a **balloon**, which has a similar effect. In fact, professional singers recommend blowing up a balloon to steady a racing heartbeat and fluttering stagefright nerves.

Get relief from cold water

- Take a few **gulps of cold water**. No one knows exactly why this helps, but some people have instantaneous results. One theory is that the swallowed water causes your oesophagus to press against your heart, and that 'nudge' restores the rhythm.
- Alternatively, **splash ice-cold water** onto your face. The shock might be enough to do the trick.

Eat, drink, but be moderate

• Eat plenty of fish. **Salmon**, **mackerel** and **sardines** are all types of oily fish, which contain particularly high levels of heart benefiting omega-3 fatty acids.

• **Avoid eating too much** at a single meal. Forcing your body to digest a huge load of food diverts blood from your heart to your digestive tract. This can lead to palpitations.

• **Cut back on alcohol, coffee and smoking**. In some people, drinking caffeinated coffee, tea or cola drinks triggers palpitations. Excess alcohol and smoking too much (and also nicotine replacement therapy) are also common causes; even chocolate can be a culprit, too.

Soothe stress and get enough sleep

• If you are experiencing palpitations, it is quite likely that stress is to blame. In fact, palpitations can be the body's way of telling you that your stress level has exceeded the safe range. **Meditating** helps to get stress levels back to normal. Try to set aside 30 minutes a day to relax and let your mind unwind.

• Calm your mind with aromatherapy. Sprinkle a few drops of relaxing **lavender oil** onto a handkerchief and inhale the lovely scent. Or try rubbing 2 drops of **bitter orange oil** (also called Seville) onto your chest or adding a little to bathwater.

• Get at least **seven hours' sleep** each night. Being tired can be another trigger for odd heartbeats.

Warm up and get moving

• Get at least 30 minutes of **aerobic exercise** three or four times a week. Walking, running and tennis are all excellent choices. Just make sure you don't become too focused on bettering your previous time or beating an opponent – that will only increase stress. Exercise at a pace that allows you comfortably to carry on a conversation.

• **Warm up** for 10 minutes before each workout and be sure to do wind down stretches for 10 minutes afterwards.

Regulate the rhythm

• Many people with irregular heart rhythms have low levels of **magnesium**. So try eating more foods rich in magnesium, such as whole grains, beans and pulses, dark green leafy vegetables

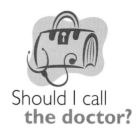

Should I call the doctor?

Unless you have a history of heart disease, there's generally no reason to see your doctor if you have palpitations unless they occur more than once a week, become more frequent or are accompanied by a feeling of light-headedness or dizziness. You should talk to your doctor if you get palpitations a lot and have other signs of increased thyroid over-activity such as weight loss, fatigue or insomnia. If you pass out or experience tightness in your chest accompanied by nausea and sweating, **dial 999 at once**. You might be having a heart attack.

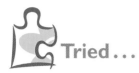

and shellfish. If you want to try magnesium supplements, take 300mg a day. (*Alert* Do not take magnesium if you have kidney disease.)

• Take **coenzyme Q$_{10}$**. This naturally occurring substance, sold over the counter in pill form, helps to keep your heart rhythm regular. Take 50mg twice a day with food. It can take a couple of months before you begin to notice any benefits.

• If you don't eat much fish, take 2g to 3g a day of **fish oil**, which is high in beneficial omega-3 fatty acids.

• The amino acid **taurine** helps to quell irregular electrical impulses in the heart. Take 2g a day. Taurine is available from chemists and health-food shops.

Check your medicines

• Many prescription and over-the-counter drugs can cause palpitations, so **read the package insert**. It might say something like, 'do not use this product if you have heart disease or high blood pressure'. Or it might give a specific warning about the drug's effect on heartbeat. Pay particular attention to over-the-counter cold and allergy medications that contain decongestants. One ingredient that is frequently implicated is pseudoephedrine.

• Some **bronchodilators** for asthma, such as terbutaline (Bricanyl), can increase the risk of palpitations. So can **antihistamines** like loratadine (Clarityn). If you've been taking these, ask your doctor about changing to different medications.

• **Avoid** any diet remedy or supplement containing the ingredient **ephedra** (also called **ma-huang**). Products containing ephedra are used to promote weight-loss and boost energy levels. However, ephedra can sharply increase your risk of irregular heartbeat or palpitations – sometimes with dangerous consequences. Weight-loss supplements containing ephedra have been banned in the USA.

Peptic ulcers

This is an ailment that makes us grateful for modern antibiotics – which are capable of wiping out *Helicobacter pylori*, the bacterium that causes most ulcers. Gone are the days when stress alone was thought to wear holes in the stomach. If *H. pylori* is the culprit in your case, you'll probably be prescribed a 10 to 14-day course of antibiotics. Complete recovery takes about eight weeks. In the meantime, there are many steps you can take to relieve discomfort and prevent a recurrence. Don't use any herbal medicines until you've finished the course of antibiotics.

Put acid in neutral

- The quickest pain relievers are over-the-counter **antacids**, such as Maalox, Asilone, Bisodol, Gaviscon and Pepto-Bismol, which will help to neutralize stomach acid, providing relief in 10 or 15 minutes. Take 2 tablespoons after every meal, at bedtime and whenever you feel your ulcer starting to play up.

- You may be prescribed **H$_2$ blockers**, such as cimetidine (Tagamet 100), famotidine (Pepcid AC) or ranitidine (Zantac 75). These drugs, sold over the counter for relief of heartburn and indigestion, reduce stomach acid secretion and help your ulcer to heal more quickly. Take prescribed H$_2$ blockers at the times recommended on the label. But don't take antacids at exactly the same time of day as your H$_2$ blockers, or the latter's effectiveness will be reduced. Allow at least an hour or two between taking the different medications. (*Alert* Don't attempt self-treatment unless you have your doctor's approval – there is a danger that self-treatment could mask symptoms of a more serious condition, such as gastric cancer.)

- **Eating** may also help temporarily to relieve your discomfort. That's because stomach acid is neutralized as food is digested. But if you have a *duodenal* ulcer, eating will actually make your pain worse, *unless* you eat a high-fibre diet. Fibre slows down the digestive process. Duodenal pain is alleviated when food travels more slowly through the stomach, allowing more time for stomach acid to be neutralized.

- Some animal studies suggest that **ginger** may help to reduce the release of digestive fluids in the gastrointestinal tract. It also

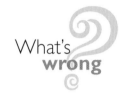

What's **wrong**

Peptic ulcers are crater-like sores in the lining of your stomach or the uppermost section of your small intestine, the duodenum. They occur when pepsin, a digestive enzyme, begins to digest your own tissue. Your gastrointestinal tract usually protects itself from digestive juices with a thick layer of mucus and natural antacids. But bacteria that might be living in the wall of your digestive tract, called *Helicobacter pylori*, can break down this defence system. So can long-term use of nonsteroidal anti-inflammatory drugs such as aspirin and ibuprofen.

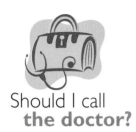

Should I call the doctor?

See your doctor if you have any of the following ulcer symptoms:
• a burning sensation in your gut;
• belching, bloating or pain;
• red blood in your stool;
• black tarry stools;
• unexplained nausea;
• you vomit blood (which looks like brown or black coffee grounds, or is bright red or maroon).

If you feel extreme pain (in which case your ulcer may have perforated, a potentially life threatening condition) **dial 999** or get to the nearest A&E department immediately.

fights inflammation. You can swallow capsules or break them open and dissolve them in water or juice. Take no more than 1 teaspoon a day, as too much can have a reverse effect and cause irritation. You can also munch crystallized root ginger. Manufactured ginger ales probably don't contain enough ginger to do much good, but real ginger beer may help.

Put on a protective coat

• Liquorice, which forms a protective coating between the stomach lining and stomach acid, has been proven to help ulcers heal. Buy the form known as **deglycyrrhizinated liquorice (DGL)**, as ordinary liquorice can send your blood pressure soaring. Chew one or two DGL wafers about 30 minutes before each meal (you need to chew wafers rather than take capsules as DGL is activated only when mixed with saliva). Don't take liquorice if you're still on antibiotics. DGL wafers are not widely available. You may be able to order them from your health-food shop or buy them online.

• Also used to coat sore throats, the inner bark of the **slippery elm** produces a lot of mucilage, a transparent, sticky, gelatinous substance, which can help to protect the stomach lining. Take it as a tea, using 1 teaspoon to a cup of hot water. Drink 3 cups a day. Other **herbal teas** that can help to soothe irritated mucous membranes are calendula, camomile, marshmallow, and meadowsweet.

• Chew and swallow a teaspoon of **flax seeds**. Like slippery elm, the seeds create a soothing mucilage in the stomach. And they have the added health bonus of being an excellent source of omega-3 fatty acids, which can also help to lower blood cholesterol levels.

• Try **aloe vera juice**. A popular European folk remedy for ulcers, the juice seems to quell gastrointestinal inflammation and may reduce stomach acid secretions. Drink one-third of a cup three times a day.

Add ulcer-fighting foods to your diet

• Drink **raw cabbage juice**. It's probably not what you'd choose to drink, but if you have a peptic ulcer, it might hit the spot. Folk healers used it for years before a US study in the 1950s showed it to be an effective treatment. The active substance in cabbage is probably glutamine, an amino acid that nourishes cells of the gastrointestinal tract. If you don't have a home juicer, you can buy raw cabbage juice in some health-food shops. Drink a litre a day for three weeks for best results.

- If you hate cabbage, **pineapple** is another good source of glutamine.
- Eat plenty of **onions**. They contain sulphur compounds that may help to neutralize *H. pylori*.
- Treat yourself to **honey**. Some studies show that honey can discourage the growth of ulcer-causing *H. pylori* bacteria. Spread honey on your morning toast, use it instead of sugar on cereal or add it as sweetener to herbal teas.

Protective plants

- **Astragalus** is an immune enhancer, natural antibiotic and anti-inflammatory that you can use when you're not taking antibiotics. Take 200mg twice a day.
- Another member of the ginger family, **turmeric**, seems to protect the gastrointestinal lining and also reduces wind. Use up to a teaspoon of the powdered root a day to season foods such as soups or rice dishes. Turmeric doesn't make a good tea because it won't dissolve in water. Because you need an awful lot of the powdered root to get any medicinal benefits, you may prefer to take a supplement. Look for one that is described as a standardized root extract, that contains 95 per cent curcuminoids and take 300mg up to three times a day with meals. Excessive turmeric can make ulcers worse, so don't overdo it.

Put the kettle on

- **Camomile tea** is an old-time favourite for soothing the stomach because it calms inflammation. Pour a cup of very hot (not boiling) water over 2 teaspoons of dried flowers. Steep for 5 minutes, then strain. Drink up to three cups a day.
- **Peppermint** is another anti-inflammatory that can relieve pain and help you to heal. To make tea, pour 1 cup of boiling water over 1 to 2 teaspoons of dried leaves, steep for 5 minutes, then strain out the leaves. (*Alert* Do not use peppermint if you have hiatus hernia as the herb relaxes gastro-oesophageal muscles and makes symptoms worse.)

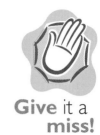

Give it a **miss!**

People say it works. It seems like it should work. It even feels as if it works. What is it? Milk. Once thought to soothe ulcer pain, milk actually increases the production of stomach acid, so in the long run, it will make you feel worse, not better.

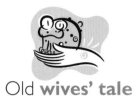

Old **wives' tale**

Doctors used to think spicy foods were no good for people with peptic ulcers. Modern research, however, has shown that this isn't necessarily the case. In fact, there's some evidence to suggest that hot peppers, which contain a chemical called capsaicin, may actually help to heal ulcers by stimulating bloodflow to the wound.

De-stress yourself

• Practise **deep breathing**, **meditate**, listen to soothing **music**, do **yoga**, inhale **calming scents** – do whatever you can to take the edge off the stress in your life. In the days before we knew about *H. pylori*, ulcers were thought to result from excessive emotional stress. Now we know that this is not the case, but doctors have found that stress can trigger pain by increasing stomach acid production. And if you already have *H. pylori* in your system, the opportunistic bacteria will take advantage of your reduced defences.

• If you're going through a particularly tough period, treat yourself to a weekly **massage**. There's no more enjoyable way to relax and melt away stress.

The power of prevention

• **Vitamin C** may slow down the growth of *H. pylori* if you have colonies of these bacteria in your stomach. Take 500mg twice a day. Citrus fruits and tomatoes are good dietary sources, but avoid these if you already have an ulcer.

• **Vitamin A** is a must. People who get plenty of the vitamin are the least likely to develop duodenal ulcers. The healthiest way to get enough vitamin A is to add a broad range of fruits and vegetables to your diet. You can also take 7mg a day of natural **beta-carotene** – the body converts beta-carotene into vitamin A.

• Eat plenty of **yoghurt** containing active cultures, especially *Lactobacillus acidophilus*, beneficial bacteria that inhibit *H. pylori*. It's an especially good idea to eat plenty of yoghurt while you're taking antibiotics, as these drugs don't discriminate between harmful and beneficial bacteria, and kill the 'good' bacteria in your gut that keep 'bad' bacteria in check.

• **Go easy on alcohol**, which can irritate the stomach lining. Two small glasses of wine a day for a man and one for a woman, is the limit.

• **Be moderate** in your use of **aspirin**, **ibuprofen** and other nonsteroidal anti-inflammatory drugs. They can contribute to ulcer formation.

• **Avoid caffeine and tobacco**. Both increase production of stomach acid, and tobacco makes antibiotics less effective.

Pregnancy ailments

As the months go by, pregnancy can start to feel more like a burden than a miracle in the making. Morning sickness is just the beginning (for ways to overcome nausea see *Morning sickness*, page 279.) When the 'blooming' you is someone with heartburn, stretch marks, back pain, swollen feet and varicose veins, you may even begin to wonder whether this was such a good idea. Here are some comforting suggestions.

Ease fatigue

- Take a **half-hour nap** each day. When you sleep, make sure that your feet are raised higher than your heart as this helps to take the pressure off your legs. Don't feel guilty about needing to rest: building a baby can be hard work. If you've got a toddler, rest when your child does, and if the child won't nap, put on a Tweenies video, put your feet up and settle down and watch it too.
- Get some **exercise** every day. Aerobic activity, such as walking or swimming, gives you more energy. And labour and delivery will be easier if you've been exercising regularly.

Deflate swollen feet

- Improve circulation to aching feet with alternating **hot and cold footbaths.** The hot water brings blood to your feet and the cold moves it back out. Fill two large bowls with water – one comfortably hot, the other cold. Immerse your feet in the hot water for three minutes, then in the cold water for about 30 seconds. Switch backwards and forwards six times, ending with the cold water.
- After your footbaths, **rest for at least ten minutes** with your feet propped up.

Get heartburn under control

- When you're pregnant, not only does the growing baby increase pressure on your abdomen but also the oesophageal sphincter (the valve between the stomach and oesophagus) is relaxed by pregnancy hormones. This combination means that stomach acids are highly likely to be forced up into the

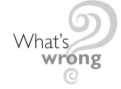

What's wrong

As a baby grows inside her womb, a mother-to-be can start feeling pretty uncomfortable. Carrying around the extra weight can cause back pain and fatigue. And as the enlarging uterus encroaches on the stomach and intestines, heartburn can result. On top of that, there are the twin unglamorous discomforts, constipation and haemorrhoids. Other side effects of pregnancy can include fluid retention – causing swollen feet – and carpal tunnel syndrome (leading to tingling or numb fingers and painful wrists). To cap it all, ropey varicose veins may develop, along with stretch marks on tummy and breasts. Hooray for pregnancy!

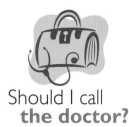

Should I call the doctor?

oesophagus, which can cause a horrible burning sensation. There are several things you can do that will help to lessen the discomfort.

- **Don't eat big meals** and leave at least an hour (and preferably three) between the evening meal and going to bed.
- Wear clothes that are **loose around the waist**.
- Avoid **excessive weight gain**.
- **Try not to bend over.** If you need to pick something (or someone small) up, bend your knees and squat.
- Eat **almonds**. Chemical compounds in these nuts help to keep stomach acid in the stomach by strengthening the oesophageal sphincter. Keep an eye on calories, though. At about 10 calories a nut, almonds are very fattening. To avoid gaining too much weight, you'll need to give up another high-calorie food in exchange.
- **Avoid** foods that relax the oesophageal sphincter. These include **coffee**, **citrus juices**, **fried foods**, **peppermint**, **tomato products** and **alcohol**.
- If all else fails, talk to your doctor about taking **antacids**, medications that help to neutralize stomach acid. Some antacids are regarded as safe for use in pregnancy but excessive use could harm an unborn child.

Combat back pain

- **Avoid standing for long periods**, particularly in the later months of pregnancy. As the baby grows and the joints in your pelvic area soften, backaches become common; standing increases the pain.
- When you must stand for any length of time, keep your weight **evenly balanced** between your feet. If you raise one of your hips, you'll put sideways pressure on your lower spine.
- When you're in a chair, **sit up straight**. Press your lower back against the chair back and repeat this several times every day to help strengthen muscles that support your back.
- If you're working at a desk, keep your feet slightly raised on a **footrest** or a **small stool**.

Control carpal tunnel syndrome

- Many women suffer numbness or tingling in the fingers during pregnancy, usually because water retention puts pressure on nerves in the wrist. To ease the discomfort, you should **exercise your arms and wrists** for 5 minutes or so every hour (see the exercises on page 109).

• If your wrist feels numb **don't bend it** in an attempt to ease the discomfort. It will actually make matters worse.

Minimize the likelihood of stretch marks

• Nearly every pregnant woman gets stretch marks – streaks on the skin that turn from purplish-red to silvery-white. They occur because the skin has to stretch to allow for the expanding abdomen and breasts. The stretching occurs in the collagen layer of skin, which lies beneath the surface, so spending a fortune on skin-care products won't help. Some women are simply more prone to stretch marks than others. But if you can **keep weight gain under control**, you'll keep marks to a minimum. On a more cheerful note, they do tend to **fade with time** and often become silvery pale streaks or virtually disappear.

Keep varicose veins at bay

• Varicose veins form because you're building up an extra volume of blood to feed the foetus. To keep them at bay, wear maternity **support tights**.

• Minimize the appearance of varicose veins by using a **cold compress** on your legs. Mix 6 drops each of essential oils of **cypress, lemon** and **bergamot** in a cup of distilled **witch hazel**. Chill in the fridge for at least an hour. Put your feet up, soak a flannel in the liquid and apply it for 15 minutes. This combination of oils helps to shrink swollen blood vessels and reduce swelling.

Combat constipation

• Pregnant women are more susceptible to constipation, so you need to **increase your fibre** intake. High-fibre foods include beans, bran and whole grain breads and cereals, ground flax seeds, leafy green vegetables, broccoli and fresh fruit.

Premenstrual syndrome (PMS)

It's not just the mood swings and headaches. Not just the pain and bloating. What's so annoying if you're a PMS sufferer is the ongoing nature of the problem – this month's symptoms repeated next month and the month after that. Many experts now agree that the best prescription of all for premenstrual syndrome is not a drug or a supplement, but exercise. Walk, dance or swim every day, if you can, boosting the level of activity before symptoms begin. And try some of these helpful ideas, too.

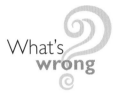

What's wrong

PMS may start a week or two before the beginning of your period. Common symptoms are breast tenderness, mood swings, headaches, backache and bloating. Experts still don't know why some women feel the effects of PMS so much more than others, but the problem is thought to be linked to out-of-balance hormones. The main culprits are oestrogen and progesterone. Levels of both can soar just before menstruation, then come crashing down. It may be that these fluctuations throw levels of the mood-regulating chemical serotonin out of kilter.

Keep moving

- Get at least 20 to 30 minutes of **aerobic exercise** every day, every month. Brisk walking and swimming are best. But if those forms of exercise seem a bit tame or boring, there's always skating, karate, kickboxing, water aerobics, dancing and much more. Try to exercise to the point of perspiration. If you keep up the good work, you will reduce the level of free-circulating oestrogen in your system. Exercise both relieves stress and enhances mood because it boosts your body's natural painkilling endorphins – feelgood chemicals that make you feel better all over – while also relaxing your muscles. Furthermore, exercise combats fluid retention.

Manage your diet

- **Eat less salt** throughout the month, but especially in the week before your period. Salt increases fluid retention, hence more bloating. Processed foods such as tinned soups, cooking sauces and packaged snacks are especially high in salt, so avoid them whenever possible. Even supermarket bread contains a lot of salt – check labels carefully, or try baking your own.
- Also **cut back on alcohol** and **caffeine**, both of which can contribute to PMS.
- **Eat lots of fibre**. High-fibre foods help to take excess oestrogen out of the body. Fill up on whole grains such as barley, oats and wholemeal breads, vegetables and beans.
- **Drink more water**. When you do, more superfluous salt leaves in your urine, and that helps to stop swelling and bloating. Aim for **at least** 8 large glasses of water a day.

- **Cut out sugary snacks**. Sweet cravings rocket when you have PMS, but sweets and biscuits send your blood sugar levels soaring. When blood sugar plummets later on, you'll feel tired and irritable. Limiting sugar intake and eating fruit when your body craves a 'sugar hit' can help to steady your mood.

Calcium and beyond

- Take 500mg of **calcium** and 250mg of **magnesium** a day. Calcium reduces headaches, mood swings and muscle cramps. It also helps make you sleepy, which is a good reason to take the supplement just before you go to bed. Many women with bad PMS symptoms are low in magnesium, which works with calcium to help control muscular activity. A combination of both minerals can help to contain symptoms.
- Take 50mg a day of **vitamin B_6** to reduce irritability and depression. Among its other powers, B_6 can help to calm jittery nerves by increasing your supply of serotonin, the mood-regulating brain chemical. It also helps with fluid retention, breast tenderness, sugar cravings and fatigue. Good food sources include protein foods (meat, poultry and fish) and fortified breakfast cereals.
- Some women take **evening primrose oil** for PMS, but due to lack of positive evidence for its benefits, doctors are no longer able to prescribe it as they once used to. If you wish to try it, the dose is 1000mg three times a day.

Balance your hormones

- Take **chasteberry** (*vitex*) supplements. This herb is prized for its ability to improve PMS symptoms by bringing hormones back into balance. Take one or two 225mg capsules a day when **not** menstruating. Give it time – it can take up to six months before you feel the full benefit.
- Use **black cohosh** for a week to 10 days before your period begins. Often prescribed for menopausal hot flushes, black cohosh also works by levelling out hormones. Take two 40mg capsules a day with food, and be prepared to give the herb four to eight weeks to begin working for you.
- **St John's wort**, a natural antidepressant, can help with mood symptoms. Take 300mg of an extract standardized to contain 0.3% hypericin three times a day.

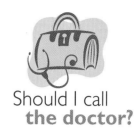

Should I call **the doctor?**

If PMS interferes with your ability to enjoy a normal life, talk to your doctor about it. He or she might be able to prescribe something to help – either some form of hormone therapy to even out hormonal fluctuations or an antidepressant such as fluoxetine that increases serotonin levels in the brain.

Old **wives' tale**

Claims that the reason women crave chocolate when they have PMS is that they're deficient in magnesium, have been dismissed by scientists. After all, wheatgerm and green leafy vegetables are high in the mineral and few people crave those. However, chocolate *does* contain mood-boosting chemicals that may explain cravings. Satisfy your desire with dark chocolate, which has less sugar and fat than milk chocolate.

Prostate problems

In later life many men begin to have urination problems – often needing to urinate more frequently and experiencing pain. Initially, it's worth checking your medicine cabinet for over-the-counter drugs, such as antihistamines and decongestants, that can make the problem worse. Then think about modifying your diet and, perhaps, trying some supplements. Many of these remedies, used alone or in combination, can make the problem more bearable. But you should see your doctor for a proper diagnosis before attempting to self-treat a potentially serious condition such as an enlarged prostate.

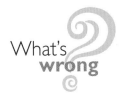

What's wrong

After 40, many men notice that their waterworks don't work as well as they once did. It is hard to pee, the flow is weak and it ends with dribbles. And annoyingly, nature calls during the night and disrupts sleep. The cause is often benign prostatic hyperplasia (BPH), a noncancerous swelling of the prostate. The prostate gland, which produces seminal fluid, is rather like a collar around the urethra (the tube that runs from the bladder out through the penis). So when it swells it blocks the flow. More than half of men over 50 have some prostate swelling.

Try these renowned herbal remedies

• Take 160mg of **saw palmetto** in capsule form twice a day. Look for an extract containing 85 to 95 per cent fatty acids and sterols. This supplement, which contains extracts of the berries of the saw palmetto plant, seems to block the action of a hormone responsible for stimulating growth in the prostate gland. There is evidence that it also decreases inflammation.

• **Pygeum**, a supplement that comes from the bark of an evergreen African tree, is the most widely used medicine in France for treating benign prostate enlargement. Pygeum has an anti-inflammatory effect and has been found to reduce swelling and help in cases of excessive night-time urination. If you wish to try this herb, you should see a qualified medical herbalist who can advise you on the correct dosage.

• Look for supplements containing extract of dried **nettle root** and take 250mg twice a day. Nettle root helps to shrink the prostate and, when taken with either saw palmetto or pygeum, it seems to help the supplement work better.

Modify your diet

• Eat lots of **tomatoes** or tomato-based products – every day if you can. US researchers found that men who ate ten or more servings a week of tomatoes cut their risk of prostate cancer by more than 45 per cent. Tomatoes are rich in **lycopene**, a carotenoid pigment. Carotenoids are natural antioxidants and potent disease fighters. Lycopene decreases inflammation and swelling of the prostate gland. **Watermelon** and **apricots** are also rich in lycopene. You can take lycopene supplements, too. The recommended dose is 10 to 20mg a day.

* A folk remedy for prostate enlargement is to eat a handful of unroasted **pumpkin seeds** each day. The seeds are a good source of zinc, a key nutrient for prostate health.

* Twice a day, mix a tablespoon of **flax seed oil** into your food. It is a rich source of omega-3 fatty acids. These and other essential fatty acids decrease inflammation in the prostate gland (and thus reduce swelling) by limiting the concentration of the hormone, prostaglandin.

Think before you drink

* Cut back on fluids in the evening, as you'll be more likely to have to get up in the night. Your body needs plenty of fluids, but **drink before supper**, not after.

* If you're already having trouble urinating, **limit** the number of caffeinated drinks you consume, such as **coffee**, **tea** and **colas**. Caffeine tends to make the outlet from your bladder tighten, creating a roadblock that interferes with urine flow. It's also a diuretic, which is exactly what you don't want if you're already getting up to pee during the night.

* Also cut out spirits – these irritate the lining of the prostate. Beer and wine are fine – but not to excess. In fact, research has shown that **moderate alcohol consumption** – two or three beers or glasses of wine a day – **can reduce your risk** of BHP and lessen symptoms.

Keep your prostate running on empty

* **Ejaculate regularly**, either when making love – or on your own. The prostate gland produces the nutrient-rich fluid in which sperm swim and ejaculation helps to relieve internal fluid pressure. It also causes the muscles around the prostate to contract, which is good for bloodflow, helping to keep the gland from becoming inflamed.

Lounge in the bath

* Sit in **warm water**. The heat increases bloodflow in the prostate gland, helping to reduce inflammation and swelling. If you can, spend 20 to 45 minutes in the bath every day.

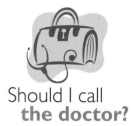

Should I call the doctor?

If you have trouble starting to urinate, a weak urine stream, a feeling that your bladder can't totally empty and a frequent need to go during the night, you should have a check-up. Your doctor can tell whether you have BPH and rule out other conditions, particularly prostate cancer. If your symptoms are more severe – you can't urinate even if you strain, for more than 8 hours – this is urinary obstruction. You need immediate hospital treatment to prevent kidney failure.

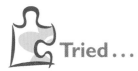

Tried...

Some men say you should get up and walk around as much as possible to help deal with a problem prostate.

...&
true

When you remain sitting you put pressure on your prostate. In fact, men who sit for long periods while they work – such as lorry drivers – or who watch more than 40 hours of television a week report more BPH than those who move around. You only need to walk for about 2 hours a week to make a difference. If you have a desk job, get up and pace every so often.

Let it flow

• Urinate **whenever you get the urge.** Some men seem to think it's best to exercise bladder control and avoid visits to the toilet. But when the bladder gets too full, urine enters the prostate, irritating it.

• When in the bathroom, **urinate as much as possible**, relax for a few minutes and then try again. Doctors call this 'double voiding'. It's a good way to guarantee that you have emptied your bladder completely.

• **Try sitting on the toilet** to urinate rather than standing. The combination of the new position and the more relaxed situation can be more effective.

• **Relax in the bathroom**. This is not a contest, no one is judging, no one is timing you. Read something, ponder something, take ten slow, deep breaths in a row. The reason for consciously relaxing is that tension and anxiety trigger stress hormones that can cause the bladder muscles to tense. If you put too much psychological pressure on yourself to 'perform', that alone can stop the performance. There's no need to turn a physical problem into a psychological one, too.

Psoriasis

There are good days and bad days, and if you're troubled with psoriasis you know the difference only too well. On good days, you hardly need to pay any attention to what your skin is doing. On bad ones, those red itchy patches are crying for attention. Here are some ways to make good days better and the bad days more bearable.

Spend time outdoors

- **Sunlight** is an excellent remedy for psoriasis. Every day, spend 15 to 30 minutes outdoors and you should see results in less than six weeks. Research shows that sunlight decreases the activity of the skin's T cells. These are specialized cells that produce substances called cytokines, which initiate a cycle of inflammation. When T cells are exposed to sunlight, it suppresses their activity, breaking the cycle.
- Protect yourself from burning by wearing **sunscreen** with an SPF of at least 15 on healthy areas of skin.

Bath solutions

- Take a good, long soak in warm water … then add some **vegetable oil**. The reason is that, while a long bath can soften scaly patches and soothe itching, it can also dry your skin and make itching worse. So lie in the water for about 10 minutes, letting your skin get thoroughly soaked. Then, about 5 minutes before you get out, add a few teaspoons of vegetable oil to the water to help seal the moisture into your skin. But be careful getting out as the oil will make the bath surface very slippery.
- To relieve itching, try a cool bath, adding **vinegar** to the bathwater. Many people find that vinegar helps psoriasis, though doctors aren't sure why. What's known is that the acetic acid in vinegar kills bacteria – and one theory suggests that psoriasis is made worse by bacteria.
- Finely-ground **oatmeal** is another good ingredient for itch relief. You can sprinkle in an oatmeal product specially made for baths, such as Aveeno (available from pharmacies). Or put ordinary oatmeal into a blender, grind it until it turns into a fine powder and sprinkle it into the water.

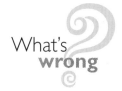

What's wrong

Your skin is growing too fast. Normally, new skin cells need about 28 days to migrate from deep within your skin to the surface, where they replace dead cells that fall away. But if you have psoriasis, the cycle is compressed into about four days. Skin cells pile up, causing distinctive red, bumpy patches covered with white scales. These frequently develop on the knees, elbows and scalp. The cause is unknown, but psoriasis seems to be more prevalent in some families than in others. People with psoriasis tend to have flare-ups – when the rashes get worse – followed by periods when the condition is far less severe.

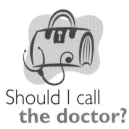

Should I call
the doctor?

If an outbreak covers a
large area of skin, or affects
the palms of your hands
and soles of your feet, then
see your doctor. You must
also see your doctor if you
see signs of infection, such
as pus or a yellow crust
on your skin. Sometimes
psoriasis is accompanied
by joint pain, a condition
called psoriatic arthritis.
Anyone with this condition
needs to be under a
doctor's care.

Put on another layer

● As soon as you get out of the bath, while the skin is still damp, smooth on a moisturizing cream to lock in its natural moisture. Make sure that you add an extra thick layer to the psoriasis patches. This helps to prevent cracking. It is best to avoid runny lotions, which dry up too quickly, and instead choose a heavy cream or ointment. Among the effective brands are **Aquadrate**, **Eucerin** or **Calmurid** which contain urea to help loosen scales.

● Try a cream that contains **camomile**. This plant has long been reputed to reduce inflammation and soothe flaky skin. Ask for it in your local health-food shop.

● Rub a few drops of **tea tree oil** into psoriasis patches several times a day. This Australian remedy is useful for relieving itching and softening psoriasis patches, especially if you have a mild case. However, because some people have an allergic reaction to tea tree oil, be sure to test it first on a small patch of skin. It is also worth remembering that skin coated in tea tree oil may be extra sensitive to sunlight.

● To soften skin and remove scaly patches, you can also use **petroleum jelly**. Apply it as often as necessary.

Add oil from the inside

● Mix a tablespoon of **flax seed oil** into your cereal, yoghurt or other food each day. This isn't for flavouring – it's for your psoriasis. Flax seed oil is high in omega-3 fatty acids, which help to block a chemical in your body called arachidonic acid, which causes inflammation.

● Oily fish are also high in omega-3s. If you like **salmon**, it's a good idea to eat it at least once a week. Other fish that are high in omega-3s are **sardines** and **mackerel**.

● You can also get these polyunsaturated fatty acids by taking 1000mg of **fish oil** three times a day, after meals. Large amounts of fish oil can thin the blood, so it is best to check with your doctor first if you're already taking a blood thinning medication such as aspirin.

● If you have an **aloe vera** plant on your windowsill, break off a leaf and apply the gel several times a day to itchy patches of skin. Aloe has anti-inflammatory compounds, and the gel contains magnesium lactate, which helps to control itching.

Avoid scratching

- **Keep your hands off** the red spots. Even minor damage to your skin can worsen your psoriasis symptoms. If you pick and scratch the itchy patches, you'll damage your skin, which can lead to more extensive outbreaks.
- Always use an **electric shaver** instead of a razor if you have psoriasis on your legs, face or other areas where you shave. A sharp razor nicks your skin, no matter how careful you are, which increases your risk of new outbreaks. Shavers are gentler.

Care for your scalp

- If you get psoriasis on your scalp, it's time to shop for special shampoos. You want a product that contains **coal tar**, such as Polytar or T Gel. Use it every day to begin with, then twice a week – alternating with ordinary shampoo – as symptoms subside. When you apply the shampoo, leave it in contact with your scalp for 10 minutes before rinsing it off.
- Keep a list of several shampoos that suit your scalp. When you finish one, choose another and rotate them. Your scalp may begin to tolerate one shampoo, which then becomes less effective the longer you use it. People report better results if they regularly **swap shampoos**.
- Consider wearing your hair in a **short hairstyle**. It will be a lot easier to treat your scalp.

Calm down

- Take regular **exercise**. It's a great stress reducer – and stress is known to contribute to psoriasis outbreaks. If you can go for a 30-minute walk every day, you may be surprised at how effectively that small amount of exercise distracts you from things that get you worked up.
- Practise a relaxing mental exercise, such as **meditation** or **deep breathing**, for a few minutes each day.

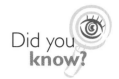

Did you know?

For reasons that are not well understood, cold temperatures aggravate psoriasis. You can't change the seasons, of course, but you might be able to keep outbreaks in check if you dress warmly and keep your skin well covered when you're out in the cold.

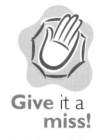

Give it a miss!

Sunlight is helpful for treating psoriasis, but keep away from tanning beds. The artificial light doesn't cover the same spectrum as sunlight and won't help your condition.

Restless legs syndrome

Of all the body's mysteries, this is surely one of the quirkiest. When you're otherwise ready for rest, why on earth do your legs want to run? When every fibre of your being says 'settle down', why are you kicking your bedmate? Since restless legs syndrome (RLS) seems to be related – at least in part – to mineral imbalances, perhaps the best place to end the night race is with supplements. You could also work on some pre-bedtime rituals to help those jumpy legs calm down.

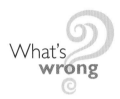

What's wrong

The name restless legs syndrome (RLS) pretty much describes what this condition is. But it fails to capture how distressing RLS can be. When you lie down to sleep or rest, you start feeling a maddening 'creepy-crawly' sensation in your legs. Generally, the only way to stop it is to move the legs or walk around. Older people, pregnant women and people with diabetes or lower back problems are more susceptible. The causes of RLS are not known, but high-risk groups all have low levels of magnesium. RLS symptoms are also associated with sugar, caffeine and alcohol consumption, as well as some prescription drugs.

Try taking supplements

• Each day, take 800mg **calcium** and 400mg **magnesium**, (some naturopaths recommend starting with lower doses, so try 500mg calcium and 250mg magnesium initially – but note that these two minerals must be taken in a 2:1 ratio); plus 800mg **potassium**. A shortage of any one of these can make legs more twitchy.

• Drink mineral water that's high in **magnesium**. The optimum magnesium level is in the range of 100mg per litre of water.

• Increase your intake of the B vitamin **folic acid** (also called folate). Folic acid helps to build red blood cells, which in turn help to oxygenate the body. That is an important benefit, as RLS is associated with a decrease in blood oxygen. Food sources of folic acid include leafy green vegetables, orange juice, whole grains and beans. You'll also find folate in most multivitamins.

• Eat **iron-rich** foods such as dark green vegetables, liver, wheatgerm, kidney beans and lean beef. Iron is part of the myoglobin molecule, which is a protein that stores oxygen in the muscles until it's needed. Without iron, myoglobin can't hold enough oxygen, and muscle problems may develop.

The home stretch

• When you get the urge to move your legs, start **rubbing** them or **stretch** them to their full length and **point your toes**. These intentional movements send signals to your brain that can override the strange tingling sensations of RLS. But be

sure to stop if the stretching causes leg cramps. These suggest a magnesium deficiency, which can't be alleviated by stretching.
* Sit on the edge of the bed and firmly **massage** your calves to give the muscles deeper stimulation.
* If these treatments don't calm your legs, get up and go for a brief **walk** around the house or the bedroom. Take long steps and bend your legs to stretch the muscles.

Before you go to bed
* Sit in a bath filled with comfortably **hot water** for 10 to 15 minutes before you go to bed.
* Chilling your legs may also help. Rub a **cold pack** on your legs before you go to bed.
* Or combine the **heat and cold** treatments. Dip your legs in a comfortably hot bath for two minutes, then apply the cold pack to your legs for a minute. Repeat several times before bed.

Relax your muscles
* After you get into bed, practise the calming ritual known as **progressive muscle relaxation**. Breathe deeply for a few minutes, then tense the muscles in your feet. Hold the tension for a few seconds, then relax. Next, tense your calf muscles, hold and relax. Then do the same with your thigh muscles. Repeat the tensing-and-relaxing pattern, working all the way up your body to your neck and face muscles. When you've finished, your whole body should feel relaxed.

Test homeopathy
* Homeopathic doctors recommend **Causticum** at the 12C dilution for legs that are restless during the night.
* Another option is a 12C dilution of **Tarentula hispanica**, three times a day until symptoms improve.

The power of prevention
* In the evening, **avoid alcoholic** or **caffeinated drinks**, which stimulate the muscles and nerves in your legs.
* Studies have found that smokers are more likely to have RLS than people who don't smoke. So **stop smoking**.
* **Avoid cold and sinus remedies**, which can make RLS symptoms much worse.

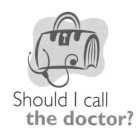

Should I call the doctor?

If RLS is causing severe sleep loss or interfering with your work or daily life, and home remedies don't help, talk to your doctor. He or she may be able to prescribe something to calm things down. If you are experiencing leg jitters for the first time, see your doctor. It could be a sign of more serious medical problems, such as diabetes, kidney disease or Parkinson's disease.

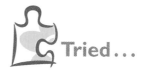

Tried...

Drinking tonic water can quench those restless feelings in the legs.

...& **true**

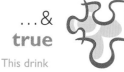

This drink contains quinine, which does relieve symptoms in some people.

Rosacea

You appear to be blushing, even when you're not. Even worse, you look like a teenager with a bad case of acne. Take heart. If Princess Diana could cope with her rosacea – you probably didn't even know she had it – then so can you. Try these approaches to prevent mild flare-ups and flushing. Should your condition get worse, ask your doctor to recommend a dermatologist to get the redness under control.

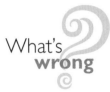

What's wrong

Sometimes rosacea looks no worse than an embarrassing blush. But the condition can gradually worsen until it resembles severe acne. If you have rosacea, tiny blood vessels in the face widen and fill with blood until areas of the face seem suffused with red. The redness fades after a few hours, but if rosacea isn't treated, the face can take on a bumpy, sunburnt look; blood vessels can become visible through the skin and the nose may become red and enlarged.

Cool your skin

- When your face gets warm and red, your first instinct is the right one – cool it down. The easiest way is to soak a clean flannel in **ice-cold water** and lay it on the red areas for about 10 minutes. The cold tightens up blood vessels.
- Camomile, applied to the skin, has anti-inflammatory effects. Don't use camomile essential oil, which is highly concentrated and might cause a skin reaction; instead use **camomile tea**. Steep 3 tea bags in 600ml (1 pint) boiling water for 10 minutes. Strain the liquid and chill it in the fridge. When your face is flushed, dip a cloth into the tea and apply it to the red area.

Wash using only the mildest soaps

- Use an unscented, moisturizing soap or cleanser designed for sensitive skin, whenever you wash your face. You need to avoid any soap that might be harsh or irritating. Afterwards, rinse your skin with lukewarm, not hot, water.
- **Avoid exfoliating skin washes** or **acne cleansers**. These contain harsh ingredients; acne treatments can actually make rosacea worse.
- Also **steer clear of** cleansers that list **salicylic acid**, **benzoyl peroxide** or **alcohol** as an ingredient – these too can make **rosacea worse**, as can any abrasive skin cleaning products.

Avoid skin reddeners

- **Give up** the spiciest of spicy foods, including **hot sauces, chilli** and **jalapeño peppers**. After you eat these foods, your face not only feels as though it's flushing – it is. The fine arteries expand in reaction to the spicy food.

- **Alcohol also enlarges blood vessels.** Take note of any flushing after you drink. If your face tends to redden when you've had a gin and tonic or a glass of beer or wine, opt for juice or sparkling water at the next social gathering.
- **Stay out of hot tubs and saunas.** Their heat can trigger flushing of the skin on your face.

Be careful of sunlight

- Stay out of the direct sunlight as much as possible, particularly in the middle of the day when the sun is at its hottest. **Sunlight can lead to flare-ups of rosacea**, as it warms your skin, dilating the blood vessels in your face.
- If you do have to be outside on a sunny day, wear a **wide-brimmed hat** that provides shade for your ears and cheeks as well as your nose. A peaked cap isn't enough.
- Use **sunscreen**, and plenty of it, all year round. For anyone with rosacea, the best sunscreens contain **titanium dioxide** or **zinc oxide**. Many rosacea patients find that other sunscreens irritate their skin but these don't increase the heat in the skin; they act by reflecting (rather than absorbing) the sun's rays. Brands include Clinique City Block Sheer, Ambre Solaire Total Screen Intolerant Skin Lotion, Delph Lotion, E45 Sunblock Lotion, RoC Total Sunblock, SpectraBan Ultra Lotion, Sunsense Ultra, Uvistat Cream and Ultrablock Cream.

Don't get angry

- When tempers flare, so do blood vessels, and that can lead to an outbreak of rosacea. One of the best ways to keep a fiery response in check is simply to **count to ten.** Take it a step further by inhaling deeply as you count. Exhale fully while you count to ten again. After you've done this a few times, you'll find that you can handle the situation much more calmly.

Shaving solutions

- Men with rosacea need to be especially careful not to irritate their faces while shaving. Use an **electric shaver** instead of razor blades. The shaver is less irritating.
- If you use aftershave, **stay away from** products that contain **alcohol**, **witch hazel** or **menthol**.

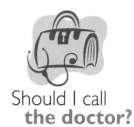

Should I call **the doctor?**

See your doctor if you have the persistent skin reddening that is a sign of rosacea. Early diagnosis and treatment with prescription medicines (metronidazole-containing creams and oral antibiotics, such as oxytetracycline) can help to prevent the condition from getting worse. Your GP may refer you to a dermatologist (skin specialist) for extra help in managing your condition.

Seasonal affective disorder (SAD)

When some people hear about the symptoms of SAD, their first reaction is, 'Oh, *that's* what my problem is!' If the depths of winter have always seemed especially gloomy, it may be reassuring to know that you're not the only one suffering the seasonal blues. If your mood turns so black that you feel as though you can't function normally, don't hesitate to tell your doctor. But if your symptoms are mild, the remedies below can help to light up your life.

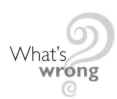

What's wrong

Seasonal affective disorder (SAD) is especially prevalent in the darkest winter months – December, January and February – when sunlight is in short supply. Symptoms include mild to severe depression, low energy levels, prolonged sleep, cravings for sugar and starch and weight gain. SAD has been linked to the hormone melatonin, produced by the pineal gland in the brain. Low levels of light result in increased melatonin production. Another theory suggests that sunlight affects levels of mood-regulating brain chemicals such as serotonin.

Brighten up!

- Do everything you can to **increase the amount of natural light** that comes into your home. Keep curtains and blinds open. If tree branches block light from your windows, cut them back. In a room that's dim, consider having a skylight installed, especially if it's the kitchen or a living area where you spend a lot of time.
- On sunny winter days, **go for walks outdoors**. Even if winter light doesn't have midsummer intensity, a dose of real sun is far more effective than indoor bulbs. In fact, one study showed that an hour's walk in winter sunlight was as effective at reducing SAD symptoms as two-and-a-half hours' walking under bright artificial light.
- Plan your longest holiday during the winter months and get away to a **warm, sunny climate** if at all possible. Just one or two weeks of escape from winter gloom can provide welcome relief from SAD symptoms.

Join a gym or stride out in the cold

- While research shows that **exercise** will help to relieve depression, it's hard to get motivated in winter. If you join a health club and set up a regular time to go, you're more likely to get the exercise you need to boost your mood.
- Better still, get your **exercise outdoors**. Walk, jog or cycle – anything you enjoy that gets you out in the fresh air and daylight. Even on grey days, you'll manage to soak up some hazy sunshine if you're outdoors exercising. If it's really too ghastly, how about setting up an exercise bike in front of a lightbox.

An anti-worry herb

● To help lift your mood, take a 300mg capsule of **St John's wort** three times a day. Once called 'God's grace' or 'the blessed herb', this herbal remedy is a mild antidepressant. Over the last 20 years, studies have shown that one of its components indirectly helps to increase the mood-boosting brain chemical, serotonin. One drawback of St John's wort, however, is that it increases the skin's sensitivity to sunlight. When you're taking it, be sure to put on plenty of sunscreen before you go outdoors. (*Alert* Don't combine St John's wort with light therapy – you risk damaging your eyes and skin. Don't take the herb with prescription antidepressants, either.)

Other mood boosters

● Take a daily multivitamin and mineral supplement that contains **vitamin B$_6$, thiamin** and **folic acid**. Studies have shown that all of these B vitamins can benefit mood.

● Don't overdo biscuits, sweets and other sugary foods. The refined sugar may give you an initial lift, but afterwards your energy plummets and so will your mood. Opt for **high protein meals** that can help to increase alertness – a boiled egg for breakfast, perhaps, and a chicken-breast sandwich for lunch.

● Tell your family and friends about your SAD and enlist their **support**. If they know that you're more susceptible to blue moods on dark days, they can help plan distracting activities.

● To prevent mood swings, **don't drink alcohol**. A drink might help to dispel anxiety for a short while. But because alcohol is a depressant, your mood will plummet when the buzz wears off.

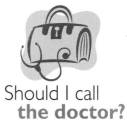

Should I call the doctor?

If you experience severe depression and changes in your eating and sleeping habits, see your doctor. Your condition may be helped by antidepressants, and also light therapy – which involves exposure to a specially-designed light fitting.

Let there be light

Beat the winter blues by boosting your exposure to light. You can buy a full-spectrum light box which emits extremely bright artificial light to compensate for lack of natural sunlight. The light is thought to alter levels of both melatonin and serotonin, so it has a positive influence on sleep patterns and feelings of wellbeing. Set the box up about ½m to 1m (2ft to 3ft) from where you are working, reading or cooking, say, and switch it on. Some people benefit from 30 minutes' exposure. Others need several hours. Try it and see: you cannot overdose on light. Light boxes are widely available online. For more information, visit the SAD Association website at www.sada.org.uk.

Shaving problems

If we didn't shave, we'd have far fewer problems with ingrowing hairs. Fortunately, a little preparation work before you apply a razor to your skin can help. So can changing the kind of shaver you use. But even with these precautions, from time to time you'll need some tricks to wrest a hair from its nest. If you've made a poor job of shaving and your skin is red and irritated, there are several ways to relieve the rash that don't involve expensive face creams or aftershave lotions.

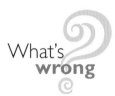

What's wrong

When you shave, you scrape cells from the skin's surface. Without its outermost protective layer, the skin beneath can get dry and irritated. Shaving too quickly or incorrectly increases the risk of razor burn, and certain people, such as Afro-Caribbeans and men with curly beards, are especially prone to bumpy reactions from shaving. For women, shaving armpits and legs can cause similar problems – irritated skin that's bumpy in places. Ingrowing hairs cause sore, red lumps. They can happen when a too-close shave damages the follicle from which the hair sprouts, or when the tip of a very curly hair grows back on itself into the follicle.

A hairy operation
- If a hair has curled back and grown into your skin, you'll probably want to remove it. First, place a **flannel soaked in hot water** over the area. Leave it on for about 5 minutes to soften the hair. Using **tweezers**, gently pull the tip of the hair away from the skin. Then use **nail scissors** to trim off the curl.

All about shavers
- If ingrowing hairs keep recurring, **changing your shaver** might do the trick. If you shave with a blade, switch to an electric shaver. If you use an electric shaver, switch to a blade.
- Many razors now feature double or even triple blades for an ultra-close shave. But when it comes to preventing ingrowing hairs, an old-fashioned **single-bladed razor** is often better. Twin-bladed razors tend to tug the stubble away from the skin before cutting it. Hairs 'snap back' a bit, and can end up embedded below the surface.
- If an ingrowing hair becomes infected and you shave with a razor, **changing blades** should speed up the healing process by helping you to avoid re-exposing your skin to the germs that caused the infection in the first place. If you want to reuse a blade, sterilize it by wiping it with **surgical spirit**.

Prepare your skin
- Before your next shave, briskly rub the area with a dry **loofah, exfoliating mitt, sponge** or **flannel**. This brushes away dead skin cells that might block hair follicles – a process called exfoliation – and lifts hairs away from their follicles.

Watch how you mow

- **Shave with the 'grain'** of your hair growth. When men shave the neck, for instance, they should go down rather than up. When shaving their legs or bikini area, women should follow the same policy. So shave your legs down, not up. This might not give the closest shave, but you won't cut the hair so short that it can burrow under your skin.
- If you shave your armpits, **don't make the mistake of pulling the skin taut** before applying the razor. That makes the hairs protrude slightly and, after you slice off the ends, they pull back under the skin's surface. For the same reason, men should not pull on facial skin when shaving.

Get rid of lumps and bumps

- **Benzoyl peroxide**, an ingredient in many acne creams and face washes, can help to minimize hair bumps.
- Lotions that contain **alpha-hydroxy acids (AHAs)** exfoliate your skin and help to cut down on the number of hairs that get trapped under your skin. Apply an AHA lotion morning and night to any skin that you shave regularly. One of these applications should be straight after you've shaved. Be careful, though – AHAs can be irritating, especially if the skin is wet. When you start using an AHA lotion, put it on every other night until you see how well you tolerate it.
- To reduce inflammation, apply an over-the-counter cream that contains the topical steroid **hydrocortisone** and follow the label directions. (*Alert* Steroid creams should be avoided if possible on the face; if you have to use one, buy the mildest topical steroid in a low dose – hydrocortisone 1% – and use it only for a short period.)

Ways not to shave

- **Give up** the quest for a close shave. The closer the shave, the greater the risk of ingrowing hairs. The only problem with this tip is that, while you may avoid ingrowing hairs, your partner will possibly end up suffering from beard rash …
- As an alternative to shaving, some women use a **depilatory lotion** or **cream**. Similar products are now available for men. Be sure to follow the instructions carefully. Use the product no more than twice a week to minimize the risk of skin irritation.

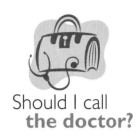

Should I call the doctor?

Few doctors will be interested in ingrowing hairs or razor burn. If, however, you get a severe 'shaving rash' that refuses to clear up, it might be an allergic reaction to your shaving cream or gel, or a bacterial or fungal infection. Your GP should be able to identify and treat the problem. And if the red spot caused by an ingrowing hair gets more painful and swollen instead of getting better, you may have an infection and will need to see your GP for antibiotics.

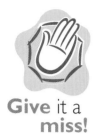

Give it a miss!

Waxing may be the best way to get a neat bikini line or super-smooth legs, but it's not a good idea if you're prone to ingrowing hairs. After waxing, hairs tend to regrow at an angle instead of straight out, so they're even more likely to grow inwards.

Soothe razor rash

- **Aloe vera** is one of the best natural ingredients for irritated or burned skin. If you have an aloe plant, snap off the tip of a branch, squeeze out some of the clear gel and apply it directly to the skin. Or use a proprietary skin care product containing the plant extract. Best is 100 per cent pure aloe vera gel.
- **Avocado** is rich in vitamins and oils that can bring relief. You can apply mashed avocado pulp directly to the skin.
- **Cucumbers** have a long history as a cure for skin problems. Apply a slice directly to the irritated area. Or peel a cucumber, whizz it in a blender and apply the purée to the area. Better still, put some avocado in the blender at the same time.
- Rub **calendula** cream onto the affected area. Creams that contain extracts of this flower have a long history of treating damaged skin, including shaving rashes.

Analyse your razor

- To avoid of minimize razor rash, **change your blade** after three or four uses. If a razor's edge is slightly dulled, you have to press harder, causing more irritation. Disposable razors should not be used more than three times – and if you have tough stubble, throw it away after a single shave.
- Better still, **alternate** between wet shaving and using an electric shaver. Use one for about a month, then switch to the other. Dermatologists don't know the reason, but by switching between the two, you reduce the chances of razor rash.

Soften bristles and wet skin

- If you shave with a blade, first ensure that your skin and hairs are **wet**. Soak in the bath or hold a warm flannel on your face for about 10 minutes before shaving. When skin is wet, the hairs stand up straighter, which makes them easier to shear off. (If you use an electric shaver, the exact opposite is true: your bristles and skin should be completely dry.)
- Choose the **right shaving cream**. Pick one designed for sensitive skin – ideally with aloe vera as one of the ingredients. Avoid scented products and products that contain benzoyl peroxide or menthol. These can irritate your skin. And don't shave with soap. Shaving creams and gels are thicker and more moisturizing and provide better skin protection.

When the can is empty

You'd be amazed at what you can – at a pinch – use as a substitute for shaving cream when you discover you've run out. Here are some that have, apparently, been tried, tested and found to be effective. All make some sense. Many are oil-based, providing the moisture and protection you want from a shave. Nevertheless, you'll probably only resort to these if you're desperate …

- cheese spread
- creamy hair conditioner
- toothpaste
- aerosol whipped-cream
- peanut butter (smooth, not crunchy)
- butter
- moisturizing cream
- mayonnaise
- cooking oil spray

- **Avoid aftershaves.** These contain lots of alcohol, which will dry your skin and make the chafing worse. A nice alternative is witch hazel, which contains just a bit of alcohol and leaves your skin feeling softer and soothed. You can also use it to clean the cut if you nick yourself with the blade.

Shingles

At the first sign of shingles see your doctor, who can prescribe an antiviral drug. This needs to be started as soon as possible. At the same time, you need relief from the pain and burning sensation. Try taking paracetamol or ibuprofen along with the remedies in this chapter. However, if the pain becomes more than you can stand, don't be a brave soldier: see your doctor who can prescribe stronger painkiller.

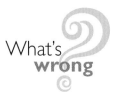

What's wrong

Shingles occurs when the dormant herpes zoster virus, which causes chickenpox, re-awakens in nerve cells and makes its way to the skin. About 20 per cent of people who had chickenpox will later develop shingles, usually when they're over 50. The infection causes a burning, blistering rash – often on the torso, face and neck – which appears as a band or patch of raised spots. Itching, tingling or pain can be mild or severe. Within a week or so, small, fluid-filled blisters form, dry up and crust over. Anything that lowers resistance to infection, such as illness or stress, can awaken the virus. On average, the rash and pain last two to four weeks, but sometimes the pain (called post herpetic neuralgia) lingers for months.

Beat blisters and soothe itching

- If you have an **aloe vera** plant on your windowsill, cut a leaf and smooth the gel over your skin. This milky liquid may help to soothe the blisters. Or use an over-the-counter aloe vera gel (buy 100 per cent aloe if you can).
- A paste of **baking powder** and water will dry up blisters and soothe the itching. Add enough water to dry baking powder to create a paste, then apply it liberally to the affected area.
- Another remedy that can help to dry blisters and soothe inflammation is a paste made from **Epsom salts** and water. Apply directly to the affected area. Repeat as often as you like.
- Brew a tea of **lemon balm**. Studies suggest that this herb from the mint family fights herpes viruses. To make it, simmer 2 teaspoons dried herb in a cup of boiling water. Allow to cool and use a cotton wool ball to dab it directly onto the affected areas. Some herbalists recommend bolstering the brew with **rose oil** or a mint such as **peppermint** or **spearmint**.
- Look in the kitchen cupboard for the ingredients for another shingles solution: **vinegar** and **honey**. Mix them together to form a paste and dab it onto your sores.

Kill the pain

- Dip a flannel or towel into **cold water**, squeeze it out and lay it over the affected area. Alternatively, you can use **cold milk** instead of water. Some people find milk especially soothing.
- If you still have pain after the blisters have healed, fill a bag with **ice** and use it to gently stroke your skin. Experts don't know why the cold treatment is helpful, but it does work.

- Some people find that eating hot, spicy foods helps with the pain. In particular, capsaicin – the hot stuff in chilli peppers – is thought to block the transmission of pain through nerve cells.

Put the brakes on breakouts

- Take 1000mg of supplemental **lysine** three times a day during the acute stage of an outbreak. This amino acid prevents viruses from replicating and may speed up healing.
- Take two 200mg **echinacea** and 125mg **goldenseal** extract three times a day to boost the immune system and help your body fight the infection.
- Try taking **cat's claw**, a herb long used by South American Indians for a variety of ailments and now considered a promising treatment for viral disorders, including shingles. Look for a preparation standardized to contain 3 per cent alkaloids and 15 per cent polyphenols and labelled *Uncaria tomentosa* or *U. guianensis* (lots of other products call themselves 'cat's claw' but are not the real thing). Take 250mg twice a day.

The power of prevention

- *You cannot catch shingles* or pass it on to anyone else. But someone with shingles could give a person chickenpox if he or she had not previously had the virus. So to protect others, wash your hands often and tell anyone with whom you are in close contact that you have the illness.

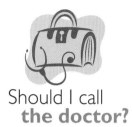

Should I call the doctor?

Yes, and quickly. You should see a doctor within 72 hours if you develop symptoms. Starting antiviral drugs immediately can help to reduce the severity and duration of an attack and may also stave off post-herpetic neuralgia, the painful after-effects of shingles. And see your GP, too, if you're unable to endure the pain of a current outbreak of shingles, or if your shingles have disappeared but the pain hasn't. If you get shingles on your nose, forehead or anywhere else near your eyes, call your doctor immediately for treatment, as there is a risk of eye damage.

Pain after the spots have gone

Many people who develop shingles experience lingering pain in the affected area months or even years after an attack. This is called post herpetic neuralgia (PHN). If you have PHN, be sure to see your doctor, who can prescribe an oral medication such as gabapentin (Neurontin) or amantadine (Symmetrel/Lysovir) or Axsain, a capsaicin cream. You may be offered an injection with local anaesthetic to block pain signals. Another treatment that may be available privately (but is very expensive) is a stick-on patch called Lidoderm, produced by the US company Endo Pharmaceuticals. The patch contains the local anaesthetic lidocaine and is designed to deliver a pain-killing drug to damaged nerves under the skin, rather than via the blood, easing pain levels more quickly.

Sinusitis

You're bunged up, your face hurts and the pressure is getting to you. If a bacterial infection is the cause of your sinusitis, your doctor can give you antibiotics that will help. Otherwise, oral or nasal decongestants can provide temporary relief. (Don't use them for more than three days, though, or the swelling in your sinuses could get worse.) You don't have to dash to the pharmacy every time your sinuses swell. There are plenty of other ways to reopen blocked passages and make yourself feel better.

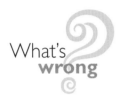

What's wrong

The sinuses – air-filled cavities on either side of the nose – are lined with a super-thin mucous membrane. When the membrane becomes inflamed and infected, it swells, blocking channels that allow mucus to drain into the nose. The resulting pressure can cause a headache, nasal congestion, yellow-green nasal discharge and cheekbone pain. Sinusitis that lasts three weeks or less (acute sinusitis) may result from a bacterial infection, a cold or flu, or swimming in contaminated water. Chronic sinusitis can be caused by a deviated septum, irritation from dust or cigarette smoke or a fungal infection.

Do some steam cleaning

- **Steam** can relieve painful sinus pressure. Take a long, hot shower, inhaling the steam and letting the water spray on your face. Then snort and swallow the hot water until your sinuses are clear.

- Give your congested sinuses a mentholated steam treatment. Pour boiling water into a basin and add a few drops of **eucalyptus oil**. Set the basin on a steady surface (not on your knee or on a bed), then drape a towel over your head and shoulders and lean forwards so that it forms a tent over the basin. Keep your face about 45cm (18in) above the water as you breathe in deeply through your nose. As the vapour rises, it carries tiny droplets of oil into your sinuses and loosens secretions. Do this for as long as is comfortable.

- If you don't have any eucalyptus oil, add a teaspoon of **Vicks VapoRub** or squeeze a **Karvol capsule** into the water instead.

Sniff a salt solution

- Another method of loosening mucus and reducing swelling is irrigating the sinuses with a **saline solution**. You can buy the solution from a pharmacy, or make your own by mixing ⅓ teaspoon of table salt and a pinch of bicarbonate of soda in a cup of warm water. Then fill a medicine syringe (sold for administering medicines to babies) with the solution. Closing one nostril with your thumb, tilt your head back and squirt the solution into one nostril while you sniff. Blow your nose gently, then repeat with the other nostril.

• You can also use a device called a **neti pot**, available online and at some health-food shops. (The neti pot is used in Ayurvedic medicine and looks like a small watering can with a narrow spout.) Pour the lukewarm saline solution into one nostril. The liquid will come out of the other nostril. Once it has drained out, blow your nose gently into a tissue. Repeat with the other nostril using the rest of the saline solution.

Clear those cavities

• Inhale freshly grated **horseradish**. The pungent root contains a fiery substance that helps to thin mucus. Wear rubber gloves to grate horseradish, and keep it well away from your eyes.

• Alternatively, mix equal amounts of grated **horseradish** and **lemon juice** and eat a teaspoon of the mixture an hour before breakfast. Take another teaspoonful an hour before dinner. It will make your eyes water.

• If you're a fan of hot, spicy foods, add some chilli peppers to your meals. The peppers contain **capsaicin,** a compound that breaks up congestion and promotes the drainage of mucus. And if you've no fresh chillis in the fridge, you can sprinkle on cayenne pepper instead; it, too, contains potent capsaicin.

• Many studies show that a substance in **garlic** called allicin has antibacterial properties. Crush a clove of garlic and stir it into 4 teaspoons of water. Then use an eyedropper or medicine syringe to draw up some of this garlic water and put 10 drops in each nostril twice a day. After three days, your infection should be well on its way to healing.

Help your body relax

• A cup of hot **tea** helps to thin nasal mucus. **Camomile tea** is an old folk remedy for sinusitis. If you like it, try it. Two other herbal teas worth sampling are rosehip and ginger. Drink several cups a day, and sniff the rising steam, too.

• **Get plenty of rest**. When you're lying down, however, be sure to keep a pillow under your head to help your sinuses drain. Lying flat on your back without a pillow will make your congestion worse.

• Apply a **warm flannel** over your eyes and cheekbones. Leave it in place until the cloth cools. Then warm it up again and repeat as often as you like until you get some relief.

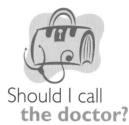

Should I call the doctor?

Usually sinusitis responds well to home treatment. It's a good idea to seek advice if sinus pain persists for more than a couple of weeks, or if you get repeated attacks.

In rare cases the condition can be serious. Call your doctor immediately if you feel pain, or have paralysis in your eyes or if they bulge or turn red. Also tell your doctor if you have nausea and vomiting. In very rare cases, sinus infection can spread to the eyes or brain, causing serious complications.

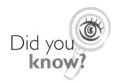

Massage your face

- Giving your sinuses a **mini-massage** will increase blood circulation to the area and help to clear the pain. Using your index fingers, press hard on the outer edge of your nostrils at the end of your nose. Then massage upwards and outwards on the bridge of the nose mid-way between the eyebrows.
- Another pressure-relieving move is to **apply your thumbs** to both sides of your nose, about halfway up, and press firmly on the cartilage. Hold for 30 seconds, then release. You can repeat this as often as you like.
- Other useful pressure points are the slight indentations on the **underside of each eyebrow** about 2cm out from the nose, and the underside of the **cheekbones** in the middle of each cheek (this last may hurt if you have sinusitis). In each case apply pressure for about ten seconds, release and repeat three times.
- Inhaling some **rosemary oil** as you do these mini massages may make them more effective. Fill a bowl with hot water and add a few drops of the essential oil so you can sniff the steam as you apply pressure to your aching face.

Bring on the herbal heavies

- **Echinacea** and **astragalus** are two herbs that can boost immunity and sometimes banish bacteria and viruses. Take 200mg echinacea four times a day and 200mg astragalus twice a day between meals. If you have the kind of sinusitis that comes on suddenly after a cold or flu, take the full dosage of

When flying causes sinus problems

Some fliers have problems with sinus pain. The air in the middle ear expands as the cabin pressure is reduced when you go up; then when you come down again it comes under increasing pressure and needs to escape rapidly – and it can't if the Eustachian tube (connecting the ear with the nose) is blocked. Some people have problems on ascent, but usually it's coming in to land that hurts. There are lots of ways to lessen the problem. Any activity that opens the Eustachian tube, such as chewing, swallowing or yawning, can help. Try sucking a boiled sweet or chewing gum. Or do what pilots do: pinch your nose, shut your mouth and try to blow out against the blockage, which forces air up the Eustachian tube. When it works you hear a 'pop' and the pressure and pain are instantly relieved. It's called the Valsalva manoeuvre. If none of these helps, use a decongestant nasal spray or ask your doctor about a prescription inhaler.

both these herbs for a few weeks or until the sinusitis gets better. For chronic sinusitis – the kind that drags on and on – alternate taking echinacea one week and astragalus the next.

- Try taking 125mg of **goldenseal** four times a day for up to five days. This herb is thought to fight infections and is sometimes combined with echinacea. Goldenseal tea can be either drunk or used as a nasal wash. To make it, boil 1g goldenseal in a cup of water.

The power of prevention

- Run a **humidifier** in your bedroom at night to keep your nasal and sinus passages from drying out. Clean the humidifier once a week so that mildew and fungi can't proliferate.
- **Cut down on** your consumption of **alcoholic beverages**. Alcohol causes swelling of nasal and sinus membranes.
- **Avoid swimming in a chlorinated pool**, and never dive. Chlorine irritates the lining of the nose and sinuses. Diving forces water from nasal passages up into the sinuses.
- **Stay away from smoke-filled rooms**. Cigarette smoke dries out nasal passages, and bacteria get trapped in the sinuses.
- If you have a cold and are worried about your sinuses becoming infected, then temporarily **cut out dairy produce**, which promotes mucus formation.

Snoring

If you're the snorer in your household, you're probably getting a lot more sleep than anyone lying next to you. For the sake of household harmony, show your partner the tips in the 'Self-defence' box (page 344). Then try the following preventative measures. Changing your sleeping position may be all it takes, but for many people a bigger project – namely losing weight – is often the real key to tranquil nights.

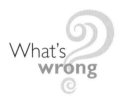

What's wrong

When you snore, structures in the mouth and throat – the tongue, upper throat, soft palate, and uvula – vibrate against the tonsils and adenoids. There are many possible causes. Overweight people are more likely to snore, and experts think it's because the extra fatty tissue compresses the air passages. Drinking alcohol before bedtime is another factor: it causes throat muscles to relax and tissues to sag. And whenever you have nasal congestion from a cold or allergies, you're more likely to snore, because inflamed tissues and extra mucus interfere with airflow.

Put yourself in a good position

● Buy yourself a few extra pillows and **prop yourself up** in bed, rather than lying flat on your back. You'll prevent the tissues in your throat from falling into your air passages.

● **Raise the head of your bed.** An easy way to do it is to place several flat boards under the legs at the top end of the bed. A couple of old phone books under each leg should also raise the bed enough to do the trick.

● **Sleep on your side.** Of course, there's no guarantee you'll stay in that position, but at least start on your side with your arms wrapped around a pillow. There's a good reason you don't want to sleep on your back: in that position, your tongue and soft palate rest against the back of your throat, blocking the airway.

● If hugging a pillow doesn't help, you can tackle the problem with using a **tennis ball.** Sew a little pouch onto the back of your pyjama top and tuck a tennis ball inside. At night, if you start to roll onto your back while you're asleep, you'll get a nudge from the ball, prompting you to get back on your side.

Unblock your nose

● If nasal congestion is causing your snoring, try taking a **decongestant** or **antihistamine** before you go to bed. But use these only as a temporary measure if you suspect that a cold or allergy is to blame. Prolonged use of either can be harmful.

● Tape your nose open with **nasal strips**, available at most pharmacies. They may look odd, but who's looking? Following the directions on the package, tape one of the strips to the outside of your nose before you fall asleep. They work by lifting and opening your nostrils to increase airflow.

• Gargle with a **peppermint mouthwash** to shrink the lining of your nose and throat. This is especially effective if your snoring is a temporary condition caused by a head cold or an allergy. To mix up the herbal gargle, add 1 drop of peppermint oil to a glass of cold water. (But *only* gargle – do not swallow.)

Chin up

• It might sound extreme, but some people have used a **neck brace** – the kind people with whiplash injuries wear – to stop their snoring. It works by keeping your chin extended so that your throat doesn't kink and your airway stays open. You don't have to use a stiff plastic brace, however. A soft foam one, available at pharmacies or medical supply stores is less restraining and will work just as well (it may have to be specially ordered).

Deal with allergies

• To relieve nasal stuffiness, alleviate bedroom allergens (dust, pet dander, mould) by **vacuuming floors and curtains**. Change sheets and pillowcases often. (See *Allergies*, page 34.)

• If your snoring is a seasonal problem – and you know you're allergic to pollen – try drinking **stinging nettle** tea. Herbalists recommend it for soothing inflammation caused by pollen allergies. To make the tea, pour a cup of boiling water over 1 tablespoon of the dried leaf (available in health-food shops). Cover the tea and let it steep for 5 minutes. Strain and drink. Drink up to 3 cups a day, 1 cup just before bedtime.

Watch what you eat, drink and inhale

• **Don't eat a heavy meal or drink alcoholic beverages** within 3 hours of going to bed. Both can cause your throat muscles to relax more than normal.

• **Losing weight** can reduce your snoring by easing any constriction of the upper airway.

• **Give up smoking.** Tobacco smoke irritates mucous membranes, so your throat swells, narrowing the airway. Smokers also have more problems with nasal congestion.

• If you regularly take any kind of **medication**, talk to your doctor about alternatives. Some drugs can make snoring worse, including sleeping pills and sedatives.

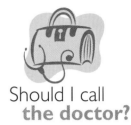

Should I call the doctor?

Loud, excessive snoring can signal sleep apnoea, a potentially dangerous condition that requires treatment. Contact your doctor if you're a loud snorer who stops breathing for short periods when you're asleep. You should also notify the doctor if you sometimes wake up gasping for breath, if you wake up with headaches, or if you're sleepy during the day. Sleep apnoea can reduce levels of oxygen in the blood, eventually leading to elevated blood pressure and an enlarged heart. In addition to lifestyle modifications (losing weight or changing your sleeping position), some doctors sometimes recommend a continuous positive airway pressure (CPAP) device to use at night. Surgery is also possible.

A short course in snoring self-defence

If you live with someone who snores, the nightly noise is probably putting a strain on your relationship. But remember, other partners have dealt with this and survived. So before you give up and escape to a single bed elsewhere, consider some practical methods to deal with the problem.

- Buy yourself a pair of earplugs. They are inexpensive and quite comfortable, once you get accustomed to them.

- A white-noise machine can make nights with a snorer more bearable. These electronic devices produce a consistent sound that muffles other noises.
- Go to bed before your snoring partner. Then, at least you could have a head start and catch some sleep before you're disturbed. Some well-practised partners manage to slumber through the full-scale thunder of a juggernaut snorer.

- Dry air can contribute to snoring. There are lots of ways to do battle with dry air. A **humidifier** or **steam vapourizer** in the bedroom can keep your air passages moist; just be sure to clean it regularly, following the manufacturer's instructions. Another tactic is to **breathe steam**. Just before bedtime, fill a bowl with hot water, drape a towel over your head, bend over the bowl so your nose is roughly 30cm (12in) from the water and breathe deeply through your nose for a few minutes.

Sore throat

An over-the-counter pain reliever like ibuprofen or paracetamol will provide temporary relief from a sore throat. Whether yours is the result of too much screaming on the touchline, an early symptom of a cold or the result of working in a dry, centrally heated office, the quickest way to soothe it is with gargles, teas or a coating of honey. Here are some effective combinations.

Get gargling

- For fast and effective relief, there's nothing to beat an old-fashioned **saltwater gargle**. Salt acts as a mild antiseptic and also draws water out of mucous membranes in the throat, which helps to clear phlegm. Dissolve ½ teaspoon of salt in a glass of warm water (use the warmest you can easily tolerate), gargle and spit out. Repeat every hour if it helps.
- For a spicier gargle, add 10-20 drops of **Tabasco sauce** to a glass of water. Tabasco is made from peppers so it works like capsaicin and it also has anti-viral properties. Don't swallow the gargle as it may irritate the stomach.
- Alternatively, gargle with a **bicarbonate of soda** solution, using ½ teaspoon of bicarb in a glass of warm water. It will soothe inflammation.

The healing power of honey

- **Honey** has long been used as a sore-throat remedy. It has antibacterial properties, which can help to speed up healing. It also acts as a hypertonic osmotic, which means that it draws water out of inflamed tissue. This reduces the swelling and discomfort. Add 2 or 3 teaspoons to a cup of hot water or herbal tea.
- **Hot lemon with honey** can also relieve pain. Combine the juice of half a lemon with hot water and add two teaspoons of honey. You can add a tablespoon or two of brandy, whisky or port to this for an appetizing and mildly numbing hot toddy.
- Blackcurrant makes another popular and soothing hot drink. The easiest way to make a blackcurrant gargle is to dilute a concentrate such as **Ribena with hot water** and sip slowly.

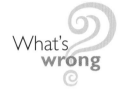

What's **wrong**

A sore throat burns, feels scratchy and may cause pain that makes it hard to talk or swallow. It may also look red and spotted with white or yellow dots. The usual cause is a virus or bacterium. Soreness brought on by viruses (such as those causing colds or flu) usually develops gradually, with little or no fever. But a bacterial infection like strep throat (from streptococcus) often comes on suddenly, accompanied by swollen glands and fever. Throat irritation from smoking, dry heat, postnasal drip (where a runny nose drips down the back of your throat, especially when you are asleep) or an allergic reaction can also cause soreness.

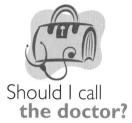

Should I call the doctor?

You can usually take care of a common sore throat, and it should clear up on its own within a day or so. However, you should see a doctor if the pain lasts more than a week, if the soreness is accompanied by a fever of 38°C (101°F) or higher for more than three days, or if you also have an earache. Also see your doctor if you find it difficult to swallow your saliva or open your mouth, if you are hoarse for three weeks or more, or if your phlegm has streaks of blood in it.

Treat it with teas

• **Horehound** reduces the swelling of inflamed throat tissue. It also thins mucus, which makes it easier for you to clear it from your throat. To make the tea, steep 2 teaspoons chopped herb in a cup of boiling water for 10 minutes; strain and drink.

• **Slippery elm** contains mucilage that coats the throat and eases the soreness. Steep a teaspoon of the inner bark in 2 cups boiling water, strain and drink.

• Like slippery elm bark, **marshmallow root** (*Althea officinalis*) contains throat-coating mucilage. To make the tea, steep 2 teaspoons of the dried herb in a cup of boiling water for 10 minutes; strain and drink. Drink 3 to 5 cups a day.

Supplementary helpers

• Take 1000mg **vitamin C** three times a day. Whether your sore throat is caused by a cold, flu or strep bacteria, this vitamin will help to boost your immune system and fight off infection. Reduce the dose if you develop diarrhoea.

• Take 200mg of **echinacea** in capsule form four times a day. This herb's antibacterial and antiviral properties will speed up healing. Make sure the echinacea you buy is standardized to 3.5 per cent echinacosides.

• As another aid to fight off infection, take 600mg of **garlic** in capsule form, four times a day. Dried garlic has potent antibacterial and antiseptic properties. Choose enteric-coated capsules – they are gentler on the digestion – and take the capsules with food.

• Take 1 **zinc** lozenge every three to four hours until your sore throat is gone – but *never* for longer than five days. In one study, people who sucked on a lozenge containing about 13mg

Could it be acid reflux?

One of the more unusual causes of a sore throat is acid reflux. If strong stomach acids come back up into your throat while you're asleep, you'll wake up with what feels just like a sore throat. To prevent this from happening, try raising the bedhead on wooden blocks or a couple of old phone books. With the bed tilted a few inches above the horizontal, reflux will flow downhill during the night – away from your throat and towards your stomach.

of zinc every two hours got rid of viral sore throats three to four days sooner than those who didn't. But too much zinc can actually damage your immune system, which is why you shouldn't take the lozenges over a long period of time. (The long-term safe upper limit for zinc supplements is 25mg a day.)

The power of prevention

● During the colds and flu season, **wash your hands often** and make an effort to keep them away from your eyes, nose, and mouth. You'll be less likely to catch a cold or flu.

● Run a **cool-mist vapouriser** or humidifier in your bedroom. Adding moisture to the air will help keep the air from drying out and prevent the lining of your throat from becoming too dry.

● If you don't have a humidifier, place a **bowl of water** on your radiator or heating vent each night. It may not look very elegant but it will work as well as any shop-bought item.

● **If you smoke, quit.** Cigarette smoke is extremely irritating to the lining of the throat.

● **Breathe through your nose** rather than your mouth. It's a natural way to humidify the air you breathe.

● If you're plagued with a sore throat that seems to come back time and time again, **buy a new toothbrush.** Bacteria collect on the bristles, and if you injure your gums as you brush, they can enter your system and re-infect you.

● **Bolster your immune system** during the colds and flu season with vitamins, herbs and good nutrition. The obvious supplement candidates are **vitamins C and E,** the minerals **zinc** and **magnesium** and immune-boosting herbs such as **goldenseal** and **astragalus.** Also cook or supplement with **garlic, ginger, shiitake mushrooms** and **reishi mushrooms,** all of which have immune-boosting properties.

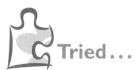

Tried...

According to folk tradition, you can cure a sore throat by taking 3 tablespoons each of honey, lemon juice and red or white vinegar, three times a day for three days.

...& true

While there's nothing special about the 'threes' in this recipe, the ingredients can soothe your throat and help to fight off infection.

TEATIME

Do you drink tea? If not, now may be a good time to start. A growing body of evidence suggests that a daily cup or two may help to prevent and control many common ailments. You may already have heard of the remarkable properties of green tea, which comes from the same shrub, *Camellia sinensis*, as your everyday cuppa (properly known as black tea). Minimally processed, green tea has been shown to boost immunity, lower cholesterol levels, fight tooth decay and even help to ward off cancer. It contains EGCG, one of the most potent antioxidants ever discovered. Ordinary black tea confers health benefits, too (see Tea, page 423).

Herbal teas have powerful healing properties all their own. They are perfect for people who want the medicinal benefits of herbs without taking capsules. Most have little or no side effects (though it's always best to check with your doctor first, especially if you're pregnant, on medication or if troublesome symptoms persist for more than a few days). Did you know, for example, that tea made with the leaves and flowers of the hawthorn plant is considered a tonic for the heart? That raspberry leaf tea helps to curb diarrhoea? Certain teas, such as camomile, are even useful in compresses to speed up wound healing and relieve inflammation.

Many herbal teas are surprisingly tasty, though some are much more drinkable with an added spoonful of honey or squeeze of lemon juice. And tea is easy to make. You simply add boiling water to some fresh or dried herb from your local grocer or health-food shop. The following recipes use dried herbs. If you use fresh herbs instead, you'll need to use three times as much.

Antioxidant tea

During World War II, pilots in the RAF were known to eat lots of bilberry jam. It seems that word had spread that the berries contained compounds that would improve their eyesight. Bilberry is a rich source of anthocyanosides, compounds that may help to protect the retina against macular degeneration, a leading cause of blindness. Because bilberries are astringent, the tea is also useful against diarrhoea. (Take some along with you on your next holiday abroad.) It also appears to strengthen veins (useful if you have varicose veins), and may lower blood sugar in people with diabetes.

Recipe *Steep 1 teaspoon of ground bilberry in hot water for 15 minutes. Drink up to 4 cups a day.*

Tummy-taming brew An aromatic blend of cardamom and three other spices makes a tasty way to stop cramps and painful wind, especially when you've overindulged at a meal. Drink it at the first sign of pain or – even better – about 15 minutes before you eat. This tea is also great for children's tummy aches.
Recipe *In a mug, mix ¼ teaspoon cardamom, ½ teaspoon ground fennel seed, ½ teaspoon ground caraway seed and half a slice of fresh root ginger. Pour in 1 cup boiling water. Steep for 10 minutes. Add a cinnamon stick if you have one to hand.*

Hot-flush help If you want to calm menopausal symptoms without resorting to hormone replacement therapy, consider black cohosh. Drinking tea made from this bitter herb helps to ease hot flushes and other menopause symptoms by lowering levels of luteinizing hormone. Talk to your doctor before taking black cohosh in the long term.
Recipe *Boil ½ teaspoon of powdered root per cup of water for 30 minutes, then strain. Take 2 tablespoons every few hours throughout the day. Honey and lemon help to tame the bitter taste.*

Before-bed beverage For occasional insomnia, there's nothing wrong with taking a sleeping pill. But why risk becoming dependent on pills when this camomile-lavender tea makes a natural substitute? You can drink the tea several times a day or once at bedtime.
Recipe *Combine 2 parts camomile flowers, 2 parts lemon balm, 1 part lavender flowers, 1 part peppermint leaf, 1 part rose petals and a pinch of nutmeg. For 1 cup of tea, put 2 teaspoons of the mixture in a cup and fill with boiling water. Steep for 5 minutes, then strain and drink.*

Cold and cough busters Hot tea is a natural choice when it comes to fighting colds and congestion. Especially good are hyssop tea for coughs, horehound tea for coughs and congestion and marshmallow tea for a sore throat.
Recipe *Use 2 teaspoons of powdered hyssop or dried horehound per cup of hot water. Add honey to offset the bitter taste. To make marshmallow tea, use 2 teaspoons of chopped root per cup of hot water, gently boil for 15 minutes, then strain.*

Queasiness calmer Ginger works so well at combating nausea that some cancer specialists now recommend it as a way to counteract the severe nausea associated with chemotherapy.
Remedy *Steep 2 teaspoons powdered dry ginger or grated fresh root ginger in a cup of hot water for 10 minutes. The tea works better at preventing nausea than at stopping nausea once it starts.*

Beneficial nettle A daily cup of refreshing nettle tea offers several benefits. For men plagued by a weak urine stream and the need to wake up repeatedly during the night to urinate – signs of an enlarged prostate – the tea can help by slowing down the growth of prostate tissue. A powerful diuretic, nettle can also help to control high blood pressure and bloating caused by premenstrual syndrome. Drinking nettle tea regularly may also help against hay fever.
Remedy *Steep 2 teaspoons of dried leaves in a cup of hot water for 10 minutes. Drink 1 or 2 cups a day.*

Splinters

You may remember as a child having a needle-wielding parent dig a splinter out of your skin while you wriggled and winced. The sharp prick of the needle was probably worse than the splinter itself. Alas, a sterilized needle and a pair of tweezers are still standard tools for splinter removal today. But try these tricks to help coax slivers out of the skin with less pain and suffering.

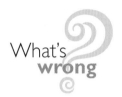

What's wrong

Almost anything can embed itself in your skin – a needle-sharp piece of wood, a sliver of glass or a piece of metal. But tiny slivers can cause a big pain, especially if they lodge in a sensitive spot, such as under a fingernail. And there's also the possibility of infection if they're not removed carefully and completely.

Try the tape trick

● If part of the splinter – however small – is protruding from the skin, try using some tape before you dive in with tweezers and needle. Put **adhesive tape** over the splinter and press down gently so the adhesive catches it. Lift the tape and the splinter might come with it. This is particularly effective if you have a number of tiny splinters that aren't very deeply embedded.

Bring splinters to the surface

● For a splinter on the tip of your finger, fill a narrow-necked bottle with **very hot water** to within 1cm of the top. Place the part of the finger with the splinter over the top of the bottle and press down lightly. As you press down, the heat from the water will 'draw out' the splinter. Be careful to set the bottle on a steady surface to avoid the risk of scalding.

● Try cutting a piece from a **wart plaster** containing **salicylic acid** (sold in pharmacies) and sticking it over the splinter area. Change the plaster every 12 hours or so. Protect surrounding skin with petroleum jelly and stop the treatment if it hurts (on sensitive areas such as fingertips). The splinter may come out, or be close enough to the surface to be grabbed with tweezers.

A woodcutters' trick

Back in the good old days when people split logs to keep the home fires burning, everyone got splinters. But woodcutters had a special way of removing them. They spread warmed pine resin onto the skin and peeled it off once it dried, lifting out the splinter at the same time. There's no reason why this shouldn't work today – you just need a source of resin or a substitute, such as PVA glue or perhaps a peel-off face mask.

Encourage it to swell

• If the splinter is a sliver of wood, it might pop out on its own if you can get it to swell up. For 10 or 15 minutes, soak the area of skin where the splinter is buried in a cup of warm water to which you've added a tablespoon of **bicarbonate of soda**. Do this twice a day. A tiny splinter might swell up so much that it pops out. If it's larger, this trick may make more of it protrude, so you can use tweezers to pull it out.

Tweezer tips

• If it looks as though the splinter isn't going to come out on its own, use **tweezers**. Sterilize them first by wiping the ends with surgical spirit or holding them over a match or cigarette lighter (but let them cool before use). Disinfect the skin with surgical spirit or iodine. Gently pull the bit of splinter poking through the skin, using a magnifying glass if you need to.

• If a splinter is buried under the skin, use a **needle** too. **Apply an ice cube** for 10 seconds first to numb the area so removal doesn't hurt as much. Sterilize the needle using spirit or by holding it over a flame (again, let it cool), then use the tip to gently lift and hold up the bit of skin that covers the end of the splinter. Then use tweezers to pull it out. This is much easier if you have **someone to help you**.

• Check to see whether you've removed the whole splinter. If you have, wash the area with soap and water, blot dry and **cover it with a plaster**. If some of the splinter remains embedded in the skin, you'll need to repeat the process.

Recipes for relief

• In the olden days, a cook who got a splinter used a kitchen remedy – **bacon fat** – to draw it out. This remedy still works. Softening the skin around the splinter, with bacon fat or any other fat or oil, helps the splinter to glide out.

• Put a blob of **mashed banana** or softened solid **soap** on the splinter, cover it with a plaster and leave it on overnight. This can draw a splinter out painlessly. Or try the same trick with a teaspoon of **bicarbonate of soda** with just enough water added to make a paste.

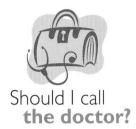

Should I call the doctor?

You can usually treat a splinter at home. But if it's very deeply embedded, or if it's underneath a nail or somewhere in the face, you should probably let a doctor deal with it. Also see your doctor if you notice an infection brewing, usually a sign that some of the splinter is still lodged in the skin. Typical signs of infection include pain, swelling, redness or red streaks. Finally, you may need a tetanus jab – though doctors now consider this unnecessary if you have had at least five tetanus injections in your life. Most children will have had four by the time they start school and get a fifth in their teens. If you were born before 1961 (when routine immunizations began) or you are unsure, have the booster.

Sprains and shin splints

Sprains would be a lot less common if all playing fields were flat. But putting a foot down awkwardly in the shallowest pothole can result in a sprained ankle. Don't ignore it; treat it. Or perhaps you've been in training for one of the big marathons – which means you've been running on a hard surface – and you've got an excruciating pain in your shin. For immediate relief, your best bets are ice and an over-the-counter pain reliever such as ibuprofen or aspirin to ease the tenderness and swelling. Both sprains and shin splints demand rest and recuperation.

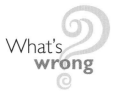

What's wrong

The most common sprain occurs in the ankle. You don't even have to be doing sport to injure yourself in this way. Just missing your footing at the bottom of the stairs or tripping on a kerbstone can result in a painful twist. Shin splints, on the other hand, is very much a sports injury. It often affects runners, ballet dancers and footballers – in fact anyone whose exercise hammers the lower leg. During exercise, muscles in the lower leg swell and press against the gap formed by the tibia and fibula, the bones that extend from the knee to the ankle. This pressure irritates nearby muscles, tendons or ligaments, causing pain.

Follow the RICE rules

● For either injury, the experts swear by the **RICE** regime: – the mnemonic stands for *r*est, *i*ce, *c*ompression and *e*levation. Raise the injured leg or joint, cool it with ice, then wrap it in a stretchy crepe bandage. If you've sprained your wrist keep it raised in a sling.

● Ice will bring down swelling and dull the pain. If you're treating a sprain, the cold will also reduce fluid accumulation in the injured area. Use a flexible **ice pack** or a bag of **frozen vegetables** wrapped in a pillowcase or tea towel and keep it on the sprain area for up to 20 minutes. The layer of fabric between the ice pack and your skin will ensure that you don't get an ice burn.

● For shin splints, you could apply a lump of ice instead of an ice pack. **Freeze water in a polystyrene cup,** then peel away the cup and press the solid ice to the shin. As the ice melts, just peel away more of the cup. If you use this method, however, limit applications to less than 8 minutes at a time. And give the chilled skin a chance to warm up before you apply that ice a second or third time.

● A sprained joint needs to be rested. It may not feel too bad, but working through the pain will only increase the damage. Allow **two days' rest** for a minor sprain. While the joint heals, wrapping it in a stretchy bandage (the 'compression' part of RICE) will restrict movement – so helping ligaments to heal – and lessen swelling by limiting the amount of fluid that accumulates in the area.

S-t-r-e-t-c-h

- For shin splints, sit or lie down with your knees slightly bent. **Flex the foot** of the painful leg up and down, in and out, and in circles. Your leg should remain still. Repeat each movement ten times.
- For a **leg stretch** that relieves pain, begin the exercise in a seated position on the floor. Keep the painful leg outstretched and the knee slightly bent. Loop a towel around the ball of your foot and, with the knee still bent, gently pull the towel towards your body. Hold for 15 to 30 seconds, then relax. Repeat the exercise three times.
- As a follow-up, stand and place your **hands against the wall** at eye level. Bring the uninjured shin forward and keep your painful shin back with the heel on the floor. Turn your back foot slightly inwards, as if you were pigeon-toed. Slowly lean into the wall until you feel a stretch in the back of your calf. Hold for 15 to 30 seconds.
- Repeat the same standing stretch, but this time **cross the back leg** behind the front one so that most of your weight is on the outside edges of your feet. Hold this stretch for 15 to 30 seconds.
- In a standing position, with one hand against a wall or chair for balance, **bend the knee** of your injured leg and grab the top of your foot. Pull the toes of that foot towards the heel to create a stretch in the front part of your shin. Hold for 15 to 30 seconds. Repeat three times.
- Holding a chair or worktop for balance, rise up **onto your toes**, hold for 5 seconds, then come down slowly. Repeat ten times. Then do two more sets of ten.
- Alternate **walking on your heels** for 30 seconds with 30 seconds of normal walking. Repeat four times.

Specially for sprains

- After a sprain, the muscles around the joint seem to seize up – partly due to lack of use and partly due to bruising. While you may be wary of stretching the joint, it is good to spend a few minutes each day **gently flexing** and easing it back towards normal mobility.
- Protect the joint and limit swelling by wearing a stretchy 'tube' **bandage**, sold at pharmacies.

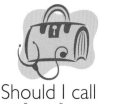

Should I call the doctor?

If a sprain is accompanied by very severe pain or a lot of swelling or bruising, then get to a hospital A&E department for X-rays as you might have fractured a bone. Any sprain that does not feel significantly better after three weeks should be seen by a doctor. You can usually treat shin splints on your own. But if the pain lingers for more than three weeks, see your doctor. You may have a stress fracture or a condition known as compartment syndrome. A stress fracture is a tiny crack in the bone, which causes pain in a small area inside the shinbone, accompanied by swelling and tenderness. It can get much worse without treatment. Compartment syndrome occurs when shin muscles become to0 big for the fibrous 'compartment' they are contained in. This may require surgical treatment.

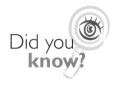

• Three days after the injury, you can begin to **apply warmth** to the joint. If you use heat any sooner, you risk increasing the swelling as heat increases circulation in the area. You can either soak in a hot bath or apply a hot water bottle or heating pad.

• **Try bromelain**, an enzyme derived from the pineapple. Taking 500mg three times a day on an empty stomach may prevent swelling, reduce inflammation and ease tenderness. It also promotes blood circulation and speeds up healing.

The power of prevention

You can reduce your risk of both shin splints and sprains by following these suggestions.

• It's vitally important to **stretch your calf muscles** before you exercise. Whether you're running, doing aerobics or playing a team sport, talk to a fitness coach or trainer to find out what type of leg stretches are most appropriate. Then make sure you do them religiously before and after each session.

• Choose the **softest available surface** for exercise. Run on a grass or clay track rather than a tarmac or concrete pavement. If you do aerobics on a hard floor (such as carpeted concrete), always put down an impact-absorbing foam mat first.

• Buy well-cushioned shoes with excellent arch support. Ask a podiatrist about **arch supports** or **heel inserts**.

• When buying sports shoes, **seek expert advice on what is best for your feet**. If, for instance, you roll your ankles inwards (known as pronation) when you run, it forces your tendons to compensate, increasing the risk of shin splints. A good sports shop will sell shoes that help to correct that tendency.

• Don't expect a sports shoe to be multi-functional – **buy the right shoe** for your sport. Running shoes, for example, don't provide the right support for squash players.

• If you are a regular runner, buy a **new pair** of running shoes before the old ones have a chance to wear out. If you run more than 25 miles a week, you will probably need new shoes every two or three months. Even if you run less than that, it's a good idea to check the wear on the sole of your shoes after four months or so.

• Anyone with **flat feet** must make sure that they have adequate arch support and shock-absorbing cushioning.

Stress

Your body is designed to handle, and even thrive on, brief periods of stress from time to time. But too much isn't good for body or soul. Fortunately, even when you can't change a stressful situation, you have some control over the way you deal with it. So, if you're pulling out your hair, biting your nails to the quick or worrying yourself into a tizzy, try these techniques to restore a sense of sanity.

Anti-anxiety herbs and supplements

- Ever since ancient Greeks began enjoying **camomile tea**, it has been praised for its healing properties. Today, when an estimated one million cups are drunk each day throughout the world, herbalists and naturopathic doctors recommend camomile as a wonderful remedy for stress. Drink 1 cup three times a day.

- You can also add camomile, along with other calming herbs such as **lavender** and **valerian**, to bathwater for a nerve-soothing soak. Wrap the dried herbs in a piece of cheesecloth and hold it under the tap while you fill the bath.

- Get more **vitamin C**. In one study, people under pressure who took 1000mg of vitamin C a day had milder increases in blood pressure and brought their stress hormone levels back to normal more quickly than people who didn't take it.

- Look to **Panax ginseng**, a herb valued for its ability to protect the body from stress. It has been shown to balance the release of stress hormones and support the organs that produce them (the pituitary gland, the hypothalamus, and the adrenal glands). Take 100 to 250mg twice a day during times of stress, starting at the lower end of the dosage range and increasing your intake gradually. Experts recommend that you stop taking it for a week every two or three weeks.

Focus your mind

- Relaxing through **meditation** has been clinically proven to short-circuit stress. Sit in a comfortable position somewhere where you won't be disturbed. Close your eyes. Now choose a word or phrase to focus on – 'it's okay', for example. As you

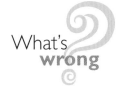

What's **wrong**

Your body is on the alert, telling you something's wrong and you need to fix it. Stress can cause your endocrine system to pump out high levels of certain hormones that weaken immunity, damage the heart and blood vessels, and increase susceptibility to colds and other illnesses. Your mind can be assaulted as well. Stress makes people irritable or easily angered; they may feel extreme anxiety and lose their ability to concentrate. They may also experience insomnia, have a chronically upset stomach, and suffer from headaches and fatigue.

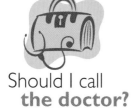

Should I call the doctor?

Seek the help of your doctor if stress-related symptoms are affecting your quality of life. Symptoms to look for include overwhelming anxiety, inability to fall, or stay, asleep, chronic or severe headaches, back or neck pain, binge eating, and the occurrence of physical signs such as eczema, irritable bowel syndrome or migraines. Long-term stress can lead to increased risk of high blood pressure, heart attack, stroke and other diseases.

concentrate on breathing in and out, repeat the phrase each time you exhale. If you get distracted by other thoughts, gently put them out of your mind and return to your word or phrase. Continue for 10 to 20 minutes. Practise at least once a day.

• Research has found that certain types of **music** can reduce heart rate, blood pressure and even levels of stress hormones in the blood. Take a break and listen to music you find soothing.

• Do a **time-travel exercise**. When you're feeling knotted up with some current anxiety, remember something that you felt just as tense about a year ago. How important does it seem today? Now try to project a year into the future and look back on your present dilemma. The chances are, that your 'leap forward' in time will give you a better perspective on what you're going through now.

Practise progressive relaxation

• When you feel especially tense, try a technique that is called **progressive relaxation**. Sit or lie down in a quiet, comfortable place. Close your eyes. Now curl your toes as hard as you can for 10 seconds. Then relax them. After your toes, tense and relax your feet, legs, tummy, fingers, arms, neck and face. In other words, progressively 'work' the tension all the way from the tips of your toes to the top of your head and then, metaphorically, 'let it go'.

The power of prevention

• Go out for a walk or do some other form of **exercise** for at least 20 minutes, three times a week. Exercise boosts feel-good brain chemicals called endorphins, which lift your mood and make you feel less anxious.

• **Limit** your consumption of **alcohol**, **caffeine** and **sugar**; and **if you smoke, quit**. All of these substances can fire up your body's fight-or-flight response, contributing to physical symptoms of stress such as a racing heart, trembling, clammy hands, anxiety and irritability.

• Take up a **calming hobby**. Gardening, knitting, doing jigsaw puzzles, reading or some other favourite pastime can help you to take a breather from the stresses of life.

Styes

Perhaps the biggest challenge when you have a stye on your eyelid is resisting the temptation to rub it. It's a natural reaction, but no amount of rubbing will get rid of that something-in-the-eye feeling, and the bacteria that infected the follicle can spread to others. Instead, use moist heat to bring the stye to a head. And follow these tips to keep your eyelids clean and clear of future irritations.

Apply warmth to the eyelid

- Apply a **warm compress** to the affected eye for 10 to 15 minutes four times a day for two or three days. For a compress, use a soft flannel, a piece of clean cotton cloth, a gauze pad or even a tea bag. Run warm water over the item, close your eye, and hold the moistened compress against the eyelid. Once you get used to the heat against your eye, you can moisten the compress a few more times with ever-warmer water. The heat will help a stye to come to a head and rupture sooner. Once you've used a compress, it should either be thrown away or (if it's a flannel) washed in very hot water before you use it again. Otherwise, you might re-infect your eye with the bacteria.
- To give a hot compress extra infection-fighting power, soak it in tea made from **calendula** flowers. Put 2 teaspoons of dried flowers in a bowl, add 2 cups boiling water, and steep for 20 minutes. Then strain out the flowers.
- There's another way to bring heat to a painful peeper. Boil an **egg** until it's hardboiled, then take it out of the hot water and wrap it in a clean cloth. Hold the hot egg against the outside of your eyelid. It stays hot longer than the compress.
- Hot **potatoes** work too. Microwave a potato, cut it in half, and put it on a cloth over your eye. It stays hot for a long time, so you can lie back and relax. Test hot potatoes on another area of skin first to avoid a burn.

Beat back bacteria

- To boost your immune system and help fight infection-causing bacteria, take 200mg of **echinacea** three or four times a day and continue until the stye goes away.

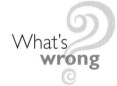

What's **wrong**

Styes are red, inflamed, painful bumps on the upper or lower edge of the eyelid that look much like pimples. They occur when an eyelash follicle gets clogged with dirt or oil, then infected by bacteria. (If a gland on the eyelid is clogged, you have a chalazion instead of a stye.) Your eye may water, or you may feel like there's something in it. Normally, a stye enlarges with pus over the course of several days, then ruptures and heals. The stye may disappear completely once the infection is over, or it may leave a small fluid-filled cyst that requires medical treatment.

When is a stye not a stye?

A chalazion – an enlarged, blocked oil gland in the eyelid – looks like a stye for the first few days, but it becomes larger and lasts longer. You can tell it's not a stye because it's further from the edge of the eyelid, and it's likely to turn into a hard, painless, round bump. Most chalazions go away with plenty of hot compresses that melt the thickened oil and allow it to drain from the pores of the eyelid. But if a chalazion lingers for weeks, you might want to see your doctor for a steroid cream or antibiotics that will help it to heal. In some cases, doctors recommend minor surgery to remove chalazions.

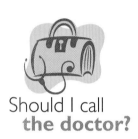

Should I call the doctor?

Although styes are painful and annoying, they're usually harmless. See your doctor if the stye starts to bleed, grows very large very quickly or doesn't begin to heal after two days. You may have a more serious eyelid infection.

• Eat one clove of fresh **garlic** a day. It may not be your favourite flavour, but it has antibacterial properties. It works best eaten raw, so grate it over a salad or mix it into adressing.

The power of prevention

• If you are prone to styes, you may want to bathe your eyelids once a day to keep the follicles clear. An easy way to do this is to gently rinse your closed eyelids with a mixture of 1 part **baby shampoo** to 10 parts **warm water**. Use a clean cotton wool pad for each eye and discard after one sweep across the eyelid.

• Every couple of days, apply a **warm compress** to your eyelids to prevent oil glands from becoming blocked.

• Take a tablespoon of **flax seed oil** every day, or take two flax seed oil capsules. This can help to prevent follicles from blocking up. If you want to get the most benefit from pure flax seed oil, add it to salads or put it on bread, but don't cook it. Heat breaks down its beneficial nutrients.

• To prevent spreading infection to other members of your family – or re-infecting yourself – when you have a stye, **wash your hands frequently** and keep them away from your eyes. For the same reason, **don't share flannels** or towels with other family members. Change your towel and pillowcase often.

• Make sure you get enough **vitamin A** – if styes are a problem for you, it may be a sign of vitamin A deficiency. Eat foods such as egg yolks, butter, offal and yellow, orange, red or dark green vegetables. These contain lots of beta-carotene, which the body converts into vitamin A. You could also take a multivitamin.

Sunburn

If you have the complexion of boiled lobster and you're in significant pain, take an over-the-counter anti-inflammatory drug such as aspirin or ibuprofen to reduce the swelling and ease the soreness. And do what you'd do for any other type of burn – cool it with cold water. You may also want to use a cooling aftersun spray that contains numbing ingredients – your pharmacist can advise you. Keep up your fluid intake as you're probably somewhat dehydrated as well as burnt. And remember to wear sunscreen next time you go out in the sun.

First, cool it down

• The most important treatment for sunburn is to cool it down, so take cooling measures before you try anything else. Soak any sunburned areas in **cold water** or with cold compresses for 15 minutes. The cold reduces swelling and wicks away heat from your skin.

• If you're burned all over, take a soak in a cool bath to which you've added **oatmeal**. You can either buy a colloidal oatmeal product such as Aveeno – which remains in suspension in the bathwater – or finely grind a cup of oats in a food processor and add it to your bath.

• Brew a pot of **green tea** and let it cool. Soak a cloth in the tea and use it as a compress. Green tea contains ingredients that help to protect the skin from ultraviolet radiation damage and reduce inflammation.

• Use the cooling, aromatic qualities of **peppermint** to soothe the scorch of sunburn. Either make peppermint tea or mix 2 drops of peppermint oil with a cup of lukewarm water. Chill the concoction and gently bathe the sunburned area using a soft cloth.

Pantry painkillers

• For extra painful spots of sunburn, rub the area gently with sliced **cucumber** or **potato**. Both contain compounds that cool the burn and help to reduce swelling.

• **Vinegar** is soothing too. It can help to ease sunburn pain, itching and inflammation. Soak a few sheets of kitchen paper

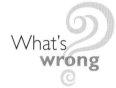

What's **wrong**

The outer layers of your skin have become inflamed by overexposure to the sun's ultraviolet (UV) rays. The vast majority of burns are first degree – though you can have associated heat stroke. Pain usually peaks around four hours after exposure and lasts for two or three days; after five to seven days the burnt skin starts to peel off. Repeated sunburn causes your skin to age more rapidly and your risk of skin cancer increases. Fair-haired people with light skin are at greater risk. Some drugs also increase sensitivity to sunlight. These include some antibiotics, tranquillizers, diuretics, contraceptive pills and oral diabetes medications.

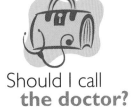

Should I call **the doctor?**

Call a doctor (or an ambulance) at once if a person affected by sunburn is confused or disorientated or too weak to stand. Call a doctor, too, if they have very large blisters (more than 1.5cm across) or signs of infection in affected skin, such as pus, red streaks or increasing tenderness.

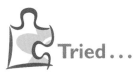

Tried…

Many people find putting milk on sunburn very soothing.

…& true

Milk has a high fat content but it doesn't seal the skin the way klard does. If milk makes your burn feel cooler, go ahead and use it. But **never, never** use any kind of oil, fat or grease on a burn as this seals the heat in and effectively fries the skin.

in white vinegar or cider vinegar and lay them on the sunburnt areas. Leave them on until the paper is dry. Repeat this treatment as often as you like.

- Break open a **vitamin E** capsule and apply it to the skin.
- If the sunburn itches, take a cool bath, adding 2 cups of **vinegar** to the bathwater before you get in.

Apply a coating

- Coat sunburn with a paste made of **barley, turmeric and yoghurt** (using equal amounts of each).
- Wipe sore pink skin with ordinary **cooled tea**.
- Apply a mix of **egg white, honey and witch hazel** (or any of these alone).
- **Toothpaste** is said to ease the pain of a small burn and is reputed to stop blisters forming.
- Apply a light coating of pure **aloe vera** to painful skin, using either a fresh piece cut from the plant or in the gel form you can buy from pharmacies. If you buy the gel, make sure it's 100 per cent pure aloe vera.
- Try applying an ointment containing **St John's wort** as a burn balm: the herb has antiseptic and painkilling properties, and was used for centuries to heal wounds and burns. If you take the herb internally, however, you must stay out of the sun, as the herb makes skin more sensitive to damaging rays.

The power of prevention

- Always cover your skin with a **sunscreen** that contains a sun protection factor (SPF) of 15 or higher, at least 30 minutes before going outdoors. And make your loved ones do the same.
- Between 11am and 3pm, **limit your exposure to the sun**. This is when the sun's rays are at their strongest.
- If you burn easily or have been diagnosed with skin cancer in the past, take no chances. **Cover up in the sun**. That means long trousers, long sleeves, a wide-brimmed hat and sunglasses.
- Finally, a 2001 study showed that eating **tomato paste** could help to prevent sunburn in fair-skinned people. It is believed that the nutrient lycopene in tomatoes helps to protect the skin against harmful ultraviolet rays.

Teething

When a baby cuts a new tooth, both baby and parents suffer. The babycare section in your local pharmacy sells teething gels, and you can buy over-the-counter infants' painkillers such as Calpol or ibuprofen syrup – but be sure to follow label directions. Here, you will find several other ways to relieve a baby's teething troubles. But whatever you try, the main ingredient will be cuddles, love and patience during those difficult days or weeks when the first teeth emerge.

Cool those hot little gums

- Pick up a water-filled **teething ring** at the pharmacy or baby shop, chill it in the fridge and let your baby chew on it. The cold temperature numbs the gums and brings pain relief. Make sure no one puts it in the freezer, though. This could cause frostbitten gums.
- Babies older than six months can chew on a **clean flannel** soaked with cold water.
- Wrap an **ice cube** in a clean muslin cloth and rub this gently on the baby's gums. Make sure that the ice itself doesn't touch the gums and keep it moving so it doesn't make any area too cold.
- If your baby is just cutting a first tooth, you can use a **chilled spoon** to help ease the pain. Chill a spoon in the refrigerator (not the freezer) and apply the rounded part of the spoon to your baby's gums. As with a cold teething ring, the chilled spoon helps to numb the areas that hurt most.
- **Cold food** can help to relieve gum pain. Cut up a bagel, put the pieces in a sandwich bag, and store it in the freezer. When your baby is uncomfortable, offer a piece of cold bagel to gnaw on. The coldness helps to numb the gums, and the edges of the bagel will massage the gums as your baby chews on it. Just be sure to stay nearby and take away the bagel when it becomes too mushy.
- Offer your baby a **frozen banana** (peeled, of course). The banana thaws quickly as your baby chews on it, and the cool fruit soothes the gums. As with the bagel, however, you want to take away the banana when it gets mushy.

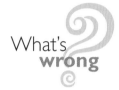

What's **wrong**

Between the ages of four and eight months, as the first teeth begin to emerge, a baby's gums can grow red, tender and swollen. Some babies sail through teething, but others become fussy and irritable and have difficulty sleeping. Most put their fingers in their mouths, and you can expect to deal with a lot of dribble. Teething problems are usually most noticeable with the first two to four teeth. But some children will have pain when their other teeth come in, which can continue up to the age of three.

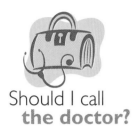

Should I call the doctor?

Contrary to common belief, teething does not cause fever, diarrhoea, vomiting or loss of appetite. If your child develops any of these symptoms, he or she is unwell rather than teething, so see your doctor or health visitor. It's especially important to see the doctor if your child has a temperature that lasts for more than two or three days.

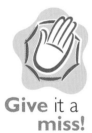

Give it a miss!

One old folk remedy for teething was to rub a spirit such as whisky or gin on the baby's gums. However, giving alcohol to babies and children isn't only unwise, it's illegal. Use a safer remedy instead.

Hold your baby close

● Sometimes giving a baby **extra affection** can ease teething pain. Give the little one some cuddling time, or carry him or her around the home with you to distract from the discomfort.

● **Massage** your baby's gums with a clean finger for a few minutes. The pressure feels good, and your attention will be comforting.

Herbal gum soothers

● Make a clove-oil gum soother by mixing two drops of **clove essential oil** with at least one tablespoon of **vegetable oil**. Before you rub it on your baby's gums, try the mixture on your own gums to make sure it's not too strong. If you feel any irritation, add more vegetable oil. Never use straight clove oil on a baby's gums; it's much too strong.

● Place 1 or 2 drops of **camomile oil** on a wet cotton bud and apply to the gums twice a day. The blue oil has a soothing effect on irritated skin and gums.

Try traditional teething gels

● Pharmacists sell various anaesthetizing teething gels such as **Calgel**, which can help to ease teething pain. Just make sure that you choose an alcohol-free painkilling gel as alcohol can sting the gums and is not recommended for use on babies. Any topical anaesthetic should be used in very small amounts. It not only numbs the gums, it also numbs the 'gag reflex', which means that swallowed food could enter the airways without producing the normal gagging or vomiting response.

Start a teeth-cleaning routine

● As soon as the teeth emerge, start **regular cleaning**. Twice a day, rub the gums very gently with a soft toothbrush or clean baby flannel. This helps to control bacteria in the mouth, which reduces teething irritation as well. Also, it's important to get your baby accustomed to the feeling of having teeth cleaned.

Toothache

Toothaches range from throbbing to excruciating, but a good dentist will ensure that the pain is short-lived. If you can't get an appointment straight away, go to your pharmacy for a pain-numbing gel such as Anbesol, which contains lidocaine, or Rinstead Adult gel, which contains benzocaine. For general pain relief, you can also take ibuprofen, paracetamol or aspirin (but don't give aspirin to anyone under 16 unless on doctor's advice). And try the following approaches.

Kill the pain with spices

- Dab some **clove oil** directly on your bad tooth. Clove oil has remarkable bacteria-slaying properties – and it also has a numbing effect, which is why it's long been used as a remedy for toothache. In the 1800s, when toothpaste was scant and dentists employed tools of torture, every doctor carried a good supply of clove oil. Today it is known that this extract from the clove bud contains eugenol, which acts as a local anaesthetic. The oil may sting at first, but then blissful relief sets in.
- You can get the same numbing effect from **whole cloves**. Put a few in your mouth, let them moisten until they soften, bruise them a bit between your non-hurting molars to release their oil, then hold the softened cloves against your painful tooth for up to half-an-hour.
- If you don't have any cloves, make a paste with **powdered ginger** and **cayenne pepper**. Pour the powdered ingredients in the bottom of a cup, then add a drop or two of water to form the paste. Roll a small ball of cotton into enough paste to saturate it, and place it on your painful tooth. (This mixture can irritate the gums, so you should be careful to keep the cotton only on the tooth.) In addition to using the spices together, you can also try them separately. Either one can help to relieve tooth pain.

Pain relieving mouthwashes

- Rinse your mouth out with a **tincture of myrrh**. The astringent effects can help with inflammation and myrrh offers the added benefit of killing bacteria. Simmer 1 teaspoon of

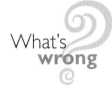

What's wrong

Cavities often cause toothache. You get cavities from bacteria in the mouth that thrive on sugary and starchy foods that cling to teeth and gums. These bacteria produce acids that damage your teeth, and when the damage reaches a nerve, misery sets in. But there can be other causes as well. You could simply have a piece of food caught between two teeth; a filling might have come loose; a tooth has cracked; there's an abscess (a pocket of infection at the gum line); or perhaps you have a sinus problem.

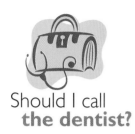

Should I call **the dentist?**

See your dentist as soon as you can, even if the problem seems to improve. The remedies in this chapter can provide temporary relief, but your dentist needs to identify what is causing your toothache. You probably have a problem that requires treatment. If you leave it, it will get worse.

powdered myrrh in 200ml water for 30 minutes. Strain and let cool. Rinse with a teaspoon of the solution in ½ cup of water five to six times a day.

- **Peppermint** tea has a nice flavour and some numbing power. Put a teaspoon of dried peppermint leaves in a cup of boiling water and steep for 20 minutes. After the tea cools, strain it, swish it around in your mouth, then spit it out or swallow. Repeat as often as needed.

- To help to kill bacteria and relieve some discomfort, rinse out with a mouthful of **20 vols hydrogen peroxide solution** diluted in equal parts with water. This can provide temporary relief if the toothache is accompanied by fever and a horrible taste in the mouth (both are signs of infection), but like other toothache remedies, it is only a stopgap measure until you see your dentist and can get the source of infection investigated and treated. Hydrogen peroxide solution should never be swallowed. Spit it out, then rinse out your mouth several times with ordinary water.

- Stir a teaspoon of **salt** into a glass of warm water and rinse for up to 30 seconds before you spit it out. Salt water cleanses the area around the tooth and draws out some of the fluid that causes swelling. Repeat this treatment as often as needed.

Compresses for comfort

- Place a small **ice cube** in a plastic bag, wrap a thin cloth around the bag, and apply it to the aching tooth for about 15 minutes to numb the nerves. Alternatively, put an ice pack on your cheek, over the painful tooth.

- A warm, wet **tea bag** is a traditional remedy for toothache that may be worth a try. Tea contains astringent tannins, which may reduce swelling and give you temporary relief.

- Another country cure advises soaking a small piece of **brown paper** in **vinegar**, sprinkling one side with **black pepper** and holding this to the cheek. The warm sensation on your cheek may distract you from your tooth pain.

A gentle brushing

- Use a **toothpaste made for sensitive teeth**. If you have a problem with shrinking gums, this could relieve a lot of the pain you probably experience from hot or cold foods. When gums shrink, the dentine beneath tooth enamel is exposed, and this material is particularly sensitive.

● Switch to the **softest-bristled brush** you can find to help preserve gum tissue and prevent further shrinkage.

Caulk it

● If you've broken a tooth or have lost a filling, you can relieve some pain by covering the exposed area with softened **chewing gum**. This might work with a loose filling, too, to hold it in place until you can get to the dentist. To avoid any further discomfort, avoid chewing anything with that tooth until you have had it repaired.

● If you can get to a pharmacy, you can also buy **temporary filling** material such as Cavit, which will protect your tooth and the inside of your mouth from scratchy edges until you can get to a dentist.

Press here for relief

● Try an **acupressure** technique to stop tooth pain fast. With your thumb, press the point on the back of your other hand where the base of your thumb and your index finger meet. Apply pressure for about 2 minutes. This will help to trigger the release of endorphins, the brain's feel-good hormones. (*Alert* Do not try this if you're pregnant.)

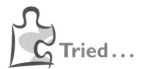

Tried...

According to folklore, if you massage your hand with an ice cube, you can help to relieve a toothache.

...& true

When nerves in your fingers send 'cold' signals to your brain, they may override the pain signals coming from your tooth. Just wrap up an ice cube in a thin cloth and rub it on the fleshy area between your thumb and forefinger.

Urinary tract infections

For women, that burning sensation when you urinate usually means one thing – a urinary tract infection (UTI). One in five women suffer at least one such infection – commonly known as cystitis – at least once a year; men suffer UTIs less frequently. If you're prescribed antibiotics, be sure to finish the course. Meanwhile, drink cranberry juice – it really works – and follow this advice to shorten the infection and ease the pain.

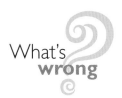

What's wrong

Women get urinary tract infections (UTIs) much more often than men. This is because women have a much shorter urethra and it's closeness to the anus and the vagina means that bugs can easily get to the bladder. Symptoms include burning during urination, a feeling of bladder fullness and frequent need to urinate and sometimes a fever. Men usually get UTIs when a swollen prostate gland obstructs their urine flow. Note that similar symptoms can arise as a result of mechanical or chemical irritation, such as after sex or due to allergies, poor hygiene or certain drugs.

Drink up

- At the first sign of infection, mix a cold, frothy drink with **bicarbonate of soda**. Dissolve ¼ teaspoon of bicarb in 125ml (4fl oz) water. Drink 2 glasses of plain water, then the mixed drink. The bicarb makes the urine less acidic, which reduces the stinging or burning sensation when you pee.
- Throughout the day, drink a **glass of water every hour** or so. When you flood your urinary tract with water, you flush out bacteria. Also, the more water you drink, the more you dilute your urine, so it's less irritating.
- It's not an old wives' tale: scientific research has shown that **cranberry juice** really does help women to get rid of urinary tract infections faster. It also helps to prevent them occurring in the first place. There's nothing in the juice to stop bacteria from multiplying, but it contains a chemical that prevents bacteria from sticking to the lining of the urinary tract. And, if bacteria don't stick, they are easily flushed away by your urine. Drink a 300ml (½ pint) glass every day, both as a way to prevent UTIs and to treat them.
- **Avoid citrus drinks, tomato juice, coffee and alcohol.** All of these drinks may make urination more painful.

Try these infection-busting teas

- Make a cup of **garlic tea**. It sounds pretty disgusting, but if you're suffering cystitis pain, you'll try anything. Garlic contains powerful bacteria-killing compounds that make it ideal for battling the bugs that cause UTIs. Peel a couple of fresh garlic cloves, mash them well, then drop them in warm water. Let them steep for five minutes.

- To help your immune system fight the infection – and boost your fluid intake at the same time – make **echinacea tea** using tea bags or by steeping 2 teaspoons of the raw root in hot water. Drink 3 cups of tea a day.
- Make a tea of **lovage** (a member of the carrot family) by pouring a cup of boiling water over 2 teaspoons of the minced, dried root. Steep for 10 minutes, then strain and drink. This garden herb contains components with anti-inflammatory and bacteria-killing powers. It's also a diuretic, which helps to flush out the system.
- Try drinking **nettle tea**. Nettle is a diuretic. It will make you urinate more, which will help to flush bacteria out of your system. Use a teaspoon of the dried herb to a cup of hot water. Drink 1 cup a day.

Herbal antiseptics

- When the urine is alkaline, as happens in strict **vegetarians**, the herb **uva ursi** is particularly recommended. Others can also use the remedy, but should, temporarily, follow a strict diet that includes plenty of fruit and vegetables and very little meat. Also called bearberry (because bears like its red berries) uva ursi is a short, woody shrub whose leaves have been used for hundreds of years to treat urinary tract infections because of their anti-septic properties. Take one or two 100-200mg capsules three times a day at mealtimes. Stop taking this herb when you feel well again, and do not take it for longer than a week, as long term high doses can cause liver damage. If you're taking uva ursi, don't also take vitamin C; it will make your urine more acidic and counteract the beneficial effects of the herb.
- **Goldenseal** is a natural weapon against the *E. coli* bacteria, the culprit behind so many cases of UTIs. It not only fights bacteria, but also stimulates your immune system and helps to heal inflammation in the urinary tract. Take 500mg to 1000mg of goldenseal-root extract once a day for up to a week.

The power of prevention

- The most important thing you can do is to **urinate regularly** – at least every 4 hours – and ensure the bladder is truly empty each time: when you think you've finished, wait (women should stand up) then try a second time.

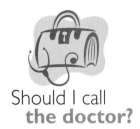

Should I call the doctor?

See a doctor if you have any symptoms of cystitis – running to the toilet every 10 minutes and an excruciating burning sensation when you urinate – that persist after 24 to 36 hours of home treatment. You also need to see the doctor if the burning sensation is accompanied by a vaginal or penile discharge; if the symptoms are accompanied by back pain, shivering or a temperature; or if there is blood in your urine. Also see a doctor if you get recurrent attacks of cystitis even after taking preventative measures, or if you are pregnant.

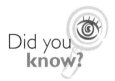

Did you know?

Even though few men suffer from urinary tract infections, any man with an enlarged prostate has a higher-than-average risk. Fortunately, there are a number of remedies that can help manage this problem. (See *Prostate problems*, page 320.)

- **Vitamin C** and **bioflavonoids** protect your bladder from clinging bacteria. Take up to 1000mg of vitamin C and up to 600mg of bioflavonoids a day.
- If you use spermicides or a 'cap' (diaphragm), consider **another type of birth control**. These can contribute to UTIs by altering the bacteria in the vagina, which can then get into the urethra. Diaphragms are also mechanically irritating.
- Use **gentle unperfumed soaps** and avoid scented bath oils and bubble baths.
- **Avoid certain foods** including asparagus, spinach, beetroot, raw carrots, tomatoes, citrus fruits, strawberries, red meat and milk – all of which can aggravate cystitis.
- Be careful to keep the genital and anal area clean. Always **wash before you make love** and **go to the toilet afterwards**. Urine will flush away any bacteria that has been introduced into the urethra during intercourse.
- After using the toilet, always wipe from **front to back** to avoid the transmission of bacteria to the urinary tract.
- When underwear is warm and damp, it's an ideal breeding place for bacteria. Instead of synthetic fibres, wear loose-fitting **cotton underwear** that 'breathes', and avoid nylon tights and tight trousers.
- For the same reason, don't hang about in a wet, tight-fitting bathing suit. Change into **dry clothes** as soon as possible after you've been for a swim.
- A recent Finnish study found that women who frequently eat cheese and yoghurt have fewer UTIs, possibly because these foods contain beneficial bacteria that help keep troublesome bacteria in check. **Eat two or three pots of bio-yoghurt**, which contains 'friendly' bacteria, *Lactobacillus acidophilus*, each day. This is an especially useful tip if you are taking antibiotics, which not only kill harmful germs but bump off the good bacteria, too.

Varicose veins

Bluish, swollen, lumpy blood vessels can ruin the look of your legs – and they can itch and hurt, too. There are several surgical methods for dealing with varicose veins that are generally considered safe and effective. But many less drastic measures can reduce the prominence of varicose veins and help to prevent them from getting worse. For a start, you could begin by eating more dietary fibre and stretching out with your feet up whenever you get the opportunity.

Put your feet up

• Lie back on a sofa or armchair, with your **legs higher than your heart**. Varicosity is the result of blood pooling in your veins, and if you prop up your feet, it lets those 'pools' drain downhill towards your heart. If you're doing the chores at home, take a break from time to time for this couch-potato assignment. Even at work, you may be able to tip back your chair and put your feet up for a while.

• For a more active approach, try this simple **yoga** move: lie on your back near a wall, propping your feet against the wall with your knees straight so that your legs are at a 45° angle. Hold the position for 3 minutes, breathing deeply and evenly.

Give your veins some help

• For three months, take 250mg of **horse chestnut** twice a day. A traditional herbal remedy for varicose veins – and one that is recommended by experts today – horse chestnut improves blood-vessel elasticity and also seems to strengthen the valves inside veins. After your third month on horse chestnut, take it just once day.

• Take 200mg **gotu kola** extract three times a day. This herb enhances the strength of blood vessel walls and the connective tissue that surrounds veins. In an Italian study, people who were taking gotu kola showed measurable improvements in the functioning of their veins. Do not take in pregnancy.

• Add some **lemon peel** to citrus drinks or to your tea. The peel contains a substance called rutin, a type of flavonoid that helps to prevent leakage from small blood vessels.

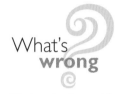

What's **wrong**

'Varicose' refers to blood vessels that are dilated, knotted and tortuous, and when your veins are varicose, that's exactly how they look. Veins are the one-way channels that transport blood towards your heart. Along these are valves that stop blood from going in the wrong direction. When these valves weaken, it's usually in the legs, where gravity causes blood to pool. The veins expand and take on a thick, lumpy appearance. Varicose veins are twice as common in women, especially pregnant women. But people who spend a lot of time on their feet – especially standing still all day – are always at risk.

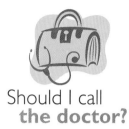

Should I call the doctor?

Varicose veins are more of a cosmetic annoyance than a health problem. However, call your doctor if you develop sores or if the skin over a varicose vein begins to peel off. See your doctor immediately if a vein ruptures and bleeds or if walking becomes painful. Blood clots may be developing if there's swelling, pain and redness in one leg, or if you detect swelling in both legs, so contact your doctor at once if you notice these symptoms.

• Take **vitamin C** with **flavonoids** daily. Vitamin C helps your body to maintain strong connective tissues that support your veins, keeping them flexible and strong. Flavonoids help the body to use vitamin C. Take 500mg vitamin C and 250mg flavonoids twice a day, but cut down the dose of vitamin C if you find you start having diarrhoea.

• Eat foods containing compounds known as **oligomeric proanthocyanidin complexes (OPCs)**. These are types of flavonoid and are found in most fruits and vegetables, but in especially high concentrations in **bilberries**, **cranberries** and **blueberries** – and also in grape seed extract, pine bark, black-currant and green tea. They are also available as supplements (take 150 to 300mg a day). OPCs appear to strengthen blood vessels and make them less prone to leakage. In one study, vari-cose veins improved in 75 per cent of people who took OPCs versus 41 per cent of those who didn't.

Be a water runner

• Run **hot and cold water** over your legs. With alternating temperatures, blood vessels expand and contract, improving blood circulation. Next time you're standing in the shower, direct the water stream onto your legs and run hot water for 1 to 3 minutes. Then switch to cold for the same length of time. Repeat three times, ending with cold.

Get support from stockings

• Women who have small varicose veins generally feel more comfortable wearing **support tights**. These tights are designed to put pressure on your legs, which helps to prevent veins from swelling. Support tights can be found in pharmacies and department stores.

• If your varicose veins are large, you'll need **elastic stockings**. These are tight at the ankle and somewhat looser further up the leg. That graduated pressure helps to push blood upwards towards the heart. These more specialized stockings are sold in medical-supply stores and some pharmacies, or you can order them from specialist catalogues or online. For women, the tights styles are the most effective. Many companies have special tights-style compression stockings that widen out at the waistline and belly for pregnant women.

● Put on your elastic stockings **before you get out of bed**. Lie on your back with your legs in the air and roll them on evenly, ensuring that they don't feel tight at calves or groin.

Keep your blood moving

● **Avoid standing or sitting still** for long periods. If you remain in either position, blood will pool in the legs.

● When you get any kind of break, spend time **walking around**. As long as your legs are moving, you're helping blood to move upwards.

● Whether you are standing or sitting, take a break about once an hour and **flex your feet**. For about 10 minutes, lift and lower the balls of your feet to work your calf muscles. Because those muscles are adjacent to your veins, flexing them helps to squeeze the vessels and move blood upwards towards your heart.

● Whenever you're sitting, make sure you **don't cross your legs**. When you put one leg on top of the other, you're putting undue pressure on your veins and blocking the return route to your heart.

● Be sure to get at least 20 minutes of **aerobic exercise** three times a week to help you stay in shape as well as lose weight. (If you're overweight, you're putting more pressure on the veins in your legs.) Walking is particularly good for varicose veins, since you help pump blood to the heart each time you contract your leg muscles.

● Give your legs a gentle **massage** to stimulate blood circulation by pressing both thumbs into the muscle (but not the veins directly) and stroking upwards towards the heart.

● Treat your legs (or other affected areas) with cloth compresses soaked in a strong tea made from **oak bark**, which is thought to stimulate bloodflow. **Witch hazel** compresses are helpful, too.

Clear up constipation

● Eat a diet rich in **high-fibre foods** such as bran breakfast cereals, apples and pears (with their skins), beans and whole grains. Straining due to constipation obstructs bloodflow from the legs and puts pressure on the veins in your lower legs.

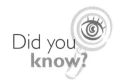

Did you know?

Wearing flat shoes instead of heels can help. In low-heeled or flat shoes, you flex your calf muscles, which helps to pump blood in your legs upwards.

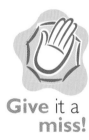

Give it a miss!

If your legs are aching at the end of a long day because of varicose veins, you might be tempted to soak in a hot bath. Resist the temptation. While alternating hot and cold water is a useful treatment, when you sit in hot water for a long time, your veins swell further.

Warts and verrucas

You don't have to touch a toad to get a wart – and you don't have to see a doctor or chiropodist to get rid of one, although there are several medical approaches to doing so. Warts and verrucas can be frozen with liquid nitrogen or burned off using lasers or an electric needle. Pharmacies sell numerous wart and verruca cures, including liquid nitrogen spray, and liquids and plasters containing salicylic acid, which has a peeling effect. (All wart treatments can be harsh, so follow label directions to the letter.) But pharmaceutical approaches are only the tip of the iceberg: we could have filled a book with folk remedies for wart removal. Here are some of the best.

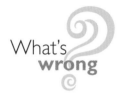

What's wrong

If you have a wart, it means the human papilloma virus (HPV) has invaded a tiny cut in the skin. HPV is really an umbrella term for many strains of a virus that can show up all over the body. Some types of warts are found singly; others, in clusters. Generally, the wart appears as a pale skin growth with a rough surface. Verrucas, or plantar warts, which grow on the soles of the feet, can be so painful that walking is difficult. Genital warts are very contagious and can increase the risk of cervical cancer.

Irritate warts to death

• Cover the wart with a small piece of **duct tape**. According to a recent study, duct tape works even better against warts than cryotherapy (using liquid nitrogen to freeze them off). Cut a piece that will just cover the wart. Stick it on and leave it there for six days. When you take the tape off, soak the area in water for a few minutes, then use an emery board or pumice stone to file down the dead, thick skin. Leave the wart uncovered overnight and apply a new patch in the morning. Repeat the procedure until you're wart-free. It seems that the mild skin irritation the duct tape causes spurs your immune system to fight off the wart virus once and for all.

• Apply freshly crushed **garlic** directly to the wart and cover with a bandage. The caustic effect of the garlic will cause the wart to blister and fall off in as little as a week. Apply new garlic every day, avoiding contact with healthy surrounding skin. (Protecting the area around the wart with **petroleum jelly** can help.) For an added effect, some herbalists suggest eating raw garlic or taking 3 garlic capsules a day to help the immune system fight the virus.

• Apply a compress or cotton ball soaked in **vinegar** and tape it down on the wart with an elastic sticking plaster for at least 1 or 2 hours a day.

• Pick a **dandelion** from the garden, break the stem and squeeze some of its milky liquid onto your wart. Do this every day. The sap is mildly irritating, so it stimulates your immune system to take care of the wart. Don't use dandelions that have been treated with weedkiller.

Acidic approaches

- Grind up a few **vitamin C** tablets, mix with enough water to make a paste, and dab it onto your wart. Cover the paste with a sticky plaster. Because the tablets are highly acidic, they can help wear the wart away and also fight the virus itself.
- If you can peel a little piece of bark from a **birch tree**, dampen it with water and tape it over your wart with the inner side of the bark facing your skin. The bark contains salicylates, which are also found in many over-the-counter wart treatments.

Kitchen cures

- Tape a piece of **banana skin**, inner side down, over a verruca every night before you go to bed. The skin contains a chemical that slowly dissolves the wart.
- Do the same with a piece of **lemon peel**. An oil in the peel seems to discourage warts.
- **Papaya** contains an enzyme that digests dead tissue. Make shallow cuts on the surface of an unripe papaya, collect the sap that runs out and let it coagulate. Mix the thickened sap with water, then apply morning and night.
- A popular folk remedy is to rub a juicy, freshly cut slice of **raw potato** over a wart. (One tradition says this remedy won't work unless you then bury the used potato but others suggest it doesn't need a funeral.) We can't vouch for the efficacy of this cure, but it can't hurt.
- Crush a fresh **basil** leaf and tape it over your wart with waterproof adhesive tape. Basil leaves contain virus-killing compounds. Replace with fresh basil daily for up to a week.

Rub-on remedies

- Several times a day, apply a tincture of **goldenseal**, a herb that contains compounds that fight off bacteria and viruses.
- **Vitamin E oil** is said to work against warts. Once a day, pierce a vitamin E capsule and rub the contents into the wart. **Cod liver oil** capsules are said to have the same effect.

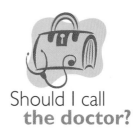

Should I call the doctor?

If you have a skin lesion and you are not sure whether or not it is a wart, get it looked at by a doctor. You want to rule out skin cancer and to make sure you don't start using wart remedies on a corn, callus or mole. If you or your partner has genital warts, use condoms and make sure you have regular cervical smears.

Imagining warts away

The power of suggestion has proved amazingly useful in making warts disappear. Odd folk remedies over the years have included rubbing the wart with dung, saliva, a penny or raw meat – and many actually seem to work. One doctor pretended to bombard a patient's warts with powerful X-rays. Although the man was in fact given no radiation at all, his warts fell off the next day. Spend a few minutes each day just imagining that the warts are shrinking. If your child has a wart, you could try making up an elaborate wart-curing ritual, such as rubbing the wart with a rock, placing the rock in a box, and then burying it. If your child believes that the ritual will get rid of the wart, it just might.

• If you have an **aloe vera** plant on the windowsill, break off a leaf and squeeze a few drops of gel onto the wart. Repeat once a day. Some people report success with this remedy, perhaps because of the malic acid in aloe vera gel.

Give feet the water cure

• Verrucas are sensitive to heat and may disappear in a few weeks if you soak your feet in **hot water** for about 15 minutes a day, according to a remedy published in a medical journal in the 1960s, but long since forgotten. For an added kick, pour 1 part **vinegar** into 4 parts hot water.

The power of prevention

• **Wear sandals or flip flops** around swimming pools and in changing rooms. Wart viruses tend to thrive in warm, moist environments.

• Be sure to **dry your verruca** carefully after a shower or bath and dry a wart on your hand thoroughly after washing, so as to reduce the chance of the virus spreading to someone else. When warts are wet, they seem to be more contagious.

• **Don't scratch** or pick at warts. You can transfer the virus when you scratch other areas of skin.

Water retention

Depending on the cause, doctors sometimes treat water retention with diuretic drugs that cause the body to excrete excess fluid. But these medications can also make the body lose important minerals which, among other jobs, keep your heart beating properly. While diuretics are necessary for some medical conditions, simple self-help remedies – modifying your diet, drinking herbal teas and getting outside for a long walk several times a week – could provide all the help you need.

Fight water with water

- It may sound strange but **drinking more water** could solve the problem of fluid retention. If you're dehydrated, your body stores water to cope with what it sees as a dry spell. Also, when you drink more water, you'll urinate more and pass more salt from your body. Put 2 litres of water in the fridge every morning and try to finish it by the end of the day.

Adjust your salt-potassium balance

- Eat less **salt**. Most of the salt we eat comes from processed foods, such as soups, sauces, packaged snacks and even shop-bought bread. Choose, instead, unprocessed fresh foods such as fruits, vegetables and whole grains that don't come in a box, bag or tin. Make your own bread if you can (a breadmaker is a worthwhile investment). When you do eat processed foods, try to get versions that are labelled 'low salt' or 'low sodium'.

- Get more **potassium**. This mineral does not work directly as a diuretic, but the right balance of potassium and sodium is crucial for regulating your body's fluid levels. Most people get too little potassium and too much sodium. Eat plenty of fruits and vegetables that are high in potassium, such as bananas, avocados, potatoes, oranges and orange juice. Potassium is also present in high levels in meat, poultry, milk and yoghurt.

Flush fluid out the natural way

- Drink 2 to 4 cups of **dandelion tea** a day. Dandelion leaf is a natural diuretic, allowing your kidneys to drain away more water. The herb is also a rich source of potassium. To make the

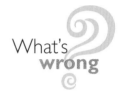

What's **wrong**

Fluid that should travel through blood vessels and lymph channels ebbs into cells and the tiny spaces between them. Sometimes the cause of fluid retention is easy to identify: too much salt in the diet is a common cause – but knee-high socks with tight elastic at the top can cause swollen ankles, too, as can standing for a long time or sitting with your legs down (as opposed to raised on a footstool). Fluid retention before menstruation is the result of fluctuating hormone levels that change the function of blood vessels and lymph glands. More rarely, fluid retention is related to kidney or liver disease. In the elderly, heart failure is a common cause.

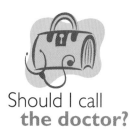

Should I call the doctor?

If fluid retention causes swelling in your abdomen or limbs that persists for more than a week, see your doctor. Also seek medical attention if water retention causes bloating so severe that poking your skin with your finger leaves a dent in it. If fluid retention is the result of congestive heart failure or another serious disease, you should be under a doctor's care.

tea, add 1½ tablespoons dried dandelion (available in health-food shops) to a litre of water and bring to the boil. Simmer for 15 minutes, strain and let cool before drinking.

• Try drinking **nettle** tea made from common stinging nettles. Nettle is a natural diuretic. To make the tea, place a heaped teaspoon of powdered root in a cup of cold water. Bring to a boil, boil for 1 minute, then remove from the heat and let steep for 10 minutes. Drink 1 cup four times a day.

• **Corn silk** is mildly diuretic, possibly because of its high potassium content. Put a teaspoon of dried corn silk (available from some health-food shops and online) in cold water. Boil for 2 to 3 minutes, then strain. Drink 1 cup several times a day.

• While you're piling up your plate with fruit and vegetables for their potassium content, save some room for **celery**, **watermelon**, **asparagus** and **cucumbers**. All contain chemicals that work as natural diuretics.

• The spice **turmeric**, an ingredient in curry powder, has anti-inflammatory qualities, and may inhibit water retention, according to research in China. Use it freely in your cooking.

Beat pre-menstrual bloating

• If you have problems with fluid retention before you menstruate, for the five days before your period take a daily dose of 100mg of **vitamin B_6**. The vitamin is a diuretic, which means it helps you to excrete more urine, thus reducing your body's water content. It also helps to balance a woman's oestrogen and progesterone levels. You can increase your intake of vitamin B_6 throughout the month by eating more spinach, fish, poultry, chickpeas, avocados and bananas. (*Alert* The recommended adult intake for vitamin B_6 is just **1.2mg a day for women**, and the Food Standards Agency warns against taking therapeutic doses of more than 10mg a day except under medical supervision. In fact, doctors say it's best not to take any of the B vitamins in isolation – take with **a B complex** as well.)

Limit swelling

• Take regular **exercise** to relieve swelling in the legs, which is a common result of fluid retention. Because gravity pulls water downwards, you may find that your lower legs and ankles become swollen, especially at the end of the day. If you do the kind of exercise that works the muscles in your calves, more fluid gets pumped up from your legs through your veins. Try to get at least 20 to 30 minutes' walking, jogging, cycling or other leg-pumping exercise most days of the week.

• Another way to help reduce swelling in your legs is to pull on a pair of **support tights** first thing in the morning. The tights fit snugly on your legs and minimize swelling.

• To help squeeze fluid from your lower legs, do a gentle **self-massage**. Start by sitting on the floor with your knees bent. Grasp your shin just below the knee with fingers on your calf and thumbs placed along your shinbone. Move your hands slowly towards your ankle while applying gentle pressure with your thumbs. Next, place both thumbs on the inside of your ankle and stroke back up towards your knee. Finally, wrap your hands around your calf and perform a squeeze-and-release massage down your leg. Repeat on the other leg.

• If you have swollen lower legs and feet, when you get home from work, **lie down** on a sofa and **put your feet up** so your legs are higher than the level of your heart. Excess fluid stored in your legs will work its way back into your bloodstream, travel to the kidneys, and pass from your body in urine. Keep your feet up for an hour or two a day if possible.

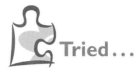

Tried...

Parsley is a traditional remedy for water retention.

...& true

Parsley has been shown to work as a weak diuretic. To make parsley tea, add 2 teaspoons of dried parsley to a cup of boiling water and steep for 10 minutes. You can drink up to 3 cups of parsley tea a day to relieve water retention.

Wind and flatulence

Just bringing up the subjects of wind or flatulence makes people snigger, but when it's you who's belching excessively or passing wind noisily, you probably don't see it as much of a joke. Instead of dashing to another room to avoid embarrassment, take the excess air out of your system by cutting out notorious gas-producing foods (such as baked beans and Brussels sprouts), munching caraway and other wind-relieving seeds after a meal and taking steps to help your body to digest food more completely.

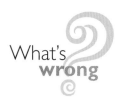

What's wrong

A burp simply means you have a build-up of air in your stomach, and your body wants to get rid of it. This air is swallowed when we eat, drink – or gulp nervously under stress. But what goes in must come out – one end or the other – of the digestive tract. The average adult passes wind at least ten times a day. This is made up of air we've swallowed plus gases – such as smelly sulphur dioxide – produced during digestion. Constipation can cause excessive flatulence, as can lactose intolerance – a condition in which a person cannot properly digest milk and other dairy foods.

Deflate your diet

- Certain foods are notorious for producing gas. Avoid them if they give you trouble. They include **beans, cabbage, bran, cauliflower, broccoli, onions, prunes, raisins** and **Brussels sprouts.** You could also add eggs to the list, as the sulphur in the yolk contributes to smelly gas.
- Before you cook beans or pulses, **soak them overnight.** The next day, pour off the old water, then replenish with fresh water for boiling. Even better than boiling for removing gas is to cook beans in a pressure cooker.
- **Avoid** sugar-free sweets and chewing gums that contain the sweeteners **sorbitol, xylitol** and **mannitol.** Your body has trouble digesting them and, when they reach the colon, the resident bacteria there feed on them and produce gas.
- **Cut down on fructose,** a sugar found in honey, fruit and fruit juices. Like other sweeteners that are difficult to digest, fructose stays in the colon, where bacteria feed on it and create gas. Don't cut whole fruit from your diet but reduce your intake of fruit juice and honey.
- If you're adding more **fibre** to your diet, do it gradually. Fibre is terrific for your health, but adding a lot to your diet all at once can increase wind.

Look at dairy produce

- Could you be lactose intolerant? Try **giving up dairy foods** for a few days and see if it makes a difference.
- If you are **lactose intolerant,** you have a low intestinal level of lactase, the enzyme needed to digest lactase, which is a type

of sugar found in dairy foods. If you can't bear the thought of giving up milk, you can buy lactase enzyme from pharmacies and add it to milk. Many people who are lactose intolerant can eat hard cheeses such as Swiss cheeses and mature Cheddar. They can usually tolerate yoghurt and buttermilk, as well. If you're lactose intolerant, you should also look out for products labelled 'low-lactose' or try soya substitutes.

Herbal digestives

- **Ginger** is available in various forms; experiment to find out which works best for you. Take a 100mg capsule two or three times a day, or 30 drops of tincture before your meals. Or eat a chunk of fresh root ginger (though it's hot, so you may find it a challenge). Or make a tasty **after dinner tea**. Finely grate a teaspoon of fresh root ginger, pour a cup of boiling water over it and steep for 5 minutes. Strain and let it cool a little before you sip. It will stimulate digestion so food won't linger in your intestines, contributing to wind. Ginger tea is also available as teabags from supermarkets.
- **Peppermint** also helps to improve digestion and minimize gas. It is also sold as teabags, or you can add a teaspoon or two of the dried leaves into a cup of freshly boiled water and steep for 5 minutes before straining. You can use this remedy three or four times daily. (*Alert* Do not use peppermint remedies if you have gastroesophageal reflux or heartburn).
- **Fennel seeds**, which have a pleasing liquorice scent, have been used for hundreds of years to reduce wind and improve digestion. (Fennel are the tiny seeds that you sometimes find in bowls at Indian restaurants.) **Caraway, anise** or **celery** seeds have a similar effect. Chewing ½ teaspoon of seeds after a meal will help to prevent after-dinner belching and expel gas from the intestinal tract. All of these seeds are available in the spice section of most supermarkets.
- **Camomile tea** is a folk treatment for stomach aches that may also help to relieve burping. Camomile is sold as teabags in supermarkets and health-food shops.
- **Cardamom tea** helps you to digest your food better so the food you eat is less likely to produce gas. Place 1 teaspoon of cardamom in 250ml (9fl oz) water and simmer for 10 minutes. Drink the hot tea with your meals.

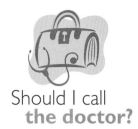

Should I call the doctor?

Chronic belching is usually an annoying habit rather than a sign of disease. But see your doctor if you cannot control your burping and it upsets you, or you develop chest pain, or if belching is accompanied by other unpleasant symptoms, such as bloating, heartburn, unexplained weight loss or changes in bowel habits. Also talk to your doctor if you develop repeated belching for the first time without any obvious change in your diet. If persistent flatulence causes you embarrassment, or is accompanied by diarrhoea and bloating, talk to your doctor. You may have irritable bowel syndrome or lactose intolerance; or you may be experiencing a reaction to a drug. Some antibiotics, anti-ulcer drugs and antidepressants can cause flatulence.

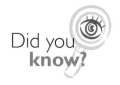

Did you know?

You're more likely to feel bloated when you fly. In an aeroplane, the air pressure around you is lower than usual – about what you'd find if you were 2,500m (8,000ft) up a mountain. Simple physics dictates that when the pressure around you falls gas inside you expands.

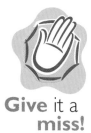

Give it a miss!

Over-the-counter antacids containing dimethicone break large gas bubbles into smaller bubbles. These medicines may decrease belching but they won't reduce the amount of wind in the gut, so you'll still have flatulence. And products that contain activated charcoal, said to absorb gas, haven't been proven conclusively to do so.

Stock up on 'good' bacteria

• Each day, eat two or three pots of **bio-yoghurt** that contains either of the beneficial bacteria **acidophilus** or **biphidus**. Or take 2 probiotics capsules three times a day on an empty stomach. These will replenish the 'friendly' bacteria that inhabit the large intestine and keep gas-producing bacteria in check.

Curl up or get moving

• If you have painful abdominal cramps, **find a private place** where you can **lie down** for a few minutes. Lie on your back and pull your knees up towards your chest. Alternatively, kneel on the bed with your head down and your bottom in the air. Either of these positions allows wind to escape more easily via the anus, relieving discomfort.

• **Walking** is a great way to encourage wind dispersal. In hospitals, it's the first thing that doctors recommend to post-operative patients to help get their bowels working again.

Not the usual suspects

It's not always what you eat that causes a build-up of air in your digestive system.

• **Poorly fitting dentures** may cause you to chew abnormally and swallow air. If you wear dentures, make sure that they are **properly adjusted**.

• **A runny nose** caused by a cold or allergy can make you swallow excessive air. An over-the-counter **nasal decongestant** can sometimes reduce belching as well as relieving the nasal symptoms (but should never be taken long term).

• In some people, **calcium supplements** that contain calcium carbonate release carbon dioxide in the stomach. If you take calcium, choose another form, such as **calcium citrate**.

• Pressure around your **midriff** can cause burping. Are you trying to squeeze into trousers or a skirt a size too small, or is

The remedy that isn't

Do you deliberately swallow air to trigger a burp, hoping that will dispense with the air in your gut? It won't. In fact, it will probably cause you to swallow more air than you expel, starting a vicious cycle of swallowing and burping. Sometimes this turns into an unconscious habit. Watch yourself to see if you do it. If so, stop.

Keep the lid shut

Certain foods can weaken an important valve that's designed to keep food and wind in your stomach. The valve, called the oesophageal sphincter, sits between your oesophagus (the tube that carries food from your mouth) and the top of the stomach. Foods that weaken the valve include peppermint, chocolate, fatty meats, fried foods and caffeine. Avoid these, and you'll be less likely to burp.

your belt too tight? You might want to **loosen up**. Tight bodyshaping underclothes can have the same effect.

The power of prevention

- To reduce the swallowed air that goes into your stomach, **avoid** drinking through **straws**.
- **Don't chew gum.** When you do, you automatically swallow more air.
- **Avoid fizzy drinks.** Have you ever opened a sparkling lemonade after it's been shaken? A similarly explosive situation will build in your stomach if you gulp down bubbly drinks.
- **Sparkling wine and beer** have the same power to remind you of their presence. If you don't want to burp, steer clear.
- If you wolf your food, you're gulping air that will eventually want to re-emerge. **Eat slowly.** If you find it hard, try putting your fork down between mouthfuls. If you empty your plate before everyone else at the table, you probably eat too fast.
- **Chew food thoroughly.** When you gulp it down, you swallow more air. Also, large chunks of food take longer to digest, which means they linger in the digestive tract, where feeding bacteria launch the fermentation process.
- Chew with your **mouth closed** so you're less likely to swallow air. For the same reason – and for the sake of good manners – don't talk with your mouth full. Finish what you're eating before you begin sharing your opinion on the nation's political future.
- Give hot drinks a few moments to **cool**. Sipping a boiling hot coffee or tea will cause you to gulp lots of air.
- Ditch that **after-dinner smoke**. When you inhale air through a cigarette, you also swallow some. (And, best of all, for your health's sake ditch smoking altogether.)

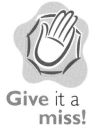

Give it a miss!

An old remedy for heartburn and belching was to down a mixture of bicarbonate of soda and water. Unfortunately, this actually *makes* people belch. The bicarb interacts with hydrochloric acid in your stomach to produce carbon dioxide – the fizz in fizzy drinks.

Wrinkles

As we age, our skin loses moisture and elasticity making it prone to wrinkles. Dermatologists have many tools for tackling those little lines that mark the passage of time. They include prescription creams, chemical peels and injections of the toxin Botox, which paralyses facial muscles temporarily so you can't wrinkle your skin when you frown, for example, or with other facial expressions. But perhaps the best option is to protect your skin just as it is, and to do what you can to keep it healthy.

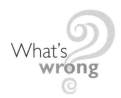

What's wrong

Nothing! But after the age of thirty or so, some of the connective tissue in your skin starts to break down, oil production slows down and wrinkles develop. Those are facts of life. But wrinkles are also caused by factors that you can control. Smoking is a major culprit; it slows down circulation, so your skin doesn't get as much oxygen. Sun exposure is another. The sun's ultraviolet rays do direct damage to connective fibres in the skin. And they promote the generation in the body of rogue oxygen molecules called free radicals, which wreak havoc on cell membranes.

Smooth fine lines with natural acids

• Use a lotion or cream that contains **alpha-hydroxy acids**, or AHAs. AHAs come from milk, fruit and sugar cane, and act by clearing away dead cells on the surface of your skin. These products encourage collagen growth, which fills in wrinkles. They also counteract free radicals – rogue oxygen molecules in your body that can damage your skin. Since AHAs can sometimes cause irritation, try rubbing a little of the product on a small patch of skin first. If the patch doesn't turn red by the next day, the moisturizer is safe for you to use.

• Soak a clean flannel in **milk** and apply it to your skin. Milk contains alpha-hydroxy acids.

• Apply fresh **aloe vera gel**, which contains malic acid. Cut off a leaf at the base and slit it open. Scrape out the gel with a spoon, taking care not to rupture the green rind, and apply.

• **Papayas** are full of enzymes that can etch away the top layer of your skin, lessening the appearance of wrinkles. Wash and peel a papaya, then thoroughly mix 2 tablespoons of the pulp with 1 tablespoon of dry oatmeal to help exfoliate your skin. Apply it to your skin and leave it on for 10 minutes. Scrub off the mixture with a flannel.

Soften and moisturize

• Apply a **moisturizer** every morning after washing to help retain moisture and make your skin feel softer. Look for the moisturizers that also contain sunscreens to protect your skin from ultra-violet rays. Don't forget to apply moisturizer to your **neck and hands** as well as your **face**.

- Try an **avocado** facial. This supplies **moisture plus vitamin E**, an antioxidant. Purée the pulp, smooth it on your face, and leave it on for 20 minutes.

Eat, sleep and move for smoother skin

- Eat fish such as **salmon, sardines, fresh tuna** and **mackerel** several times a week. These are rich in omega-3 fatty acids, which are very nourishing to your skin.
- Another good way to get omega-3s is to eat a teaspoon of **flax seed oil** a day. Mix it with juice or pour it over a salad.
- Pile your plate with plenty of **fruits**, **vegetables**, **nuts** and **seeds**. These provide vitamins A, C, and E – antioxidants that block harmful free radicals before they can cause skin damage.
- As well as getting more **vitamin C** in your diet, you could go a step further by putting it onto your skin. Recent French research found vitamin C skin cream to be as effective as the current 'gold standard' vitamin A-based retinol creams. Both vitamins A and C are ingredients in several skin creams; if you want to give vitamin C a whirl, look for Reti-C corrective day cream and Reti-C night concentrate.
- Get in the habit of **sleeping on your back**. When you sleep on your side or stomach, you bury your face in the pillow, 'ironing in' wrinkles and crevices.
- **Exercise** for 20 to 30 minutes most days of the week. You've probably noticed that exercise can make your skin flush – a sure sign that oxygen and nourishment in your blood are reaching the capillaries in your skin.

The power of prevention

- **Don't smoke.**
- Drink enough **water** to make your urine very pale. This really does help to keep your skin moist.
- On sunny days, apply a broad-spectrum **sunscreen** to your face, neck and other areas of exposed skin before you go outdoors, and head for the shade in midday sun.
- **Never use a tanning salon.** Half-an-hour on a sunbed does more harm than lying on the beach all day without sunscreen.
- Wear **sunglasses** to avoid crow's feet – wrinkles that come from screwing up your eyes. Even **existing crow's feet can fade** after several months of consistently wearing sunglasses.

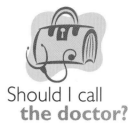

Should I call the doctor?

If you'd like to see more improvements than you're getting from self-help treatments, talk to your doctor about medical options for treating wrinkles.

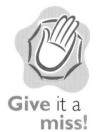

Give it a miss!

Will pulling funny faces treat wrinkles, as some beauty writers claim. Sadly, no. Smiles, grimaces and other facial contortions only contribute to further wrinkling.

PART TWO

20 TOP HOUSEHOLD HEALERS

People are increasingly opting for **gentler methods of healthcare** – and using natural medicines and simple kitchen cures is one way to achieve this. How about using **lemons** to prevent kidney stones, strengthen veins and ward off skin cancer? You may already know that **aloe vera** soothes sunburn, but did you know you can also use it for acne and psoriasis? Or that **garlic juice** can kill the fungi that cause ear infections? Here you'll discover the **amazing healing properties** of 20 common herbs, foods and kitchen staples. Find out how to use **camomile tea** to soothe inflamed gums, **Epsom salts** to treat sprains and bruises and soothe tired feet, **ginger** to short-circuit migraines and ease arthritis pain, **lavender** to take the itching out of insect bites and **mustard** to get rid of athlete's foot. And learn myriad uses for **bicarbonate of soda**, **honey** and **vinegar** and nine other healers.

Aloe vera

Every kitchen should have one or two potted aloe vera plants on the windowsill. The plant has been used medicinally since prehistoric times. Today the clear jelly inside aloe vera leaves is a popular herbal remedy for sunburn, minor wounds and other skin problems. It has even been used to treat haemorrhoids and insect bites because it is rich in anti-inflammatory agents and the gel forms a cool, soothing coating on itchy, irritated tissues.

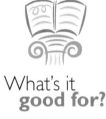

What's it good for?

- acne
- age spots
- athlete's foot
- blisters
- dry hair
- dry skin
- heat rash
- psoriasis
- shaving rash
- shingles
- sunburn
- warts
- wrinkles

Researchers are studying aloe vera for its potential benefits when taken orally, but so far have reached no definite conclusions. However, aloe vera enthusiasts are convinced that the gel – or a juice containing a high concentration of aloe vera – can be taken by mouth as a treatment for arthritis, diabetes and peptic ulcers. It is probably wise to take such claims with a large pinch of salt, but one thing that is known is that aloe vera is one of the best natural skin remedies ever discovered.

Powerful skin healer

Scientists are not exactly sure how aloe vera works, but they have identified many of its active components. The gel contains gummy substances that form soothing natural emollients. It is rich in anti-inflammatory compounds as well as a chemical called bradykininase that acts as a topical painkiller. The magnesium lactate in aloe vera soothes itching and the gel contains substances that promote healing by dilating blood vessels and increasing bloodflow to injured areas.

Aloe vera is helpful for a variety of skin conditions, including:

• **Minor burns** A quick application of aloe vera gel reduces pain, moistens the skin and keeps germs and air out. It soothes the pain of sunburn as well. To relieve the pain of widespread sunburn, add a cup or two of aloe vera juice to a bath of lukewarm water and have a cooling soak.

• **Cuts and grazes** Aloe vera gel dries to form a natural bandage over skin and speed up healing. However, it's not a good choice for serious wounds. Researchers at a Los Angeles hospital found that the gel actually increased the time it took such wounds to heal.

● **Psoriasis** The gel soothes inflammation and softens the itchy skin scales that characterize this chronic skin condition. One four-week study found an 83 per cent rate of skin clearing in those who used aloe vera, compared to only 6 per cent of those using an inactive cream.

● **Acne** Apply aloe vera when you have a painful outbreak. One study found that 90 per cent of skin sores completely healed within five days using aloe vera – nearly twice the success rate of those applying conventional acne medications.

● **Shingles** Painful lesions caused by the herpes virus heal more quickly when aloe vera is applied to the skin. The gel appears to have some antiviral effects. In addition, aloe vera dilates tiny blood vessels known as capillaries, allowing more blood to reach the area so speeding up healing.

The inside story

Doctors are unanimous that aloe vera gel is helpful for minor skin ailments, but what about taking the gel or juice by mouth? Nothing has been proved yet but a number of studies suggest some intriguing possibilities. For example, a scientific study found that volunteers who took aloe vera juice twice a day for up to 42 days had significant reductions in blood sugar, suggesting that it's potentially helpful for treating diabetes.

Japanese researchers report that the active ingredients in aloe vera inhibit stomach secretions and sores, giving credence to aloe vera's reputation as an ulcer remedy. In fact, two of the active chemical compounds in aloe vera appear to inhibit or destroy *Helicobacter pylori*, the bacterium that causes most ulcers.

Finally, a chemical compound called acemannan, found in the outer skin of aloe vera, may have antiviral activity. But much more work must be done before scientists are able to determine its usefulness.

Too strong for comfort

Aloe is a very effective – too effective, really – laxative. Aloe latex, which is extracted from the leaf's rind, is classified as a stimulant laxative. It stimulates intestinal contractions that promote bowel movements. As with other stimulant laxatives,

Aloe vera

however, doctors rarely recommend it. It can cause severe cramping or diarrhoea, along with loss of fluids and vital electrolytes – minerals that play critical roles in the body.

How to use aloe vera

You can buy skincare products containing aloe vera from supermarkets and pharmacies, but it isn't clear whether the 'stabilized' form of aloe vera in these products has the same beneficial effects as the natural gel. If you do buy prepared creams or lotions, make sure that aloe vera appears near the top of the ingredients list. For internal use, buy juices that contain at least 98 per cent aloe vera.

To get the full benefits of aloe vera, there's no substitute for the real thing. The plant is easy to grow – even for the most inexperienced and least greenfingered gardener. It thrives on neglect, needing little water and tolerating shade and poor soil. However, aloe vera should not be exposed to temperatures below 5°C and is therefore best suited to growing on windowsills or in greenhouses.

To soothe sunburn, cuts, piles and minor burns, wash the area thoroughly with soap and water. Then cut a chunk off a large leaf, slice it lengthwise and squeeze out the gel. Apply a generous coating to the injured area and repeat the treatment two or three times a day.

Aloe vera

Arnica

Don't be fooled by arnica's pretty face. The attractive daisy-like flowers of this mountain herb contain toxic compounds that could send blood pressure sky high and cause permanent heart damage. So neither distilled oils from arnica nor infusions made from its dried flowers should ever be taken by mouth. But for external use, arnica is surprisingly effective for muscle soreness, bruises and sprains. So if you've had any sort of minor accident or sports injury, arnica is a good herb to turn to for relief.

Banish bruises, eliminate aches

Arnica has received the stamp of approval from Germany's Commission E – regarded as the world's leading authority on the safety and effectiveness of herbs – as an external treatment for bruises as well as muscle aches and pains. Never take arnica internally (unless as a homeopathic remedy when it is too diluted to cause any harm), or use near the eyes or mouth, or near an open wound: it's poisonous.

You can buy arnica in gel, cream, ointment and tincture forms. Alternatively, you can make an arnica compress. First brew a strong tea using 2 teaspoons of arnica flowers per cup of boiling water. Let the tea cool, then soak a clean cloth in it and apply. This herb is most effective for:

* **Healing bruises** Arnica erases bruises by helping the body to reabsorb blood that has seeped into the tissues. A cream or ointment containing 5 to 25 per cent arnica extract, applied several times a day, reduces pain and swelling – along with that ugly dark purple bloom. If you prefer to use the tincture form, mix 1 part tincture with 3 to 10 parts water, soak a clean cloth in the liquid and apply to the bruise. Two of the chemicals in arnica, helenalin and dihydrohelenalin, have painkilling and anti-inflammatory properties when absorbed through the skin. You can also take 1 or 2 tablets of the homeopathic remedy Arnica 30c as soon as possible after you've bumped yourself to minimize bruising. Follow the dosage instructions on the label.
* **Soothing sprains and strains** Because it curbs inflammation, arnica is perfect for treating mild sprains. It may also improve circulation, increasing the flow of healing nutrients into sore

What's it
good for?

* bruises
* bursitis and tendinitis
* carpal tunnel syndrome
* foot pain

muscles while removing certain by-products of injury – such as lactic acid – that cause pain. It also helps to relieve pain. Because arnica is toxic when taken internally, don't use it on broken skin.

● **Looking after the footsore** Do your feet hurt at the end of the day? Try soaking them in a warm footbath to which you've added a tablespoon of arnica tincture. The improved bloodflow almost instantly results in less pain.

Watch out for rashes

Most people can enjoy the benefits of arnica without any side effects. However, if you are allergic to helenalin, one of the active chemicals in arnica, then regular use of the herb can result in contact dermatitis, a harmless but extremely irritating skin rash. This is most likely to occur in people who use the herb often or apply an overly strong tincture to the skin.

If you are allergic to chrysanthemums or other members of the aster family (*Asteraceae*), you need to avoid arnica, which is a member of the same flower family.

Arnica

Bicarbonate of soda

Whole books have been written about the healing powers and other uses of bicarbonate of soda. It is renowned as a household cleanser. It's also used as a raising agent in baking, because it produces carbon dioxide bubbles that give cakes, muffins and some breads and pastries their 'lift'. And on top of all that, it has wide-ranging healing properties.

Bicarbonate of soda, also known as sodium bicarbonate or simply 'bicarb', is among the fastest-acting antacids. It stops itching from insect bites and stings. It helps to remove dental plaque and neutralizes tooth-damaging acids. It eases the symptoms of bladder infections. Doctors even use it to reduce blood acids during dialysis for kidney disease. So don't take that little plastic drum on your baking shelf for granted.

Nature's neutralizer

All chemicals can be rated according to their pH, a measure of acidity and alkalinity. Water, with a pH value of 7.0 is neutral. Anything above 7.0 is alkaline and anything below 7.0 is acid. With a pH of 8.4, bicarbonate of soda is mildly alkaline and takes the edge off potentially harsh acids.

Look at heartburn, for example. This usually occurs when highly corrosive hydrochloric acid in the stomach finds its way upwards into the oesophagus causing a temporary chemical burn. You can obtain relief by taking a sodium bicarbonate tablet or a teaspoon of bicarbonate of soda with a few drops of lemon juice mixed in a glass of water. (Lemon juice helps to dispel some of the gas bicarbonate of soda can form when it combines with stomach acid.) When you drink this fizzy medicine, it neutralizes hydrochloric acid by converting it to harmless sodium chloride and carbon dioxide. The effects last about 30 minutes, but they occur almost instantly. (*Alert* Only use this bicarbonate of soda remedy three or four times a year as it is high in sodium, which may raise your blood pressure.)

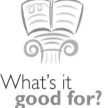

What's it good for?

- athlete's foot
- bites and stings
- body odour
- chickenpox
- dry mouth
- foot odour
- gum problems
- heartburn
- heat rash
- hives
- indigestion
- itching
- mouth ulcers
- sore throat
- splinters
- sunburn
- urinary tract infections

Bicarbonate of soda

There are many other ways to take advantage of bicarbonate of soda. For example, you can:

• **Reduce tooth-damaging acids** Acids produced by bacteria in the mouth erode tooth enamel. You can neutralize them by rinsing out your mouth with a bicarbonate of soda solution several times a day. Or damp your toothbrush with water, dip it in bicarbonate of soda, and brush. Bicarb (now added to lots of toothpastes) is slightly abrasive and polishes teeth without damaging the enamel.

• **Make feet smell sweet** Added to a footbath, bicarb can neutralize bacterial acids that cause foot odour. You can also use it when you wash to combat underarm smells. And a bicarb and water paste can help to clear up athlete's foot.

• **Take the bite out of stings** Don't scratch yourself raw when mosquitoes or other insects have made you their dish of the day. Instead, mix a little water with bicarbonate of soda and apply the paste to the itchy areas. A bicarb paste can also help to ease the itching of chickenpox.

• **Soothe tender bottoms** Infants with nappy rash feel better after a bicarb soak. Add a little powder to baby's bathwater. It decreases itching and helps irritated skin to heal more quickly.

• **Ease bladder infections** Bacteria thrive in the slightly acidic environment inside the bladder. When you have an infection, a cocktail of bicarbonate of soda and water is the perfect after-dinner drink.

• **Cool down sunburn** Added to a warm bath, bicarbonate of soda 'softens' the water and makes a soothing soak.

• **Ease a sore throat** Add ½ teaspoon of bicarb to a glass of water and gargle every 4 hours to reduce pain-causing acids. Swishing the solution around your mouth will ease mouth ulcers too.

Bicarbonate of soda

Camomile

With its agreeable taste and appley scent, camomile makes a comforting tea. A cup of camomile tea at bedtime soothes frayed nerves and promotes sleep. But camomile's benefits don't end there. Scientists have identified more than a dozen active chemical compounds within its daisy-like flowers that not only take the edge off stress but can soothe a stomach upset almost as fast as you can say Pepto Bismol.

A chemical in camomile called apigenin calms the central nervous system and makes it easier to fall asleep at night. If you feel really wound up, drink a cup of camomile tea or relax in a warm bath doctored with several cups of camomile tea, 10 drops of camomile oil or a handful or two of camomile flowers. The essential oil penetrates the skin and takes the edge off anxiety and stress.

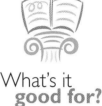

What's it good for?
- belching
- boils
- conjunctivitis
- foot pain
- gum problems
- hives
- indigestion
- inflammatory bowel disease
- menstrual problems
- peptic ulcers
- psoriasis
- rosacea
- stress
- teething

More uses inside and out

Camomile doesn't just help you to calm down. Several of its chemical compounds, especially one called bisabolol, act as antispasmodics: this means that they relax the smooth muscles that line the digestive tract and uterus, easing after-meal stomach ache or soothing menstrual cramps. A cup or two of camomile tea a day may also reduce the stomach-eroding effects of aspirin and related drugs – useful for people with arthritis or other painful conditions who need to take painkillers every day.

Because of its anti-inflammatory and antiseptic powers, camomile is also very useful for a number of other minor health complaints.

Rashes and burns Camomile can benefit your skin as well as your intestinal tract. When camomile is applied externally in the form of camomile cream or a compress made with strong camomile tea, it helps cuts, burns and rashes to heal more quickly. If you have mild sunburn, mix camomile oil (sold in health-food shops) with equal parts almond oil or another neutral carrier oil. Apply it to reddened skin to reduce the inflammation that causes itching.

Camomile

Skin irritation In Germany, where herbs are widely used in mainstream medicine, doctors often recommend a camomile-based cream called Kamillosan for wounds or inflammation caused by eczema, contact allergies and post-radiation treatment skin damage. Small amounts of camomile oil can be applied to treat skin ailments such as boils.

Infections A wash of camomile kills some of the bacteria and fungi that cause eye or skin infections. Camomile tea can be used as a mouthwash to soothe inflamed gums, help fight gum disease and speed up the healing of mouth ulcers.

Buying and using camomile

You can buy camomile tea bags or look for the dried flowers in health-food shops. Some people have successfully grown camomile in the garden by simply sprinkling the contents of a bag of camomile tea on the soil. Note that there are two different camomile plants: Roman camomile (*Chamaemelum nobile*) and German camomile (*Matricaria recutita*), also known as Hungarian camomile. While the two plants may look almost identical, German camomile is more popular and is thought to have greater healing powers.

You can find camomile cream in health-food shops, but it's just as easy, and less expensive, to make your own skin-healing brew. Pour a cup of boiling water over a heaped tablespoon of camomile flowers. Let it steep for 10 minutes, wait until it cools to room temperature, then soak a cloth in the tea and apply it to a cut, rash or burn for about five minutes.

A media uproar followed a report in the US *Journal of Allergy and Clinical Immunology* that camomile tea might cause a potentially fatal allergic reaction in people allergic to ragweed. But when scientists looked at the available data, they were able to identify only a handful of reactions (and none of them fatal) to German camomile, the variety commonly used in the UK. If you are allergic to plants of the *Asteraceae* family – asters and chrysanthemums – then do not use camomile.

Camomile

Cranberries

Cranberries are traditionally associated with Christmas dinner and roast turkey. They are used in many recipes – both in sauces and desserts – and are eaten fresh or dried or squeezed for their juice. In addition to their culinary uses, cranberries are increasingly recommended by doctors and complementary practitioners as a treatment and prevention for people who suffer from frequent bladder infections.

The cranberry, a shrub native to peat bogs and forests in North America, is now widely cultivated in Europe. You can grow it at home from cuttings, but it likes a damp acid soil. The shrub will survive extreme cold, though frosts can kill buds and warm sun is needed to ripen the berries.

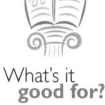

What's it good for?

- incontinence (deodorizes urine)
- urinary tract infections

The small dark red berries have been used medicinally for hundreds of years. As well as being prescribed for urinary infections, cranberries have been used for blood disorders, liver problems, stomach complaints and poor appetite. Cranberries reduce the odour of urine, so the juice is useful for those who suffer from incontinence. Constituents in cranberries also help to prevent tooth decay by stopping bacteria from sticking to the teeth so inhibiting plaque build-up.

The phytochemicals in cranberries include tannins and antioxidant anthocyanins (which aid night vision), and the seed oil contains omega-3 fatty acids. The fruit is also a rich source of vitamin C. Pure cranberry juice is very acidic and so strong that it can erode dental enamel, which is one reason why cranberry drinks are usually diluted – often with sugar.

Combating bladder infection

Cranberries fight urinary tract infections in several ways. In the past it was thought that cranberries acidified urine, raising the level of hippuric acid, a substance that creates an inhospitable environment for *E. coli* and other bacteria that can colonize the urinary tract. But although cranberry is acidic, it does not seem to acidify the urine. Research is now focusing on other constituents of cranberries, particularly fructose and the fruit's antioxidants. These ingredients have been shown to prevent

Cranberries

bacteria not only from colonizing the urinary tract, but also from sticking to the bladder wall where they could otherwise reproduce. The berries' high vitamin C content may also boost the body's immune system for fighting infection.

Research has proved that drinking a lot of cranberry juice can reduce the incidence of urinary tract infections in susceptible people. It also appears to shorten the duration of symptoms but, if you already have an infection, ask your doctor or pharmacist for advice. In this instance, cranberry is best used to bolster prescribed medication rather than as a cure.

Blood benefits

Research has shown that cranberry juice can increase the levels of 'good' (HDL) cholesterol and blood antioxidants. Cranberry juice could thus help to prevent heart disease, but the amounts needed to show a beneficial effect in this study were quite large – 3 glasses of full strength juice a day for three months. Doctors also think that cranberries may help both to reduce the severity of strokes and aid recovery from them.

How much, how often?

Most scientific studies looking at the prevention of urinary tract infections use 800mg cranberry extract a day. This is equivalent to drinking 500ml (18fl oz) undiluted cranberry juice twice a day. The juice sold in supermarkets is really too dilute to be effective. You can make your own using a juicer or buy full-strength juice from a health-food shop. If you find the juice too sour when undiluted, try mixing it in equal parts with pure bilberry juice, which has similar beneficial ingredients. Or mix the day's allocation of cranberry juice with an equal amount of apple juice, which is naturally sweet.

Cranberries, even in large amounts, are usually very safe. But unfortunately, blood clot patients on warfarin must not take cranberry, either in drink, concentrate or capsule form, as cranberry can increase warfarin's anticoagulant effect, causing severe bleeding. Also, check with your doctor if you have prostate problems or severe kidney disease before taking cranberry juice. Drinking more than a litre a day for prolonged periods may also increase your risk of kidney stones because cranberries contain oxalates.

Cranberries

Epsom salts

You wouldn't think that a common mineral could do so much. Magnesium sulphate, better known as Epsom salts, is popular for adding to bath water – whether to reduce stress, soften skin or relieve aches and pains. Outside the remedy arena, gardeners swear by it because it helps roses to thrive, while potters sometimes add Epsom salts to clay to improve its elasticity.

Epsom salts are found anywhere mineral or seawater evaporates. The name comes from a mineral spring in Epsom, Surrey. Not long ago Epsom salts were given as part of the spring round of purgatives to cleanse the body of 'toxins' that supposedly built up over the winter. One reason was probably their laxative effect. Until a few decades ago, when proprietary laxatives began to occupy pharmacy shelves, Epsom salts were a popular shortcut to regular bowel movements. The active ingredient in milk of magnesia, Epsom salts are a saline-type laxative: the magnesium draws fluids from the blood into the intestine, making stools softer, while triggering intestinal contractions that stimulate bowel movements.

Some people still take one or two teaspoons of Epsom salts in a glass of water to ease constipation. The problem with this remedy is that it's often too powerful, causing diarrhoea or abdominal cramps. And it can interfere with the body's absorption of essential nutrients. So it's best not to use Epsom salts as a laxative unless advised to do so by your doctor.

Soaks and softeners

External uses of Epsom salts, on the other hand, are entirely safe – and incredibly useful. Among other things, Epsom salts can be used to:

- **Draw out splinters and stings** Epsom salts draws toxins from insect stings and brings splinters to the skin's surface. Add water to Epsom salts to make a paste and apply it to the affected area; it will usually begin working in about 10 minutes. You can also soak in an Epsom salts bath to soften the skin and help draw out a splinter.

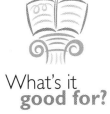

What's it good for?

- acne
- calluses and corns
- dry skin
- foot odour
- haemorrhoids
- muscle cramps
- ringworm
- shingles

Epsom salts

- **Deep-clean pores** Add a teaspoon of Epsom salts to ½ glass of warm water and rub your skin with the solution to dislodge blackheads, cleanse open pores and freshen skin.

- **Ease muscle aches** An Epsom salts solution draws fluid out of the body and helps to shrink swollen tissues. As it draws fluid through the skin, it also draws out lactic acid, the build-up of which can contribute to aching muscles. Add a cup or two of the salts to a hot bath and enjoy a relaxing soak.

- **Sprains and bruises** Epsom salts will reduce the swelling of sprains and bruises. Add 2 cups of Epsom salts to a warm bath, and soak.

- **Help haemorrhoids** Because it shrinks swollen tissues, Epsom salts makes an excellent soak for haemorrhoids. Just add some to your bath or bidet and immerse the tender area.

- **Soften skin** Massage handfuls of Epsom salts onto your skin while bathing. The massaging action will exfoliate the skin – in other words remove dead skin cells – leaving your skin looking and feeling smoother and refreshed.

Fabulous foot soak

This recipe for 'fabulous feet' comes from the Epsom Salts Industry Council.

Mix the following ingredients in a foot bath or large washing-up bowl:

2 cups Epsom salts
1 cup Dead Sea salt
1 tablespoon olive oil
½ teaspoon peppermint oil
2 tablespoons oatmeal
Enough warm-to-hot water to fill the basin

Soak your feet until the water turns cold, then, using a pumice stone, buff all the rough areas of skin. Rinse your feet in cold water and dry thoroughly. Then rub petroleum jelly into your feet and put on a pair of thick socks. Don't try to walk around until you've put the socks on: petroleum jelly makes your feet very slippery. Keep the socks on overnight for best results. Repeat as often as you like.

Epsom salts

Evening primrose oil

The evening primrose, a native of North America, began to find its way round the world during the seventeenth century. The seeds hitched a ride in the ballasts of ships travelling from North America to Europe, where they took root. From Europe, the evening primrose spread to Asia. Traditionally, the plant and its root were used to treat bruises, piles, coughs and stomach aches, but it is in fact the seeds that contain the therapeutic oils.

Evening primrose oil comes from the seeds of this biennial plant. These are reddish in colour and produced during the plant's second year (it bears only leaves during its first year). The light yellow, sweetly scented flowers don't open until dusk, hence the plant's name.

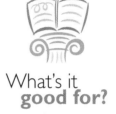

What's it good for?
- arthritis pain
- eczema
- premenstrual syndrome (PMS)

The seed oil contains a special fatty acid known as gamma-linolenic acid (GLA). This substance is the active ingredient in evening primrose oil, making up 7 to 10 per cent of its fatty acids. GLA is converted in the body to a variety of hormone-like compounds – prostaglandins and leukotrienes – that fight inflammation.

GLA can be made in the body from other types of fat such as linoleic acid, which is found in vegetable oils and poly-unsaturated margarines and spreads. However, some people do not have enough of the enzyme to be able to do this. Evening primrose oil can be used to compensate for the missing enzyme and encourage the body to make these anti-inflammatory compounds. Its anti-inflammatory activity makes evening primrose oil useful for several conditions.

Soothe eczema irritation Eczema and itchy skin can develop if the body has trouble converting the fats in foods into GLA. Taking evening primrose oil for three to four months has been found to alleviate itching and reduce the need for topical steroid creams and drugs.

Ease menstrual problems Evening primrose oil can be effective for menstrual disorders such as pre-menstrual syndrome (PMS), the breast tenderness that some women experience before their periods, and menstrual cramps.

Evening primrose oil

- **Reduce rheumatic pain** Some people find that taking evening primrose oil reduces symptoms of rheumatoid arthritis pain. Try taking it in combination with omega-3 fatty acids, found in fish oil or flaxseed oil.
- **Other inflammatory conditions** Conditions that involve inflammation such as rosacea, acne and sprains may also benefit from evening primrose oil.

Hyperactive children and fatty acids

There is a lot of interest in the role of essential fatty acids, including GLA and omega-3 fatty acids, in children with attention deficit hyperactivity disorder (ADHD). It is thought that some of these children may be deficient in these fatty acids. Supplements containing GLA and omega-3 fatty acids are available and are worth a try. Buy one which is made especially for children and follow the dosage instructions on the package label.

When not to take it

Evening primrose oil is safe for most people. It can sometimes cause mild side effects, including headache and mild stomach upsets or bloating. There has been some concern that evening primrose oil might increase the chance of problems during pregnancy, so do not use it if you are pregnant or breastfeeding. Evening primrose oil may slow down blood clotting, so avoid taking it with other medicines that also delay blood clotting, because it might increase the chance of bruising and bleeding. It can also increase the risk of seizures, so do not use it if you have epilepsy or are taking any medication that increases the risk of seizures (such as the phenothiazine group of anti-psychotic drugs).

Garlic

Garlic's therapeutic benefits have been so exaggerated by enthusiasts that it can be hard to distinguish fact from fantasy. The history of this pungent herb undoubtedly suggests its broad potential, and medical historians have identified more than 100 non-culinary uses for garlic. The Egyptians, for example, gave it to the pyramid builders to boost their strength and prevent dysentery. Europeans ate it to protect themselves during the plague. Battlefield doctors in both World Wars used garlic to disinfect wounds. It has been used to treat athlete's foot, tuberculosis and high blood pressure, not to mention colds and coughs. It is even rumoured to have aphrodisiac properties.

In the last few decades research has caught up with folklore and garlic is the subject of more than 1,000 pharmacological studies. Most of these focus on its roles in cardiovascular disease and cancer, along with its antibacterial and antioxidant properties. It seems fairly clear that garlic is a medicinal herb worth considering – and one that may, in some cases, even rival the effects of prescription drugs.

Help for the heart

Garlic contains more than 100 chemically active compounds. One of the most important is alliin, a sulphur compound that is transformed into allicin when the bulbs are crushed or chewed. Scientists think that allicin is responsible for garlic's antibiotic properties as well as many of its heart benefits. What is known is that in countries where people eat lots of garlic, there seem to be unusually low rates of heart disease.

Consider garlic's effects on platelets, cell-like structures in blood that tend to stick together and form clots in the coronary arteries. One study discovered that the rate of platelet aggregation, or clumping, in men given the equivalent of 6 cloves of fresh garlic dropped anywhere from 10 to 58 per cent. Certain chemicals in garlic may be as effective as aspirin at inhibiting the formation of blood clots.

Garlic appears to function somewhat like prescription drugs that inhibit the liver's production of cholesterol, the fatty stuff that contributes to plaque formation and increases the risk of

What's it good for?

- bites and stings
- colds and flu
- coughs
- cuts and grazes
- diarrhoea
- ear problems
- fungal infections
- high blood pressure
- high cholesterol
- sinusitis
- sore throat
- styes
- urinary tract infections

Garlic

heart disease. Reviews of dozens of scientific studies suggest that eating garlic every day can lower cholesterol levels by between 9 and 12 per cent.

Garlic improves bloodflow throughout the body, not just in the coronary arteries. It's a vasodilator, which means it causes blood vessels to expand and blood pressure to drop. It also appears to improve the flexibility of arteries.

A cancer fighter

Dozens of studies suggest that garlic blocks cell changes that can lead to cancer – and may destroy cancer cells that have already formed. In one study, eating less than a clove a day was shown to cut the risk of prostate cancer in half. A study of women in Iowa in the USA found that those who ate garlic every week were about a third less likely to get colon cancer than those who never ate it.

A Chinese study found garlic consumption to be associated with a significantly reduced risk of stomach cancer. The incidence in high garlic-eaters was only 8 per cent of that in minimal garlic-eaters – but the garlic consumption was very high, amounting to about 20g (at least a whole bulb) a day.

No one is certain exactly how garlic combats cancer. Allicin and other compounds it contains seem to work directly against tumours. Garlic may also block the formation of cancer-causing compounds. It neutralizes dangerous molecules called free radicals, by-products of the oxidation process that contribute to cell ageing and also damage DNA and initiate carcinogenic cell changes. It inhibits the formation of nitrites, chemicals involved in triggering stomach cancer. And it boosts the immune system.

An edible antibiotic

Raw garlic that has been crushed and applied to wounds kills a variety of infection-causing organisms, including the fungi that cause athlete's foot, vaginal yeast infections and many types of ear infection. It kills many different sorts of bacteria, including the one that causes tuberculosis and the dreaded *E. coli*, the culprit behind many urinary tract infections. It may even kill some bacteria that are resistant to standard antibiotics.

Garlic

Garlic destroys germs both on the outside and inside of your body. Eating it may help to protect the lining of your gut from *H. pylori*, the bacterium that causes most peptic ulcers. And because garlic's essential oil is excreted through the lungs, it is particularly useful when you have a respiratory ailment.

How much to take

One to two cloves of raw or lightly cooked garlic a day are probably enough to obtain most of its healing and preventative benefits. Raw garlic packs more healing punch, as cooking inhibits the formation of allicin and eliminates some of the other healing chemicals.

You should bruise, chop or chew the clove to make sure the alliin in raw garlic is converted to allicin. Interestingly, according to the US National Cancer Institute, a delay of about 15 minutes between peeling and cooking garlic allows enzyme activities to take place which may help to preserve some of the healing properties normally lost in cooking.

The problem (for some people) with fresh garlic is its powerful aroma and flavour. If you want to get rid of 'garlic breath', munch a few sprigs of parsley after eating garlic.

Doctors agree that fresh garlic offers the greatest healing and preventative properties. But if you really can't stand the taste, then you could take enteric-coated garlic supplements instead. These won't give you garlic breath because they pass through the stomach undigested. Doctors advise taking 400 to 600mg of garlic in supplement form a day – but you can take this dose four times a day if you're fighting a cold or flu. Look for a supplement standardized to contain 4000mcg of allicin potential per tablet.

(*Alert* Do not take therapeutic doses of garlic if you take the blood thinning medication warfarin.)

Ginger

Ginger, a gnarled root with a distinctive hot pungent flavour, is among the most widely used and best studied of all kitchen cures. Closely related to the spices turmeric and cardamom, ginger has been used medicinally and as a seasoning for at least 5,000 years. It is renowned worldwide for its ability to alleviate nausea, vomiting, morning sickness and other digestive complaints – conditions that aren't always helped by modern drugs. And in the last few decades, the potential uses for ginger have extended far beyond the gut.

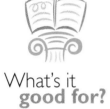

What's it good for?

- arthritis
- bursitis and tendinitis
- colds and flu
- coughs
- headache
- heartburn
- high cholesterol
- hives
- indigestion
- irritable bowel syndrome
- itching
- menstrual problems
- migraines
- morning sickness
- nausea
- peptic ulcers
- toothache
- wind, bloating and flatulence

Whether you have an upset stomach or feel shivery and have a cold, ginger can help. You can take it as a tea, a capsule or crystallized in sugar. Or you can add it to food or simply munch gingernuts. Many healing herbs have to be taken in huge amounts to provide health benefits. Ginger is different because the amount you'd add to a curry or stir-fry can easily match or exceed the amount used in supplements.

Stomach soother

Ginger is among the most potent remedies for motion sickness as well as common-or-garden tummy upsets. In fact, some studies have shown that it works just as well as certain nausea-stopping drugs. In one famous piece of research, scientists strapped volunteers in rotating chairs and took them for a ride. Those given a pharmaceutical anti-nausea medication lasted only about 4½ minutes before begging to stop. Half of the people given ginger, on the other hand, lasted 6 minutes, with less nausea than the medicated group.

The chemical compounds that give ginger its zesty taste – mainly gingerol and shogaol – appear to reduce intestinal contractions, neutralize digestive acids and inhibit the 'vomiting centre' in the brain. Doctors often recommend ginger to prevent nausea because it doesn't cause drowsiness the way anti-nausea drugs can. It has even been used to lessen chemotherapy-induced nausea and post-operative nausea.

Ginger is much better at preventing nausea than stopping it. If you're susceptible to motion sickness, for instance, the time to take ginger is before you get in the car or board a cross-channel ferry. Take about a ¼ teaspoon of powdered ginger, 1g of ginger in capsule form or a 1cm slice of fresh root ginger at least 20 minutes before leaving.

Whole-body protection

Ginger is most popular for nausea and stomach upsets, but there is evidence of many other benefits. For example, it can:

• **Short-circuit migraines** Danish researchers report that a ⅓ teaspoon of fresh or powdered ginger, taken at the first sign of migraine, may reduce symptoms by blocking prostaglandins, chemicals that cause inflammation in blood vessels in the brain. Unlike aspirin and related drugs, ginger blocks only the types of prostaglandins that cause inflammation, not the ones that have beneficial roles, such as strengthening the stomach lining.

• **Ease arthritis pain** The same prostaglandins that contribute to migraine pain also cause joint swelling in people with rheumatoid arthritis or osteoarthritis. A study of 56 people found that ginger eased symptoms in 55 per cent of people with osteoarthritis and 74 per cent of those with rheumatoid arthritis. Repeatedly applying crushed root ginger to the skin may provide additional relief by depleting stores of substance P, a neurotransmitter that carries pain signals to the spinal cord and, ultimately, the brain.

• **Reduce blood clots** Doctors often advise patients to take aspirin every other day because it 'thins' the blood by inter-fering with the action of platelets, cell-like structures that cause blood clots and increase the risk of heart attack. Ginger has similar effects but without the stomach upset often caused by aspirin (unless, of course, your stomach is sensitive to ginger or you eat too much of it).

• **Take the stuffiness out of colds** Ginger can block the body's production of substances that contribute to bronchial constriction, as well as fever. The gingerols in ginger also act as natural cough suppressants.

• **Lower cholesterol** Laboratory studies suggest that ginger reduces the absorption of cholesterol by the body and also promotes its excretion.

• **Relieve menstrual cramps** Chemical compounds in ginger act as antispasmodics. They inhibit painful contractions of the uterus, as well as the smooth muscles of the digestive tract.

Ginger's many guises

The active ingredients in ginger retain their potency when they're processed into almost any form. Many people prefer ginger capsules because they're easy to take and provide a concentrated (and predictable) source of ginger's chemical compounds. The usual dose is 100 to 200mg, three times a day. Here are healing amounts of other forms of ginger:

- A 1cm (½in) slice of root ginger. Grating the ginger will release more of the active ingredients than slicing or chopping. It is also important to buy ginger when it's fresh. Avoid root ginger that has soft spots or mouldy, wrinkled skin.
- 1 teaspoon of powdered ginger.
- 1 or 2 pieces of crystallized ginger.
- 1 cup of ginger tea, made with a ginger tea bag or half a teaspoon of grated root ginger. Steep in a cup of hot water.
- A 350ml (12fl oz) glass of natural ginger beer. But check the label to make sure it contains real ginger, not simply ginger flavouring.

Ginger

Honey

We are regularly advised to cut our consumption of sweet foods, but there's something special about honey. Honey is the unique product of swarms of bees that cover a six-mile radius during nectar collection. Anything that takes so much work to make must be good! Honey is sweeter than sugar, with 65 calories per tablespoon, as opposed to white sugar's 48. Calories apart, it has some surprising health benefits.

Honey is not a nutritional powerhouse. It contains trace amounts of B vitamins, amino acids and minerals, but it's really no more nutritious than plain sugar. If honey gets attention from doctors, it's for other reasons. Its thick syrupy texture makes it a natural for easing sore throat pain, especially when it's added to hot lemon or a soothing tea such as camomile.

But honey does much more. It kills bacteria and helps cuts and wounds to heal faster. It is a natural laxative. It appears to reduce the pain of stomach ulcers. And it is a quick-acting energy source that can reinvigorate tired muscles faster than you can say 'Lucozade sport'. Scientists have actually found that athletes perform better when they eat a little honey.

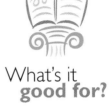

What's it good for?

- acne
- age spots
- allergies
- coughs
- insomnia
- laryngitis
- peptic ulcers
- sore throat

A sweet antiseptic

Infection was the greatest health threat in the days before antibiotics. Even small cuts or grazes could turn deadly, which is why doctors often carried a little honey in their black bags. Honey contains hydrogen peroxide and propolis, a compound in nectar that kills bacteria. Even today, when antiseptic creams are found in every medicine cabinet, some doctors believe that honey might be a superior wound dressing in some cases. Indeed, it works so well that a number of manufacturers sell honey-impregnated dressings for hard-to-heal wounds.

The high sugar content of honey pulls moisture from wounds and denies bacteria the moisture they need to survive. It also locks out harmful external contaminants. And because honey is inexpensive, it can be the ideal choice in countries without access to modern wound creams.

Honey

Where honey comes from

Bees sip a little nectar when they make their flowery rounds, but they carry most of it back to the hive and stash it in the hexagonal wax cells of the honeycomb to nourish young bees. The liquid nectar turns into honey when moisture evaporates. The finished product is mainly sugars – fructose and dextrose – plus a little bit of pollen, wax, proteins, vitamins and minerals. The clover honey that occupies most of the shelves in supermarkets is the blandest variety. More flavoursome honeys come from lavender, citrus blossoms and raspberry flowers.

Back in the 1970s, surgeons reported that women who had gynaecological surgery had shorter hospital stays and showed no signs of infection when incisions were coated with honey. Studies in India show that burns dressed with honey heal more quickly and with less pain and scarring than burns coated with silver sulphadiazine, a conventional burn treatment.

Honey has even been used to treat superficial eye problems, including conjunctivitis and chemical burns. In a study of more than 100 patients with eye disorders that didn't respond to conventional treatments, doctors tested a honey ointment. Eighty-five per cent of cases reported an improvement. Applying honey to the eyes (don't do it without asking your doctor first) may cause a brief stinging sensation and some redness, but is unlikely to cause other side effects.

Sweet digestion

Traditional healers used honey to treat a variety of gastro-intestinal complaints. Now there's good evidence that it works. For example:

● **It soothes stomach ulcers** Honey may reduce ulcer symptoms and speed up the healing time. Honey appears to reduce inflammation, stimulate bloodflow and enhance the growth of epithelial cells, the ones exposed along the interior of the stomach or intestine. Studies have also shown that honey kills *H. pylori*, the bacterium responsible for most ulcers. Raw honey (from farm shops or farmers' markets) is probably the best choice as high-heat processing used to create pasteurized honey may neutralize some of the active compounds. A form of honey called Active Manuka Honey, produced in New Zealand from the manuka tree and available in health-food stores, appears to be more effective than other types.

It promotes regularity Honey's high concentration of fructose makes it just the thing for occasional constipation. Undigested fructose provides nourishment for normal intestinal bacteria. The resulting fermentation brings water into the large intestine and has a laxative effect.

A word of warning

Never give honey to children under the age of 1, as it may contain a small number of spores called *Clostridium botulinum*, the organism that causes botulism. The spores don't thrive in the intestines of adults and older children. But they are able to multiply in babies, possibly causing a serious form of food poisoning known as infant botulism.

Lavender

Who would have thought that a medicine could smell so lovely? The oils in lavender, long valued for making perfumes, soaps and scented sachets, also aid digestion, ease anxiety and help to dismiss insomnia. There's even scientific evidence that one of the oils in lavender, perillyl alcohol, may one day play a role in treating cancer.

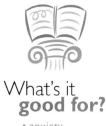

What's it good for?

- anxiety
- athlete's foot
- bites and stings
- body odour
- dandruff
- ear problems
- foot odour
- headache
- head lice
- insomnia
- oily skin
- wind

A perennial shrub with spikes of purple or light blue flowers, lavender has a long history of healing. The dried flowers can be sewn into a pouch and tucked under the pillow to restore restful sleep. The lavender aroma comes from airborne molecules of linalyl esters, oils that stimulate the olfactory nerve in the brain and calm the central nervous system. The mere smell of lavender may be as effective for setting the stage for peaceful rest as more powerful (and potentially habit-forming) sleep drugs.

Lavender is also the herb to look to when you're feeling anxious or tense. Researchers have discovered that lavender increases the type of brain waves associated with relaxation. Add some lavender oil to a diffuser to disperse the scent throughout a room. If you don't have a diffuser, add 3 drops of lavender oil to a bowl of steaming water and inhale the steam. When you have the luxury of time, add lavender bath oil or a handful of dried lavender flowers to bathwater for a stress-busting soak.

It's no coincidence that massage oils are often infused with lavender. The essential oils in lavender are easily absorbed through the skin and their sedative effects on the central nervous system can help you to feel relaxed. Unlike other essential oils, lavender oil (sold in health-food shops) can be applied directly to the skin. But it can cause severe sensitivity and should be used with caution. You can also mix it with a light carrier oil such as olive oil. Other uses for lavender are:

● **Headache medicine** Apply a little oil to each temple when you have a headache and massage it in for remarkable relief.

● **Tummy tamer** German doctors often recommend lavender tea as a digestive aid. The oils relax the smooth muscles of the digestive tract and soothe after-meal cramps in the stomach and intestine. Lavender also helps to ease intestinal wind. To make an infusion, steep a heaped teaspoon of lavender flowers in a cup of boiling water for 10 minutes and strain.

● **Infection fighter** The tannins in lavender kill bacteria and help to prevent minor cuts and grazes from becoming infected. Soak a clean cloth in a lavender infusion and apply the compress to the wound.

● **Ear soother** The same chemical compound in lavender that fights skin infections will knock out the itch and irritation of swimmer's ear.

● **Pain reliever** Lavender oil has minor painkilling properties. It appears to reduce the transmission of nerve impulses that carry pain signals. Mix a few drops of the oil into a tablespoon of carrier oil and rub it in. Lavender also relieves itching, thanks to its anti-inflammatory action. It's the perfect remedy for insect bites and stings.

How lavender may, one day, combat cancer

Cancer specialists have observed that a class of chemical compounds in lavender called monoterpenes appear to inhibit the development of cancerous cells and may help to prevent them from multiplying. Early laboratory research suggests that monoterpenes such as perillyl alcohol may inhibit soft-tissue cancers, such as those in the liver, breast and prostate gland. These compounds have even been shown to slow down the growth of colon and liver tumours.

It is too early to say for definite that lavender has beneficial effects on cancer. But early results are so promising that the essential oils are being tested in clinical studies for possible anti-cancer potential.

Lavender

Lemon

You get more than a sharp tang when you suck a lemon wedge or drink fresh lemonade. Lemons are an extraordinarily rich source of healing chemical compounds that improve immunity, strengthen blood vessels, help skin to heal and may even block certain cell changes that can lead to cancer. A quick rub of lemon in the armpits helps to combat unpleasant smells. A squeeze of lemon added to hot water and honey is the perfect sore-throat elixir. And lemon is a vital ingredient when it comes to making homemade cough mixtures.

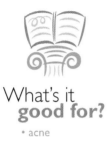

What's it good for?

- acne
- age spots
- body odour
- calluses and corns
- colds and flu
- cold sores
- coughs
- dry mouth
- greasy hair
- head lice
- heartburn
- hiccups
- kidney stones
- laryngitis
- morning sickness
- oily skin
- pregnancy ailments
- sore throat
- varicose veins
- warts

Centuries ago, British sailors ate lemons by the boatload to prevent scurvy, a deadly disease caused by vitamin C deficiency. A single lemon contains 40mg vitamin C, the full recommended daily target intake. We don't worry about scurvy anymore because there are so many sources of vitamin C in our diet. But lemons provide a host of other benefits.

Citrus power

Never underestimate the power of vitamin C – or the tried and trusted advice to drink lemony drinks when you have a cold. The vitamin C in lemons reduces levels of histamine, the chemical that contributes to stuffed noses and runny eyes. The vitamin is a powerful antioxidant that also reduces levels of unstable cell-damaging molecules known as free radicals, and helps to guard against heart disease. (Several studies have shown that low levels of vitamin C increase the risk of heart attack. When cholesterol becomes oxidized – attacked by free radicals – it's more likely to turn into artery-blocking plaque.) The body uses vitamin C to boost the activity of immune cells and manufacture collagen, the tissue-building substance that assists in wound healing.

Here are more reasons to enjoy the zesty pleasure of lemons:

● **Fewer kidney stones** Lemons are loaded with citric acid, a chemical that reduces calcium excretion and helps to prevent the formation of these painful little stones. Two litres (3½ pints) of lemonade daily, made with fresh lemon juice – with as little added sugar as possible – are as effective as citrate medications.

* **Stronger veins** Lemon zest is rich in a bioflavonoid (a group of antioxidant plant chemicals) called rutin, which strengthens the walls of veins and capillaries and reduces the pain – and even the occurrence – of varicose veins.

* **Breast protection** Another chemical, found in lemon peel and the white membrane beneath it, is limonene. Experiments suggest that limonene has significant anti-tumour activity. Researchers are now investigating limonene for its potential application as a cancer treatment and preventative, especially breast cancer. Scientists tested the substance – in the laboratory – on human breast cancer cells and found that it inhibited their growth. Limonene also causes oestrogen to break down into a weaker form in the body, which is important because raised oestrogen levels are linked with a higher risk of breast cancer. Limonene also boosts the liver's ability to remove potential carcinogens from the blood.

* **Beauty benefits** If applied often enough to age spots, lemon juice will eventually fade these marks of maturity. You can also dab it onto acne for faster healing.

* **Lemon tea reduces skin cancer risk** A study of 450 people found that those who regularly drink black tea, and especially those who usually add lemon to their tea, have a reduced risk of certain types of skin cancer. It may be that lemon works by boosting the activity of an enzyme (called glutathione S-transferase), which detoxifies cancer-causing compounds.

Mustard

Scientists have known for a long time that mustard's pungent heat thins mucus and makes it easier to breathe when you have a cold or flu. But this versatile kitchen condiment has turned out to be more than a feel-good remedy. A close relative of broccoli, cabbage and other cruciferous vegetables, mustard contains a variety of chemical compounds with impressive healing credentials.

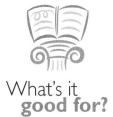

What's it good for?

- athlete's foot
- back pain
- colds and flu
- fever
- headache

Let's begin with mustard's role as an expectorant. When your nose is so blocked up that you can hardly breathe, a dollop of mustard – on a hot dog, for example – delivers a hefty dose of myrosin and sinigrin, chemicals that make mucus watery and easier to expel from the body.

A traditional congestion remedy is to apply a mustard poultice – made by crushing a few tablespoons of mustard seeds and adding them to a cup of flour along with a little water to make a paste – to your chest. The aroma unblocks stuffed nasal passages, while the 'heat' increases blood circulation in the chest and makes it easier to breathe. Be sure to protect the chest skin by applying a thick coating of petroleum jelly *before* you put on the plaster. And don't leave the plaster on for more than 15 minutes or it will burn the skin. Finally, wash your hands thoroughly after handling a mustard poultice and before touching your eyes, nose or mouth.

Another way to benefit from mustard's congestion-busting properties is to add a little ground mustard seed to your bath.

That's just the beginning of mustard's magic. It's also used for:

● **Easing Raynaud's symptoms** For people who periodically suffer from the painfully cold fingers that characterize this circulatory problem, a mustard plaster has been found to help. Mustard plasters have long been used to treat Raynaud's disease. Applied to the skin, the mustard causes mild irritation that increases the local blood supply creating a warm tingling sensation – a perfect antidote to frigid fingers. Mix 100g (3½oz) fresh ground mustard seed with hot, but not boiling, water to make a thick paste. Spoon it onto a piece of gauze large enough to wrap round the affected fingers. Apply the plaster and remove it after 1 minute. If the skin reddens (which is very likely) rub in a little olive oil. Rubbing some Vaseline into the hands *before* you apply the plaster will help to stop the mustard from burning the skin.

● **Stimulating appetite** Adding mustard to your food increases the flow of saliva and digestive juices – natural ways to stimulate appetite when you've been under the weather and aren't eating as well as you should be.

● **Knocking out athlete's foot** A bit of mustard powder added to a footbath can help to kill athlete's foot fungus.

● **Rubbing out back and joint pain** Herbalists call mustard a rubefacient, which means that it stimulates soothing warmth when applied to the skin. Like cayenne pepper, it also appears to deplete nerve cells of substance P, a chemical that transmits pain signals from the back to the brain. In fact, mustard oil is the main ingredient in at least one proprietary arthritis liniment. To use mustard for pain, either mix up a mustard plaster (see above) or soak a cloth in a strong mustard infusion made by pouring a cup of boiling water onto 1 teaspoon of ground mustard seed and infusing for 5 minutes. Apply this compress to the sore area. One arthritis sufferer suggested massaging a mixture of warm mustard oil and camphor into aching joints – but mustard oil is simply too strong to use on the skin, so we don't recommend this approach.

● **Easing headache, fever and congestion** Soaking your feet in hot water with a little mustard powder added can accomplish a number of goals. It can unblock a head cold, help to reduce a fever and soothe a headache. Drawing blood to the feet helps to disperse congestion, increases circulation and eases pressure on the blood vessels in your head.

There are several varieties of mustard including black, brown and white (also called yellow). White mustard seeds aren't quite as hot as other varieties. If you take mustard seeds by mouth, beware: they have a laxative effect if you eat enough of them. Mustard powder is also used to induce vomiting; eating more than a teaspoon is likely to have this effect.

Mustard

Omega-3 fatty acids

You may think that fat is bad for you. But there is one type, known as omega-3 fatty acids, that you should try very hard to eat more of. Found mainly in fish, omega-3s – a collective name for a group of polyunsaturated fats that include the unpronounceable eicosapentaenoic, docosahexaenoic and alpha-linolenic acids – play a key role in many vital body processes, from controlling blood clotting and blood pressure to reducing inflammation.

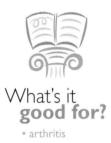

What's it good for?

- arthritis
- asthma
- bursitis and tendinitis
- depression
- dry skin
- eczema
- gout
- high blood pressure
- high cholesterol
- hives
- inflammatory bowel disease
- memory problems
- menstrual problems
- nail problems
- palpitations
- prostate problems
- psoriasis
- wrinkles

Scientists first began looking at omega-3s when they noticed that the Inuit (Eskimos) seldom suffered from rheumatoid arthritis or heart disease, even though their diet was a veritable slick of fish, seal and whale oils. As it happens, all of these foods are high in omega-3s, so it didn't take doctors long to realize that this class of fats is essential for good health.

Reduce your risk of heart disease

Heart disease is the number-one killer of British adults today. Most heart attacks occur when blood clots form in the arteries and block the flow of blood and oxygen to the heart. Study after study has shown that a diet rich in omega-3 fatty acids can reduce the risk of heart attack and also stroke. How do omega-3s help?

- They lower blood pressure by inhibiting the production of prostaglandins, leukotrienes and thromboxane – substances in the body that cause blood vessels to narrow.
- They make cell-like structures in blood called platelets less likely to clump together and form clots.
- They reduce levels of triglycerides, blood fats related to cholesterol that have been linked to heart disease.
- They reduce inflammation in the arteries and also appear to strengthen the heart's pumping rhythm.

Omega-3s clearly play an important role in prevention. There is also good evidence that they provide a valuable treatment option for people who already have heart disease. When taken in large amounts, they help to prevent restenosis, the reblockage of arteries that often occurs after a person has undergone angioplasty to open up a blocked blood vessel.

If you already have heart disease or want to make sure you never get it, doctors advise eating oily fish, which are rich in omega-3s, every week. These include salmon, mackerel and fresh tuna (but not tinned, as the oils are lost in processing), fresh or tinned sardines and pilchards. The Food Standards Agency has recently issued safety guidelines for oily fish intake: up to four times a week for men and for women past child-bearing age; for girls and women of childbearing age, the limit is two servings a week. Significantly, the FSA advises that children under 16 and women of childbearing age avoid marlin, shark and swordfish altogether, because high levels of harmful pollutants accumulate in the fat of large predatory fish.

If you really can't stand fish, take fish oil capsules.

Oil away bone and joint pain

You can think of omega-3s as WD-40 for the joints. Because they inhibit the effects of inflammatory chemicals such as prostaglandins, they're a great choice for people who suffer from joint pain and stiffness caused by rheumatoid arthritis. They work so well, in fact, that people who depend on aspirin or other anti-inflammatory painkillers are often able to lower their dose once they start taking fish oil supplements.

What's good for the joints also seems to be good for the bones, especially in postmenopausal women who either have osteoporosis or are at risk of getting this bone-depleting condition. One small study found that those given omega-3 fatty acids for 18 months had denser bones and fewer fractures than those who didn't take omega-3s.

Myriad other applications

Research results show that omega-3s help to:

* **Reduce gut pain** A one year study of people with Crohn's disease, a painful type of inflammatory bowel disease, found that 69 per cent of those who took fish oil supplements stayed symptom-free, compared with just 28 per cent of those who didn't take the oil.
* **Improve mental health** Some scientists suspect that the increasing incidence of depression in the USA is due in part to declining levels of fish eating. Low levels of omega-3s may weaken cell membranes and the production of certain neuro-

Omega-3 fatty acids

transmitters in the brain. When scientists looked at 44 people with bipolar disorder (or manic depression), they found that nearly two out of three improved if they were given fish oil.

● **Manage lupus** This serious auto-immune disease appears to improve somewhat in those who take fish oil supplements, probably because omega-3s reduce inflammation and also help to stop the immune system from overreacting.

● **Ease menstrual pain** Women who take omega-3s generally experience less cramping during their periods, probably because the supplements can lower levels of prostaglandins, chemicals that increase cramps and discomfort.

● **Possibly prevent cancer** There is some preliminary evidence that fish oils may help to prevent breast and colon cancers.

Facts about fish oil

● Omega-3s from non-fish sources don't provide the same benefits as those found in fish oil or cod liver oil.

● Always store fish oil supplements in the fridge to stop them going rancid.

● The recommended dose of fish oil supplements is usually 3,000 to 5,000mg a day. You can avoid common side effects – bloating and flatulence, diarrhoea or a slightly fishy body odour – by dividing the dose into two or three smaller doses and taking them throughout the day. Or freeze the pills and take them with food. Or try switching brands.

● Some naturopaths advise getting your omega-3s from fish oils in the summer and cod liver oil in the winter, because cod liver oil is rich in vitamin D. (In summer, we get enough vitamin D through exposure to sunlight.) The advantage of cod liver oil is that taking a couple of teaspoons (10ml) a day is as beneficial as taking anything up to about 15 fish oil capsules a day. (*Alert* Pregnant women shouldn't take cod liver oil as it is high in vitamin A.)

● Excess fish oil can interfere with blood clotting: don't take more than 6,000mg a day. (*Alert* Consult a doctor before taking fish oil supplements if you take a blood thinner such as aspirin or have a bleeding disorder. If you have diabetes, limit your intake to 2,000mg a day as larger doses may raise blood sugar levels. Do not take fish oil if you are allergic to fish.)

Peppermint

There's good reason your local pizzeria has a bowl full of peppermints next to the till. They are a nice post-prandial sweet and also make good short-term breath fresheners. Peppermint, in the right form, also combats indigestion and reduces wind and bloating. Peppermint not only makes an ideal digestive sweet: its healing powers are more powerful than you might imagine.

Intestine protection

Peppermint is among the best herbs for digestive problems and intestinal pain. The oils it contains, especially menthol and menthone, relax the smooth muscles that line the intestinal tract, helping to relieve cramping. British gastroenterologists who sprayed diluted peppermint oil on endoscopes – the tubelike instruments used in colonoscopy – found that it stopped painful spasms in less than 30 seconds.

The herb's antispasmodic properties make it a natural choice for easing irritable bowel syndrome (IBS), a condition that causes unpredictable cramping, indigestion and alternating bouts of constipation and diarrhoea.

In a study conducted in Taiwan, IBS patients who were given peppermint oil capsules 15 to 30 minutes before meals had a significant reduction in bloating and wind. Abdominal pain was reduced or disappeared completely in some cases.

Doctors who have an interest in herbal medicine now recommend peppermint for a variety of digestive complaints:

• **Wind** Because it aids digestion, peppermint can help you to avoid flatulence.

• **Gallstones** Preliminary evidence suggests that peppermint helps to dissolve gallstones and could potentially reduce the need for surgery.

• **Nausea** Peppermint slightly anaesthetizes the stomach lining and reduces mild nausea.

• **Stomach ulcers** Peppermint can help to relieve the pain and aid healing. (*Alert* Don't use peppermint if you have frequent heartburn. Peppermint can relax the oesophageal sphincter, the ring of muscle that prevents harsh stomach acids from backing up into the oesophagus.)

What's it
good for?

- bites and
  stings
- body odour
- foot pain
- headache
- indigestion
- inflammatory
  bowel disease
- irritable
  bowel
  syndrome
- morning
  sickness
- nausea
- oily skin
- peptic ulcers
- snoring
- sunburn
- toothache
- wind

Peppermint

Less congestion and pain

Whether you choose to drink the tea or sniff the aromatic vapours, you will find peppermint an effective decongestant that thins mucus and reduces nasal inflammation. It may even reduce bronchial constriction and the tightening of the airways that accompanies asthma attacks.

If you get frequent headaches, try dabbing a little diluted peppermint oil on your forehead and temples. A small study of 32 headache patients found the oil an effective painkiller.

The menthol in peppermint has significant painkilling powers. Whether you're an athlete or a weekend warrior, keep some peppermint oil (or a menthol-containing ointment) in your medicine chest to rub into sore muscles. As it's too strong to use neat, mix a few drops with a tablespoon of a neutral carrier oil, such as sunflower or olive oil.

Because of its numbing properties, peppermint is also useful against toothache.

Like many essential oils, peppermint kills certain viruses and bacteria. Add a few drops of peppermint oil to a cup of water to make a minty, germ-killing mouthwash. Or to freshen your breath, place a drop or two of the oil on your tongue. (*Alert* Do not take more than this by mouth: it's not just that the oil may upset the stomach; just a couple of teaspoons can be fatal.)

Teatime

Most people like the aroma and refreshing taste of peppermint tea. Drink a cup or two a day to ease or prevent digestive discomfort. You can also take enteric-coated capsules between meals, following the directions on the label (enteric-coated capsules pass through the stomach and are broken down in the intestines instead). Or add 10 to 20 drops of peppermint tincture, which is much less potent than the oil, to a glass of water and drink it as needed.

Petroleum jelly

Petroleum jelly, better known by the brand name Vaseline, is the pharmacy equivalent of a can of oil – you can use it for just about everything. It is a superb moisturizer; petroleum jelly takes the soreness out of chapped lips; it eases skin disorders such as eczema; and as if that weren't enough, you can also use it to coat car battery terminals to prevent corrosion.

As you can tell from the name, petroleum jelly is made from petroleum, the same basic stuff that lubricates a car engine and goes in the petrol tank. The reason that petroleum jelly smears instead of pours is that it's made from heavier petroleum products, including mineral oils and paraffin wax. It makes an excellent base for salves and ointments and is also useful by itself.

Doctors will often recommend petroleum jelly as a winter moisturizer because it's heavier and traps more moisture than ordinary lotions. It's perfect for dry hands and feet, especially when you put on an extra-thick coating and cover up with gloves or socks before going to bed. To get the best skin protection, apply petroleum jelly after a shower or bath. This traps moisture next to the skin where it's needed. At the same time, the oils seep into the skin and make it supple and soft.

What else is petroleum jelly good for? Plenty. For instance, you can use it to:

● **Prevent windburn** Petroleum jelly makes an excellent protective barrier between your skin and the wind.

● **Get relief from psoriasis** Apply petroleum jelly to dry skin patches caused by this chronic skin disorder. It lubricates and helps to remove hard, itchy scales.

● **Eliminate lice** Irritating head lice that are resistant to over-the-counter lice medications might succumb to a thick layer of petroleum jelly, applied to the scalp. Leave it on overnight and repeat several nights in a row. When you remove it with baby oil, you get rid of lice at the same time. Note that this treatment does *not* eliminate the need for nit-combing. Some mums find this remedy more trouble than it's worth, as the petroleum jelly can be difficult to remove. If baby oil doesn't

What's it good for?

- allergies
- blisters
- chapped lips
- cold sores
- cuts and grazes
- dry skin
- eczema
- head lice
- haemorrhoids
- nosebleeds
- psoriasis

work, try the trick one mother uses: apply a runny paste made from washing-up liquid and cornflour. Let it set hard, then wash it out with shampoo.

• **Soothe chapped lips** Rub petroleum jelly on the lips to stop rapid evaporation, which has a drying effect. It's an ideal moisturizer and makes a nice lip gloss, too.

• **Protect cuts and grazes** A layer of petroleum jelly keeps moisture in and air and bacteria out.

• **Moisturize healing burns** Do not apply petroleum jelly immediately when you have a burn, because it will trap heat and increase skin damage. However, after three days or so, when the skin is starting to heal itself, moisturizing with petroleum jelly can be useful for reducing dryness and promoting better healing.

• **Trap pollen** Dab a little petroleum jelly just inside your nostrils to trap pollen spores that are wafting around before they make it further into your airways.

• **Prevent nosebleeds** If you want to avoid nosebleeds, keep your mucous membranes moist by dabbing the insides of your nostrils with petroleum jelly. This is an especially useful tip when flying.

Multi-purpose gloop

Canny householders keep a tub of Vaseline in the toolbox as well as in the medicine chest. When you're painting, apply a coating to door handles and hinges to prevent paint from sticking. Mechanics often coat their hands with petroleum jelly to seal the skin and keep oil and grease out. You can even use petroleum jelly to slide stuck chewing gum from hair, slip off too-tight rings and remove make-up.

Petroleum jelly

Tea

It's the most popular hot drink in the world. With half as much caffeine on average as coffee, tea offers a refreshing pick-me-up without giving you the jitters. But drinking tea is far more than just a civilized habit; it could actually be a lifesaving one. Researchers have found that tea drinkers may have a lower risk of heart disease, stroke, cancer and – oddly – even tooth decay.

In the early 1990s, researchers noted that Japanese women who practised the art of chanoyu, the traditional tea ceremony, had much lower mortality rates than other women. It didn't take scientists long to work out that the chemical compounds in tea – mainly polyphenols, which make up nearly 30 per cent of tea's dry weight – are among the most potent antioxidants ever discovered. Antioxidants are chemicals that block the effects of free radicals, the rogue oxygen molecules that damage cells throughout the body and increase the risk of serious diseases such as cancer.

Incidentally, don't confuse herbal teas such as camomile with real tea that comes from *Camellia sinensis*, the tea plant. The green tea popular in Asian countries is simply the steamed and dried leaves of this plant. The everyday tea we drink here, properly called black tea, undergoes a process of fermentation that gives it a stronger flavour and darker colour – and may reduce its levels of health-protective chemical compounds.

What's it good for?

- athlete's foot
- diarrhoea
- fever
- foot odour
- gum problems
- haemorrhoids
- headache
- itching
- mouth ulcers
- sunburn
- toothache

Brew some cancer prevention?

Tea has long been recognized in the laboratory as an antioxidant, but study results involving humans have been contradictory. Some epidemiological studies, comparing people who drink tea with those who don't, claim that drinking tea prevents cancer; others do not. There have been more studies based on drinking green tea, so the evidence to date is better for green. Studies in China, for example, showed that regular consumption of green tea significantly reduced the risk of stomach and oesphageal cancers. However, a study in the

Netherlands found no link between tea consumption and protection against cancer. Because the production process reduces the amounts of antioxidants in black tea, it seems likely that green tea is a more powerful cancer-fighter than black tea, although both teas offer protective benefits.

Green tea is high in substances known as catechins. These are potent antioxidants – 100 times more powerful than vitamin C – that appear to protect DNA in cells from cancer-inducing changes. Black tea also contains catechins but in much smaller amounts.

In skin-cancer studies, laboratory animals that were given green tea developed one-tenth as many tumours as animals that were given water instead. When it comes to preventing skin cancer, green tea seems to be equally effective whether it's sipped from a cup or applied to the skin. Many cosmetics manufacturers have started adding green tea to skin-care products because its antioxidant effects may reduce wrinkles or other evidence of skin damage.

The US National Cancer Institute is researching green tea as a preventative agent against skin cancer. One study is investigating the protective effects of a pill form of green tea against sun-induced skin damage; another is looking at the topical application of green tea in shrinking precancerous skin changes.

While green tea is mainly valued for its cancer-preventing powers, there is some evidence that it may help people who already have cancer. The catechins in green tea inhibit the production of urokinase, an enzyme that cancer cells need in order to grow. It also seems to stimulate the process of programmed cell death, or apoptosis, in cancer cells. In a seven-year study of breast cancer patients, women who drank five cups of green tea a day were less likely to have their cancers spread to lymph nodes than women who drank less.

Heart health and more

Because tea's polyphenols are such potent antioxidants, they play a protective role throughout the body in any areas that free radicals cause damage, including the arteries. Tea also has antibacterial properties that benefit dental health. Your everyday cuppa may offer:

Tea

• **Less heart disease** The chemicals in tea help to prevent cholesterol from oxidizing. Oxidization occurs when cholesterol is bombarded by free radicals. The process makes the cholesterol more likely to stick to artery walls, a step on the road to heart disease. Dutch researchers reported that men who consumed the most flavonoids – a chemical family that includes tea's polyphenols – had a 58 per cent lower risk of dying from heart disease than men who got the least. The healthiest men in the study drank about 4 cups of tea a day.

• **Reduced stroke risk** Women who drink tea frequently appear to have lower rates of stroke than those who drink less, probably because the polyphenols in tea reduce damage to vulnerable blood vessels in the brain.

• **Stronger teeth** Tea contains a modest amount of fluoride, the mineral that strengthens teeth and reduces tooth decay. Moreover, the tannins and polyphenols in tea inhibit bacteria that damage the teeth. There's even evidence that tea improves the ability of tooth enamel to resist the onslaught of oral acids.

• **Soothe sunburn and more** Because tea contains astringents that help to reduce inflammation, a wet tea bag can provide soothing relief for sunburnt skin and well as haemorrhoids and mouth ulcers. (Tea is alkaline, so it neutralizes acids that eat into tissue exposed by an ulcer.)

Drink to your health

Two to three cups of tea a day is probably enough to provide most of its health benefits. Green tea supplements, sold in health-food shops, also appear to be effective. The usual dose is 250 to 400mg taken once a day.

One caveat: if you usually drink tea with milk, you might be missing out on some of the health protection. Proteins in milk may bind to tea's polyphenols and block their beneficial effects.

Tea

Vinegar

As tart as an unripe apple, vinegar combats bacteria and fungi, takes the itch out of mosquito bites and soothes sunburn. It can also settle an upset stomach, prevent swimmer's ear, make hair shinier and skin softer. Some people say that vinegar mixed with honey and warm water can ease the pain of leg cramp. Others use vinegar to dry up cold sores. And if someone faints, vinegar is a useful alternative to smelling salts.

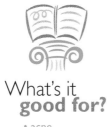

What's it good for?

- acne
- bites and stings
- body odour
- bruises
- dandruff
- dry mouth
- ear problems
- foot odour
- greasy hair
- headaches
- head lice
- hiccups
- hives
- indigestion
- nappy rash
- psoriasis
- sunburn
- warts

Put a drop of vinegar on your tongue and you will instantly taste its sourness. Vinegar's sharp flavour comes from its high concentration of acetic acid, which is formed when bacteria digest fermented liquids. Acetic acid may be kind to your body, but it is also an industrial-strength product: millions of tonnes of it go into the making of photographic films and artificial fibres such as rayon.

The power of acid

Vinegar is an effective weapon against bacteria. Infectious bugs have been wiped out again and again with vinegar cures. In World War I, the wounds of soldiers were cleaned with vinegar and even today, if you can stand the sting, it is a perfectly adequate disinfectant if you have a scratch or a sore. It's equally malevolent towards fungal infections. Most will retreat when tackled with a dose of vinegar.

Vinegar is also good for the hair and skin. As an acid, vinegar reacts with chemical bases to produce neutral H_2O (water), along with some salts. When spread on skin or used as a final hair rinse, it can spirit off soap, shampoo or conditioner residue. Rinsing the hair with vinegar may also help to reduce dandruff and calm an itchy scalp.

Here are some of vinegar's other uses:

Stomach settler If you suffer from indigestion because of a lack of stomach acid, a teaspoon of vinegar after meals may be just what you need. (Of course, if your problem is *too much* stomach acid, vinegar won't be any help and will probably make things worse.)

Vinegar

• **Gentle coolant** Spread on skin, it evaporates quickly, which provides a friendly chill that can take the burn out of sunburn. Vinegar also helps to counter the inflammation that causes sunburnt skin to itch.

• **Bacteria slayer and fungus fighter** When bacteria or fungi flourish in the warm, moist hollows of an ear canal, the condition is called swimmer's ear. Vinegar does double duty – fighting both kinds of invaders – which is why, when mixed in equal parts with surgical spirit and dropped into the ear, it may help to cure the condition (but never drop anything into the ear if there is any chance that the eardrum is ruptured and, if in doubt, always get a doctor's advice).

• **Between the toes** Soaking your feet in vinegar is an effective treatment for athlete's foot.

• **Odour eater** The high acid content gives it a nice, sharp scent that can override less lovely odours. A vinegar rinse will banish the smell of cigar smoke from clothes, freshen a baby's nappies when added to the final rinsing water or expurgate unpleasant pongs from armpits or feet.

• **Sting stopper** Both jellyfish stings and mosquito bites can be relieved with vinegar, which neutralizes pain-causing substances that get in the skin. Vinegar can also relieve the itching of hives: water it down slightly and dab it onto the skin with a cotton wool ball.

• **Headache tamer** Vinegar is one of the most popular folk remedies for headache. The traditional approach was to soak brown paper with cider vinegar and apply it to the forehead – as happens in the nursery rhyme Jack and Jill. You can also soak a clean cloth in vinegar and tie it tightly around your head. No one is sure why it works but many people swear by it.

• **Throat soother** Vinegar is also a trusted folk remedy for sore throats. Some people recommend gargling with a tablespoon of vinegar in a glass of warm water. Others make a homemade cough syrup by combining equal amounts of honey and cider vinegar and stirring or shaking until dissolved.

More than sour grapes

If you travel the world in search of varieties of vinegar, you will find brews made from sugar cane in the Philippines, coconut in Thailand, and in China red, white and black rice wine vinegars that have flavoured stir-fries for more than 5,000 years. Elsewhere you may come across vinegars yielded by honey, potatoes, dates, nuts and berries. But if you shop nearer home, the most common kinds you'll find are brown malt vinegar (great with chips), cider vinegar (made from apples), wine and sherry vinegars (made from grapes) or plain distilled white vinegar that's produced from grain and is as useful as a household cleaner as it is in cooking.

Cider vinegar is often recommended for its health benefits in preference to any others. There are two good reasons. Firstly, fermented apples are rich in pectin, a type of fibre that is very good for digestion. And secondly, apples contain malic acid, which combines with magnesium in the body to help fight aches and pains.

You can make your own vinegar quite easily, but you must use sterilized jars and utensils to avoid bacterial contamination. Starting with cider or wine, fermentation is speeded up by addition of a 'mother' – in other words, a slosh of existing vinegar that triggers the process. When you become a more experienced vinegar maker, you'll begin to recognize the moment when the brew is ready.

Once it's been bottled, capped and stored, homemade vinegar will remain usable for months. But you can use any commercial vinegar for home remedies.

Vinegar

Witch hazel

Along with paracetamol, disinfectant and sticky plasters, witch hazel is a medicine-cabinet staple. A liquid extract made from an American plant (*Hamamelis virginiana*), it is used externally to calm itching, take the sting out of haemorrhoids and freshen the skin. It has nothing to do with witches, although forked hazel branches were used by 'witchers' to find underground water and are still valued by dowsers today. The herb's name comes from the Middle English word *wych*, which means pliable. The wood is so springy that Native Americans once used it to make bows.

The active ingredient in traditional witch hazel is tannin, a chemical compound with astringent properties: it tightens skin pores much as skin toners do. Tannin also shrinks blood vessels and can reduce bleeding from shaving nicks and other minor wounds. Because of its tannins, witch hazel was once taken internally to combat diarrhoea. But the distilled preparation sold as witch hazel or hamamelis water in pharmacies today is a different remedy altogether.

In the late 1800s manufacturers abandoned the traditional steeping method and switched to a steam distillation process. The new technique was more efficient, but the high heat involved in the steaming process means that modern witch hazel is virtually devoid of tannins. Its mildly astringent action comes from its alcohol content. However, you can still buy proper herbal witch hazel preparations including liquid extract, dried leaf (which can be used to make an infusion) or tincture. It is also an active ingredient in many skin care preparations.

A cooling astringent

Even though the witch hazel sold in pharmacies today has little in common with the traditional remedy, the alcohol content (about the same as table wine) makes it a safe and effective astringent useful for:

Shaving cuts Dab on a little witch hazel to disinfect the cut and possibly slow down bleeding. (But don't use witch hazel on serious cuts: the alcohol may increase skin damage.) Even if you haven't cut yourself, witch hazel leaves your skin feeling softer and soothed when used as an aftershave.

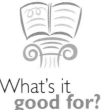

What's it good for?

- body odour
- bruises
- haemorrhoids
- hives
- itching
- oily skin
- shaving rash

Witch hazel

• **Fresher skin** Soak a gauze pad or cotton wool ball in witch hazel and dab it onto your face to remove surface oils, tighten pores and tone the skin. Witch hazel is an ingredient in a number of skin-care products.

• **Take the sting out of stings** As a mild astringent, witch hazel is useful for sunburn, skin inflammation and insect bites. In the summer, keep witch hazel in the fridge so that it's cold – and all the more soothing – when you apply it to sunburned skin.

The real witch hazel

Benefit from witch hazel's healing tannins by brewing your own infusion or using liquid extract from a health-food shop:

• **Make a skin spray** Mix it with rosewater and geranium as a soothing spray or lotion for skin conditions.

• **Bruise balm** Apply tincture to bruises and sprains.

• **Haemorrhoid relief** Pour some strong witch hazel infusion or liquid extract onto a cotton wool ball and apply it to the tender area. The tannin shrinks blood vessels and the liquid provides a soothing, cooling sensation as it evaporates. Witch hazel is an ingredient in Preparation H and several other over-the-counter haemorrhoid treatments.

• **Soothe itchy rashes** Keep a mixture of witch hazel and camomile infusions in the fridge to spray on itchy rashes, eczema, dermatitis, chickenpox or measles.

• **Freshen breath** Use a weak infusion as a mouthwash. Witch hazel extracts have been shown to inhibit oral bacteria and may be useful for treating periodontal disease. Swish it round and spit it out – don't swallow.

• **Soothe raw rashes** The herb's anti-inflammatory, hydrating and antibacterial effects make it useful for treating intertrigo (an inflammatory condition that can occur in damp skin folds) and some forms of dermatitis. Apply the infusion to the affected area using a fine mist plant sprayer or on a soft cloth or cotton wool pad.

• **An after-sun balm** Its anti-inflammatory properties make witch hazel a good after-sun soother. Because one of its constituents, hamamelitannin, is thought to protect against UV irradiation, witch hazel is used as an ingredient in some after-sun lotions.

Yoghurt

Did you know that there are more bacteria in your body than there are human cells? About 500 species of bacteria inhabit the digestive tract alone. Don't shudder. The vast majority of intestinal organisms – *more than a kilo of them* – are beneficial. They strengthen immunity, digest milk sugars (lactose), assist in the absorption of nutrients and generally maintain digestive health. But some intestinal bacteria, along with organisms in the vagina and urinary tract, can cause all sorts of problems. That's why it's a good idea to keep the fridge stocked with live yoghurt.

Yoghurt is milk to which cultures of bacteria are added. The bacteria consume the sugar in the milk for energy and excrete lactic acid (the same acid that builds up in muscles during exercise), which curdles the milk. Yoghurt that contains 'active cultures' – meaning live bacteria – is the one that's brimming with health benefits. That's because organisms such as *Lactobacillus acidophilus*, *Streptococcus thermophilus* and *Lactobacillus bulgaricus* – collectively known as probiotics – protect your body from harmful bacteria by using up resources that those bacteria need in order to thrive. And some bacteria in yoghurt produce acids that kill other bacteria, including the germs that cause botulism, among other ailments.

Eat for digestive health
When you're healthy, about 85 per cent of bacteria in the large intestine are *Lactobacillus* organisms. The other 15 per cent consist largely of other beneficial strains. But if you're taking antibiotics, the drugs wipe out the 'good' bacteria along with the 'bad' ones responsible for your infection. This can lead to diarrhoea, stomach cramps, wind and bloating, fungal infections and less efficient absorption of nutrients.

Yoghurt can protect. US researchers found that patients who ate two 250g servings of live yoghurt a day suffered half as much antibiotic-associated diarrhoea as non-yoghurt eaters.

Other studies show that the beneficial bacteria in live yoghurt (or probiotic supplements) reduce infant diarrhoea, suppress symptoms of inflammatory bowel disease and irritable

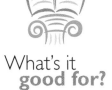

What's it good for?
- athlete's foot
- cold sores
- diarrhoea
- fungal infections
- inflammatory bowel disease
- irritable bowel syndrome
- mouth ulcers
- urinary tract infections
- wind

Yoghurt

bowel syndrome and ease some types of food poisoning. There's even evidence that yoghurt's healthy organisms, in combination with a high-fibre diet, can prevent diverticulosis, a painful and potentially serious condition in which small pouches form on the colon wall.

Can't live without them

Yoghurt has been used for centuries as a multi-purpose healer but it's only within the last decade or so that scientists have discovered just how beneficial yoghurt really is. Here are some of the things it can do:

● **Knock out thrush** The yeast fungus, *Candida albicans*, that normally inhabits the vagina is usually kept in check by other organisms. It's only when it multiplies that it causes the miserable itching and burning of thrush. A US study found that the rate of infections dropped considerably in women who ate 250mg of live yoghurt a day. Eating live yoghurt – or using acidophilus supplements in pessary (vaginal suppository) form – can treat infections that are already underway. Just make sure its really is a yeast infection; treating a bacterial infection with yoghurt will make the problem worse.

● **Protect the bladder** Yoghurt can make a real difference if you are one of the many women who suffer from recurrent urinary tract infections. Finnish researchers report that women who eat at least three servings of yoghurt and cheese a week are almost 80 per cent less likely to suffer from urinary tract infections than women who eat these dairy foods less than once a week.

● **Strengthen immunity** Medical researchers in California found that eating two pots of live yoghurt a day can quadruple levels of gamma interferon, a protein produced by white blood cells that assists the immune system in fighting off germs.

● **Combat cancer** The acidophilus in yoghurt isn't a cancer cure but it has been shown to help prevent recurrences of tumours in patients treated for bladder cancer. It seems that the beneficial bacteria may prevent harmful bacteria from creating cancer-causing substances in the body when those bacteria react with foods.

Yoghurt

Build strong bones Many people are lactose intolerant (they lack the enzyme needed to digest lactose), and therefore keep off milk – and the bone-strengthening calcium it provides. Live yoghurt can be an easy-to-digest alternative because the organisms it contains digest the lactose before you eat it. So people with lactose intolerance can usually eat yoghurt without suffering from wind or other uncomfortable symptoms. Yoghurt is even higher in calcium than milk, with more than 400mg in a single serving.

What to look for

Don't assume that all the yoghurt products sold in the super-market contain beneficial bacteria. Look for products with the words 'live', 'active' or 'bio' on the label. And to ensure that you get as many live organisms as possible, buy and eat yoghurts as far ahead of their 'use-by' date as you can.

Even if you're not a yoghurt fan, you can get most of the benefits by taking probiotic supplements. Optimal doses haven't been determined, but researchers suspect you need about 10 billion organisms daily. That sounds like a lot, but it's actually only a capsule or two. Be sure to keep supplements in the fridge, as probiotics are living organisms. Don't put them in the freezer, though; freezing temperatures (as well as high heat) can easily kill the cultures.

Yoghurt

Cautions and side effects

Supplements are helpful for many health problems but, as with drugs, you need to be careful when taking them. Even herbs and other harmless-seeming substances can have unwelcome side effects if you use them inappropriately. Before taking a herb or supplement recommended in this book, check the cautions listed below. If you experience any side effects while taking a supplement, stop taking it and talk to your doctor. *ALERT* If you are pregnant or breastfeeding do not take *any* herb or supplement without first talking to your midwife or doctor. Likewise, if you are on prescribed medication, talk to your pharmacist or doctor.

ACIDOPHILUS At first, may increase wind or bloating. If taking antibiotics, wait at least 2 hours before taking acidophilus.

ANISE Avoid in pregnancy (though the amounts in cooking are fine). Do not take with iron. May trigger sensitization to sunlight – do not sunbathe. Do not use if taking hormone preparations.

ARGININE Take only under a doctor's supervision. Excess may cause nausea and diarrhoea. Avoid if you have genital herpes: may increase outbreaks. Long-term effects unknown. Take at least 1½ hours before or after food. Do not take if you have heart disease, kidney problems or cancer, unless advised to by your doctor.

ARNICA Do not apply to broken or bleeding skin. Avoid in pregnancy. Can cause an allergic rash in sensitive people or with prolonged use.

ASTRAGALUS Do not take if you are taking cyclophosphamide. Do not take with acute infections, such as those that cause a high fever or pronounced swelling.

B COMPLEX Do not exceed the dosage recommended on the label.

BETA-CAROTENE Avoid if you have hypothyroidism, if you are a smoker or if you are pregnant. Best taken as a mixed carotenoid supplement. Large doses can turn skin orange and may cause harm.

BLACK COHOSH Recent research indicates a strong link between black cohosh and adverse liver reactions. Avoid if pregnant or breastfeeding, if you have heart disease or are on blood pressure medication. If on oestrogen therapy, consult a doctor before taking. Do not use for more than 6 months. May cause headache, upset stomach, reduced heart rate and raised blood pressure. Excess can cause vertigo, nausea, impaired vision, vomiting and impaired circulation.

BROMELAIN May cause nausea, vomiting, diarrhoea, rash and heavy menstrual bleeding. May increase the risk of bleeding in people taking aspirin or blood thinners. Do not take if you are allergic to pineapple.

CALCIUM Do not exceed 1,500mg daily except under a doctor's supervision. Avoid calcium derived from oyster shells, bone-meal and dolomite: it may be contaminated with lead. Excess may cause constipation. Check with your doctor if you have had calcium oxalate kidney stones before taking.

CAMOMILE Taken by mouth can cause a reaction if you are allergic to related plants, such as aster and chrysanthemum. Camomile contains an anticoagulant: use with caution if you have a blood-clotting disorder or take anticoagulant drugs.

CARNITINE Take the 'L' form only (L-carnitine), and only with consent of your doctor. The 'D' form may displace the active form of carnitine in tissues and lead to muscle weakness. Doses above 2g may cause stomach pain, nausea and diarrhoea. May require monitoring of levels in blood/urine in long term use. Use with caution in kidney disease. The use of individual amino acids in large doses is experimental and long-term health effects are unknown.

CASCARA Avoid if pregnant or in a weakened condition. Do not take for more than eight days, except with a doctor's guidance. Do not use if you have intestinal inflammation or obstruction or abdominal pain. Can cause laxative dependency an diarrhoea. Do not take with anti-coagulant medicines such as warfarin.

CAT'S CLAW Do not use if you have haemophilia or are pregnant. Do not take with immuno-suppressant drugs. Side effects may include headache, stomach ache or difficulty in breathing. Cat's claw may impair fertility.

CELERY SEED Do not take if pregnant. Use with caution if you have a kidney disorder; may have diuretic effects, so do not take if already on diuretics. Avoid with blood-thinners (aspirin or warfarin). May sensitize skin to sunlight; don't sunbathe.

CHASTEBERRY Do not take if pregnant. May impair action of oral contraceptives. Read label carefully if you have high blood pressure: capsules may contain liquorice or Siberian ginseng, which can raise blood pressure. May cause stomach upset, headache, itching, rash and menstrual irregularities.

CINNAMON Do not take large amounts during pregnancy.

COENZYME Q$_{10}$ Do not take for more than 20 days at daily doses exceeding 120mg without medical supervision. Side effects such as heartburn, nausea and stomach ache can be avoided by taking with food. May decrease action of warfarin.

COPPER Do not take with Wilson's disease. Do not exceed 1mg a day on a regular basis. High doses may cause stomach pain, diarrhoea and nausea and long term could damage liver and kidneys.

CRANBERRY Do not take if on blood thinning drugs.

CURCUMIN May cause heartburn in some people.

DANDELION Do not use as a diet aid. Seek advice from a medical herbalist before using to treat gallstones. Avoid if you have blockage of the bile duct. If you have gallbladder disease, do not use root preparations.

DEGLYCYRRHIZINATED LIQUORICE (DGL) Avoid in pregnancy. Do not take with blood pressure, antiarrhythmic, corticosteroid, diuretic or antihistamine drugs. Take only DGL, if you have high blood pressure, never straight liquorice. Use caution if you have high blood pressure; heart rhythm abnormalities; cardiovascular, liver or kidney disorders or low potassium. Do not use DGL more than three times a week for more than 4 to 6 weeks. Overuse may lead to water retention, high blood pressure, or impaired heart or kidney function.

DIGESTIVE ENZYMES Alpha-galactosidase supplements alter the way you process sugar: don't use without a doctor's consent if you have diabetes. Do not use if you have galactosaemia. Do not take if you are sensitive to mould or penicillin (these supplements are often made from a type of mould).

ECHINACEA Avoid if you have a chronic immune or auto-immune disease such as tuberculosis, lupus, multiple sclerosis or rheumatoid arthritis. Also avoid if taking HIV medications, anti-anxiety drugs, immunosuppressants, cholesterol-lowering or anti-cancer drugs. Avoid using in conjunction with drugs that are toxic to the liver, such as anabolic steroids, amiodarone, methotrexate and ketoconazole, as it may worsen liver damage. Do not take echinacea if you are allergic to closely related plants, such as chrysanthemums, asters or ragweed. Don't use for more than eight weeks at a time.

ELDER, ELDERBERRY Do not use when pregnant. Seeds, bark, leaves and unripe fruit may cause vomiting or severe diarrhoea. Seeds of raw berries are toxic – eat ripe and cooked.

FALSE UNICORN This herb is best known as a uterine tonic and small doses may be recommended for morning sickness and for the prevention of miscarriage but you should not take during pregnancy except under medical supervision. Do not take if you are emaciated or experiencing acute inflammation. May cause gastrointestinal irritation.

FENNEL Do not use medicinally for more than six weeks.

FENUGREEK Not to be taken during pregnancy, though the amounts used in cooking are fine. Check with your doctor if diabetic or on blood thinners.

FEVERFEW Avoid with warfarin and MOAI antidepressants.

FISH OIL Do not take if you are pregnant except under a doctor's guidance. Do not take more than 2 teaspoons fish oil a day (too much can interfere with blood clotting). If taking blood thinners or aspirin regularly, do not take fish oil unless advised to by your doctor. Avoid if you have a bleeding disorder, high blood pressure or an allergy to any kind of fish. Avoid if you have liver disease. If you have diabetes, check with your doctor before taking fish oil because of its high fat content. Fish oil increases bleeding time, possibly resulting in nosebleeds and easy bruising. May cause upset stomach.

5-HTP Experimental. Avoid if pregnant. May cause stomach upset, muscle pain, lethargy and headache. Do not take with antidepressants, other serotonin altering drugs, weight control drugs or substances known to cause liver damage. Also don't use for more than three months without medical advice.

FLAXSEEDS Do not use if you have bowel obstruction or thyroid problems. Always take with water. May decrease the absorption of medications. Do not heat the oil.

FOLIC ACID Do not exceed 1,000mcg a day without medical supervision. Taking more than 400mcg can mask vitamin B_{12} deficiency; excess can cause nerve damage if you have a B_{12} deficiency. Can impair action of anti-epileptic drugs. Don't use if you have cancer except with medical advice.

GAMMA LINOLENIC ACID (GLA) Do not take borage oil or evening primrose oil (both of which contain GLA) if you are pregnant or breastfeeding. Do not use without asking your doctor if you take aspirin or blood thinners, have a seizure disorder or take epilepsy medication such as phenothiazines. May cause headache, indigestion, nausea and softening of stools.

GARLIC Avoid garlic supplements with anticoagulants (warfarin) and medications for diabetes.

GINGER If you are pregnant, ask your midwife or doctor before using ginger. Do not use the dried root or powder if you have gallstones.

GINKGO BILOBA Rarely, ginkgo can cause headache, stomach ache, restlessness or irritability (these side-effects usually subside). Do not use with MAOI antidepressants; aspirin or other non-steroidal anti-inflammatory drugs; blood-thinning drugs like warfarin. Can cause rash, diarrhoea and vomiting in doses above 240mg concentrated extract.

GINSENG If you have a heart condition, high blood pressure or an anxiety disorder, consult your GP before taking ginseng. Do not take with warfarin. May cause insomnia, nervousness, diarrhoea, headaches and high blood pressure. Has been reported to cause menstrual bleeding in post-menopausal women. Korean, Chinese and American ginsengs should not be used if you have acute illness, fever or swelling. Avoid Siberian ginseng if you have high blood pressure or high fever. Do not take ginseng with any other herbal stimulant, particularly ephedra, and restrict caffeine intake.

GLUCOSAMINE May cause nausea or heartburn: if so, try taking it with food. Check with your doctor if diabetic (animal studies have shown that glucosamine increases insulin resistance).

GLUTAMINE Do not take if you have end-stage liver failure or kidney failure.

GOLDENSEAL Should not be used for more than one week because it decreases the absorption of vitamin B_{12} leading to deficiency. Do not take if you are pregnant or have high blood pressure, hypo-glycaemia (low blood sugar) or weak digestion. Avoid if you have an auto-immune disease such as multiple sclerosis or lupus, or if you are allergic to plants in the daisy family such as camomile and marigold. Never take more than 2g a day: goldenseal is poisonous if taken in excess.

GOTU KOLA Do not take if you are pregnant or breastfeeding. Do not use with medications for diabetes or high blood pressure. Talk to your doctor if you are thinking of taking it for an extended period of time. Rarely, it may cause rash or headache.

HAWTHORN Do not take if you are on digoxin. If you have a cardio-vascular condition, do not take regularly for more than a few weeks. Do not use if you have low blood pressure caused by heart valve problems. Large amounts may cause drowsiness (do not drive).

HOPS Avoid in pregnancy. Do not take if prone to depression. Handle fresh or dried hops carefully as they occasionally cause skin rashes.

HOREHOUND Not to be used during pregnancy.

HORSE CHESTNUT Avoid in pregnancy. Avoid if suffering from kidney disease. May interfere with other drugs, especially blood-thinners. May irritate the gut.

HORSERADISH Not to be taken if you have gastric ulcers, thyroid conditions or a kidney disorder. Do not give to children under four years.

LYSINE Experimental; long-term effects are unknown. Use only under the supervision of a doctor. Do not take lysine and arginine at the same time, as they cancel each other out.

MAGNESIUM Do not take if you have impaired kidney function. Avoid if you are taking tetracycline antibiotics as it may reduce their effectiveness, and if you are taking diuretics or any other prescription drugs, unless recommended by your doctor. May cause diarrhoea. Do not take doses exceeding 400mg a day.

MARSHMALLOW May slow the absorption of other medications taken at the same time.

N-ACETYLCYSTEINE (NAC) Do not use if you have peptic ulcers or use drugs known to cause gastric sores.

NETTLE Not to be taken during pregnancy. Can cause mild stomach upset or a skin reaction.

PAPAYA May affect blood sugar: do not use if you have diabetes. If taking warfarin seek medical advice: both papaya fruit and enzymes may interact with this drug.

PARSLEY Do not use excessively large amounts (several handfuls a day!) if you have kidney disease; it may increase urine flow. Not to be used therapeutically during pregnancy, but safe in normal amounts as a garnish or in sauces.

PEPPERMINT May relax the oesophageal sphincter, increasing the risk of heartburn: use the herb cautiously if you are prone to acid reflux.

POTASSIUM We get plenty of this mineral in our food. Only take supplements if prescribed by a doctor.

PROBIOTICS May increase wind or bloating at first, which is a sign that the good bacteria are fermenting. Within a week or two, your body will adjust to the change.

PSYLLIUM Always take this fibre supplement with plenty of water. May cause bloating or constipation. Talk to your doctor before taking if you have difficulty swallowing or have diverticulitis, ulcerative colitis, Crohn's disease, bowel obstruction or if you are taking insulin (for diabetes) or any other medicines.

PYGEUM AFRICANUM Avoid in pregnancy. Avoid if you have high blood pressure. Talk to your doctor before using pygeum to self-treat an enlarged prostate.

ROSEMARY In large amounts may cause excessive menstrual bleeding. Not to be taken during pregnancy.

ST JOHN'S WORT Do not use when pregnant. Can make skin light-sensitive so wear sunscreen and don't sunbathe. Check with your doctor before taking *any* medication with St John's wort as it reacts with many drugs including: oral contraceptives; theophylline; digoxin; HIV medications; tamoxifen; prescribed antidepressants; alcohol and over-the-counter cold cures. May cause high blood pressure if taken with ephedra compounds. Do not use to self-treat clinical depression, a serious condition requiring a doctor's help.

SAM-E (S-ADENOSYLME-THIONINE) May increase blood levels of homocysteine, a risk factor for cardiovascular disease.

SAW PALMETTO If you have prostate problems, see your doctor *before* trying this supplement. Do not take with anticoagulants. Rarely, stomach problems have been noted.

SELENIUM Avoid in hypo-thyroidism. Do not exceed 200mcg a day. Excess may cause fragile, thickened nails; stomach pain; nausea; diarrhoea; a garlic taint on the breath and skin; a metallic taste in the mouth; loss of sensation in the hands and feet; irritability and fatigue. Doses of 800mcg have been known to cause tissue damage. Works best taken with vitamin E.

SENNA Not to be taken during pregnancy. Don't use for more than eight to ten days. Take 1 hour after other drugs and always with water. Do not use if you have abdominal pain, diarrhoea, haemorrhoids, intestinal obstruction or any inflammatory condition of the intestines. Not to be used by children under 12. Discontinue use if you have diarrhoea or watery stools. Excess amounts can lower levels of digoxin, so don't take if you are on this drug without consulting your doctor first.

TAURINE This is sometimes advocated for ulcers and diabetes but best not taken except under medical supervision. May increase stomach acid or cause diarrhoea.

VALERIAN Avoid with drugs such as diazepam or amitriptyline. Do not drink alcohol. May intensify the effects of sleep-enhancing or mood-regulating drugs. Discontinue use if you experience palpitations, nervousness, headaches or insomnia.

VITAMIN A Do not take if you are pregnant or trying to conceive. Do not exceed 1,500mcg per day. Possible side-effects include weight loss, skin problems, bone pain, bleeding, vomiting, diarrhoea, fatigue, dizziness, blurred vision, hair loss, joint pain and enlargement of the liver and spleen.

VITAMIN B$_6$ The UK safe upper limit for long-term supplementation is 10mg daily. In the short term, do not take more than 100mg a day. Reduce the dose if you have tingling fingers or toes, your limbs ache or feel weak and numb, or you feel depressed and tired.

VITAMIN C More than 1,000mg a day may cause diarrhoea. Pregnant women should not take more than 200mg of vitamin C a day. Consult a doctor if you have chronic renal failure or are on haemodialysis. Always cut back to 100mg a day at least three days before a medical examination; high levels can affect certain tests, particularly for blood in the stool and sugar in the urine. Large doses may interfere with anticoagulant drugs. People who are allergic to corn may react to supplements in a corn base.

VITAMIN E If on aspirin, or taking warfarin or other blood-thinners, then talk to your doctor before taking vitamin E.

WILLOW BARK Avoid if allergic to aspirin or taking a blood-thinner such as warfarin. May trigger asthma or allergies or cause gastrointestinal bleeding, liver dysfunction, blood-clotting disorders, kidney damage or anaphylactic reactions. May interact with barbiturates or seda-tives such as anobarbital or alpra-zolam, and it can cause stomach irritation when taken with alcohol.

YARROW Rarely, handling flowers can cause a skin rash. Do not use during pregnancy. In large doses may cause headache and dizziness. Can sensitize skin to sunlight – don't sunbathe.

ZINC Do not take more than 25mg a day unless advised to by a doctor. Zinc supplements should always include copper. Excess zinc intake can impair immunity.

Index

A

Aaron's rod 267, 268
abdominal breathing 51
acetyl-L-carnitine 142
aches and pains 258
aciclovir 123
acidophilus 146, 380, 434
acid reflux 346
acne 30–31, 305, 387
acne cleansers, and rosacea 328
acupressure 298–9
    for constipation 130
    for food poisoning 176
    for headaches 199, 299
    for morning sickness 280
    for motion sickness 284
    for nausea 297, 298
    for neck and shoulder pain 300
    for sinusitis 299, 340
    for toothache 365
adhesive tape, for splinters 350
aerobic exercise *see* exercise
aftershave 329, 335
age spots 32–33, 413
air baths, for nappy rash 293
air filters 36, 37
air travel 282–4, 340, 380
alarms, bedwetting 66
alcohol: and anxiety 41
    and depression 140
    and dry mouth 151
    and dry skin 155
    and fatigue 172
    and gout 189
    hangovers 197–8
    and heartburn 207
    and high blood pressure 216
    for high cholesterol 222
    and hot flushes 275
    and incontinence 231
    and infertility 241
    and insomnia 251
    and jaw problems 260
    and palpitations 309
    and peptic ulcers 314
    and premenstrual syndrome 318
    and prostate problems 321
    and restless legs syndrome 327
    and rosacea 329
    and seasonal affective disorder 331
    and sinusitis 341
    and snoring 343
    and stress 356
    and urinary tract infections 366
    and wind and flatulence 381
alcohol wipes, for oily skin 307
alginic acid 156
allergies 34–37
    asthma 49–51
    conjunctivitis 127
    ear problems 161
    eczema 163–4
    hives 223–5
    and nosebleed 304
    and snoring 343
almonds 316

aloe vera 18, 386–8
    for acne 31, 387
    for age spots 32
    for athlete's foot 53
    for blisters 72
    for burns and scalds 93, 386
    for cuts and grazes 386–7
    for dry hair 149
    for dry skin 153
    for heat rash 210
    for mouth ulcers 285
    for peptic ulcers 312
    for psoriasis 324, 387
    for razor rash 334
    for shingles 336, 387
    for sunburn 360
    for warts 374
    for wrinkles 382
alpha-hydroxy acids (AHAs) 30, 153, 305, 333, 382
Alzheimer's disease 269, 271
anal fissures 131
anal itching 256–7
anaphylaxis 69, 224
angina 38–39
animals: allergens 36–37, 164
    bites 71
    and high blood pressure 217
    ringworm 186
anise 62, 205, 280, 379, 434
ankle exercises, for arthritis 47
ankles, sprains 352–4
antacids 285, 311, 316, 380
antibacterial cleansers 75, 78
antihistamines 223, 240
    for allergies 34
    for chickenpox 112–13
    for colds and flu 119
    for conjunctivitis 127
    for inflammatory bowel disease 245
    and palpitations 310
    for snoring 342
antioxidants 48, 383
antiperspirants 74, 75, 178
anxiety 40–42
appetite loss 415
apples 307
apricots 92, 321
arginine 123, 227, 434
arm exercises 109
arnica 389
    for bruises 91, 92, 389
    for bursitis and tendinitis 98
    for carpal tunnel syndrome 106
    cautions and side effects 434
    for foot pain 181, 390
    for sprains and strains 389–90
aromatherapy 22–23
    see also individual oils
arrowroot 176
arteries, high cholesterol 219–22
arthritis 43–48, 115, 259, 405
aspirin: for acne 30
    and asthma 51
    for bruises 92
    for cold sores 122
    for corns 104
    and gout 187
    for headaches 199, 200
    and infertility 240

    for insect stings 68
    and nosebleed 304
    and peptic ulcers 314
asthma 49–51
astragalus: for bronchitis 88
    cautions and side effects 434
    for colds and flu 117, 121, 347
    for peptic ulcers 313
    for sinusitis 340–1
athlete's foot 52–54, 256, 415, 427
avocados 148, 220, 334, 383
Ayurveda 64, 126, 134, 192, 205

B

babies: hiccups 214
    infant colic 236–8
    nappy rash 293–5, 392
    teething 361–2
baby powder 295
back pain 55–60, 298, 316, 415
bacon fat 351
bacteria 314, 402–3, 407, 431–2
    see also probiotics
bad breath 61–63, 64
baking powder 336
    see also bicarbonate of soda
balloons, blowing up 308
bananas 166, 197, 248, 351, 361, 373
bandages 90, 97, 352, 353
barley 221, 360
barrier cream 294
basil 269, 373
baths 258–9
    for anxiety 40
    for arthritis 259
    for boils 77
    for chickenpox 112
    for dry skin 153, 154
    for eczema 162
    for fevers 173
    for food poisoning 175
    for haemorrhoids 194
    for heat rash 211
    for hives 223
    for insomnia 249
    for itching 256
    and jaw problems 260
    for menopause 274
    for menstrual problems 276
    for muscle cramps 288
    for nappy rash 294
    pets 37
    for prostate problems 321
    for psoriasis 323
    for restless legs syndrome 327
    for stress 355
    for sunburn 360
bay leaves 139
beans 221, 378
bearberry 367
beds 36, 250–1, 342
bedwetting 66–67
beer 81, 123, 214
bee stings 68–69, 71
beeswax 110
belching 378–81
benzoyl peroxide 30, 78, 179, 328, 333
bergamot oil 317
beta-blockers 229
beta-carotene 156, 314, 434

X, Y, Z

Picture credits

18-19 (all) RD ©/Sarah Cuttle; 64-65
RD©/Richard Surman; 115 Getty
Images/Romilly Lockyer; 156-157,
Science Photo Library/ Maximilian
Stock Ltd.; 208-209 Getty
Images/Photodisc; 248-249 Getty
Images/Photodisc; 258-259 Getty
Images/Photodisc; 299 Punchstock

Concept code	US4467/G
Book code	400-180 UP0000-13
ISBN	978 0 276 43015 2
Oracle code	250007691H.00.24